D1619458

Full View of Yangtze River Pharmaceuticals Group (Taizhou,Jiangsu,China)

扬子江药业集团全景（中国·江苏·泰州）

A Newly Compiled
Practical English-Chinese Library
of Traditional Chinese Medicine
（英汉对照）新编实用中医文库

General Compiler-in-Chief Zuo Yanfu
总主编 左言富
Translators-in-Chief
Zhu Zhongbao Huang Yuezhong Tao Jinwen Li Zhaoguo
总编译 朱忠宝 黄月中 陶锦文 李照国（执行）

Compiled by Nanjing University of
Traditional Chinese Medicine
Translated by Shanghai University
of Traditional Chinese Medicine
南 京 中 医 药 大 学 主编
上 海 中 医 药 大 学 主译

CHINESE TUINA(MASSAGE)

中 国 推 拿

Compiler-in-Chief	Jin Hongzhu
Vice-Compiler-in-Chief	Zha Wei
Translator-in-Chief	Yang Hongying
Translators	Pei Huihua Liu Shengpeng

主　编　金宏柱
副主编　查　炜
主　译　杨洪英
译　者　裴慧华
　　　　刘升鹏

PUBLISHING HOUSE OF SHANGHAI UNIVERSITY
OF TRADITIONAL CHINESE MEDICINE
上海中医药大学出版社

Publishing House of Shanghai University of Traditional Chinese Medicine

530 Lingling Road，Shanghai，200032，China

Chinese Tuina(Massage)

Compiler-in-Chief　Jin Hongzhu　Translators-in-Chief　Yang Hongying

(A Newly Compiled Practical English-Chinese Library of Traditional Chinese Medicine General Compiler-in-Chief　Zuo Yanfu)

ISBN 7 - 81010 - 651 - 1/R · 617　paperback

ISBN 7 - 81010 - 682 - 1/R · 647　hardback

Printed in Shanghai Xinhua printing works

图书在版编目(CIP)数据

中国推拿/金宏柱主编;杨洪英主译 . —上海：上海中医药大学出版社,2002

(英汉对照新编实用中医文库/左言富总主编)

ISBN 7 - 81010 - 651 - 1

Ⅰ.中... Ⅱ.①金...②杨... Ⅲ.推拿学-英、汉 Ⅳ.R244.1

中国版本图书馆 CIP 数据核字(2002)第 082863 号

中国推拿　　　　　　主编 金宏柱　　主译 杨洪英

上海中医药大学出版社出版发行　　　　（蔡伦路 1200 号　邮政编码 201203）

新华书店上海发行所经销　　　　　　　上海新华印刷有限公司印刷

开本　787mm×1092mm　1/18　印张 22.444　字数 536 千字　印数 3 601—6 600 册

版次 2002 年 12 月第 1 版　　　　　　印次 2004 年 3 月第 2 次印刷

ISBN 7 - 81010 - 651 - 1/R · 617　　　　　定价 62.90 元

《（英汉对照）新编实用中医文库》编纂委员会

名誉主任　张文康

总 顾 问　陈可冀　徐镜人

顾　　问　（按姓氏笔画为序）

干祖望　尤松鑫　刘再朋　许芝银　孙 桐　宋立人　张民庆　金 实

金妙文　单兆伟　周福贻　施 震　徐景藩　唐蜀华　曹世宏　符为民

外籍顾问

萨利姆（爱尔兰）　亚历山大·古丽（意大利）　卡塞拉·塞肯多（意大利）

雷蒙特·凯·卡罗（澳大利亚）　汤淑兰（英国）　马万里（英国）

大卫·莫罗尼（美国）　施祖谷（美国）　石上博（日本）　赫尔木特（德国）

主　　任　项 平

执 行 主 任　左言富

执行副主任　马 健　杜文东　李照国

副 主 任　黄成惠　吴坤平　刘沈林　吴勉华　陈涤平　蔡宝昌

编　　委　（按姓氏笔画为序）

丁安伟	丁淑华	于 勇	万力生	王 旭
王旭东	王玲玲	王鲁芬	卢子杰	申俊龙
刘 玉	刘跃光	严道南	杨公服	闵仲生
吴昌国	吴拥军	吴建龙	何文彬	何树勋（特邀）
何贵翔	汪 悦	汪受传	沈大庆	张 庆
陈永辉	陈廷汉（特邀）	邵健民	林显增（特邀）	
林端美（特邀）	岳沛平	金宏柱	周礼杲（特邀）	
赵 霞	赵京生	胡 烈	胡 葵	查 炜
姚映芷	袁 颖	夏有兵	夏登杰	倪 云
徐恒泽	郭海英	唐传俭	唐德才	凌桂珍（特邀）
谈 勇	黄桂成	梅晓芸	曹贵珠	蒋中秋
曾庆琪	翟亚春	樊巧玲		

Translation Committee of the Library

Approval Committee of the Library

Foreword I

As we are walking into the 21st century, "health for all" is still an important task for the World Health Organization (WHO) to accomplish in the new century. The realization of "health for all" requires mutual cooperation and concerted efforts of various medical sciences, including traditional medicine. WHO has increasingly emphasized the development of traditional medicine and has made fruitful efforts to promote its development. Currently the spectrum of diseases is changing and an increasing number of diseases are difficult to cure. The side effects of chemical drugs have become more and more evident. Furthermore, both the governments and peoples in all countries are faced with the problem of high cost of medical treatment. Traditional Chinese medicine (TCM), the complete system of traditional medicine in the world with unique theory and excellent clinical curative effects, basically meets the need to solve such problems. Therefore, bringing TCM into full play in medical treatment and healthcare will certainly become one of the hot points in the world medical business in the 21st century.

Various aspects of work need to be done to promote the course of the internationalization of TCM, especially the compilation of works and textbooks suitable for international readers. The impending new century has witnessed the compilation of such a

序 一

人类即将迈入 21 世纪，"人人享有卫生保健"仍然是新世纪世界卫生工作面临的重要任务。实现"人人享有卫生保健"的宏伟目标，需要包括传统医药学在内的多种医学学科的相互协作与共同努力。世界卫生组织越来越重视传统医药学的发展，并为推动其发展做出了卓有成效的工作。目前，疾病谱正在发生变化，难治疾病不断增多，化学药品的毒副作用日益显现，日趋沉重的医疗费用困扰着各国政府和民众。中医药学是世界传统医学体系中最完整的传统医学，其独到的学科理论和突出的临床疗效，较符合当代社会和人们解决上述难题的需要。因此，科学有效地发挥中医药学的医疗保健作用，必将成为 21 世纪世界卫生工作的特点之一。

加快中医药走向世界的步伐，还有很多的工作要做，特别是适合国外读者学习的中医药著作、教材的编写是极其重要的方面。在新千年来临之际，由南京中医药大学

series of books known as *A Newly Compiled Practical English-Chinese Library of Traditional Chinese Medicine* published by the Publishing House of Shanghai University of TCM, compiled by Nanjing University of TCM and translated by Shanghai University of TCM. Professor Zuo Yanfu, the general compiler-in-chief of this Library, is a person who sets his mind on the international dissemination of TCM. He has compiled *General Survey on TCM Abroad*, a monograph on the development and state of TCM abroad. This Library is another important works written by the experts organized by him with the support of Nanjing University of TCM and Shanghai University of TCM. The compilation of this Library is done with consummate ingenuity and according to the development of TCM abroad. The compilers, based on the premise of preserving the genuineness and gist of TCM, have tried to make the contents concise, practical and easy to understand, making great efforts to introduce the abstruse ideas of TCM in a scientific and simple way as well as expounding the prevention and treatment of diseases which are commonly encountered abroad and can be effectively treated by TCM.

This Library encompasses a systematic summarization of the teaching experience accumulated in Nanjing University of TCM and Shanghai University of TCM that run the collaborating centers of traditional medicine and the international training centers on acupuncture and moxibustion set by WHO. I am sure that the publication of this Library will further promote the development of traditional Chinese med-

主编、上海中医药大学主译、上海中医药大学出版社出版的《(英汉对照)新编实用中医文库》的即将问世,正是新世纪中医药国际传播更快发展的预示。本套文库总主编左言富教授是中医药学国际传播事业的有心人,曾主编研究国外中医药发展状况的专著《国外中医药概览》。本套文库的编撰,是他在南京中医药大学和上海中医药大学支持下,组织许多著名专家共同完成的又一重要专著。本套文库的作者们深谙国外的中医药发展现状,编写颇具匠心,在注重真实,不失精华的前提下,突出内容的简明、实用,易于掌握,力求科学而又通俗地介绍中医药学的深奥内容,重点阐述国外常见而中医药颇具疗效的疾病的防治。

本套文库蕴含了南京中医药大学和上海中医药大学作为 WHO 传统医学合作中心、国际针灸培训中心多年留学生教学的实践经验和系统总结,更为全面、系统、准确地向世界传播中医药学。相信本书的出版将对中医更好地走向世界,让世界更好地了解中医产生更

icine abroad and enable the whole world to have a
better understanding of traditional Chinese medicine.

为积极的影响。

Professor Zhu Qingsheng
Vice-Minister of Health Ministry of the
People's Republic of China

Director of the State Administrative Bureau of
TCM

December 14, 2000 Beijing

朱庆生教授
中华人民共和国卫生部副部长

国家中医药管理局局长

2000 年 12 月 14 日于北京

Foreword Ⅱ

Before the existence of the modern medicine, human beings depended solely on herbal medicines and other therapeutic methods to treat diseases and preserve health. Such a practice gave rise to the establishment of various kinds of traditional medicine with unique theory and practice, such as traditional Chinese medicine, Indian medicine and Arabian medicine, etc. Among these traditional systems of medicine, traditional Chinese medicine is a most extraordinary one based on which traditional Korean medicine and Japanese medicine have evolved.

Even in the 21st century, traditional medicine is still of great vitality. In spite of the fast development of modern medicine, traditional medicine is still disseminated far and wide. In many developing countries, most of the people in the rural areas still depend on traditional medicine and traditional medical practitioners to meet the need for primary healthcare. Even in the countries with advanced modern medicine, more and more people have begun to accept traditional medicine and other therapeutic methods, such as homeopathy, osteopathy and naturopathy, etc.

With the change of the economy, culture and living style in various regions as well as the aging in the world population, the disease spectrum has changed. And such a change has paved the way for the new application of traditional medicine. Besides,

序 二

在现代医学形成之前,人类一直依赖草药和其他一些疗法治病强身,从而发展出许多有理论、有实践的传统医学,例如中医学、印度医学、阿拉伯医学等。中医学是世界林林总总的传统医学中的一支奇葩,在它的基础上还衍生出朝鲜传统医学和日本汉方医学。在跨入 21 世纪的今天,古老的传统医学依然焕发着活力,非但没有因现代医学的发展而式微,其影响还有增无减,人们对传统医学的价值也有了更深刻的体会和认识。在许多贫穷国家,大多数农村人口仍然依赖传统医学疗法和传统医务工作者来满足他们对初级卫生保健的需求。在现代医学占主导地位的许多国家,传统医学及其他一些"另类疗法",诸如顺势疗法、整骨疗法、自然疗法等,也越来越被人们所接受。

伴随着世界各地经济、文化和生活的变革以及世界人口的老龄化,世界疾病谱也发生了变化。传统医学有了新的应用,而新疾病所引起的新需求以及现代医学的成

the new requirements initiated by the new diseases and the achievements and limitations of modern medicine have also created challenges to traditional medicine.

WHO sensed the importance of traditional medicine to human health early in the 1970s and have made great efforts to develop traditional medicine. At the 29th world health congress held in 1976, the item of traditional medicine was adopted in the working plan of WHO. In the following world health congresses, a series of resolutions were passed to demand the member countries to develop, utilize and study traditional medicine according to their specific conditions so as to reduce medical expenses for the realization of "health for all".

WHO has laid great stress on the scientific content, safe and effective application of traditional medicine. It has published and distributed a series of booklets on the scientific, safe and effective use of herbs and acupuncture and moxibustion. It has also made great contributions to the international standardization of traditional medical terms. The safe and effective application of traditional medicine has much to do with the skills of traditional medical practitioners. That is why WHO has made great efforts to train them. WHO has run 27 collaborating centers in the world which have made great contributions to the training of acupuncturists and traditional medical practitioners. Nanjing University of TCM and Shanghai University of TCM run the collaborating centers with WHO. In recent years it has, with the cooperation of WHO and other countries, trained about ten thousand international students from over

就与局限又向传统医学提出了挑战,推动它进一步发展。世界卫生组织早在20世纪70年代就意识到传统医学对人类健康的重要性,并为推动传统医学的发展做了努力。1976年举行的第二十九届世界卫生大会将传统医学项目纳入世界卫生组织的工作计划。其后的各届世界卫生大会又通过了一系列决议,要求各成员国根据本国的条件发展、使用和研究传统医学,以降低医疗费用,促进"人人享有初级卫生保健"这一目标的实现。

世界卫生组织历来重视传统医学的科学、安全和有效使用。它出版和发行了一系列有关科学、安全、有效使用草药和针灸的技术指南,并在专用术语的标准化方面做了许多工作。传统医学的使用是否做到安全和有效,是与使用传统疗法的医务工作者的水平密不可分的。因此,世界卫生组织也十分重视传统医学培训工作。它在全世界有27个传统医学合作中心,这些中心对培训合格的针灸师及使用传统疗法的其他医务工作者做出了积极的贡献。南京中医药大学、上海中医药大学是世界卫生组织传统医学合作中心之一,近年来与世界卫生组织和其他国家合作,培训了近万名来自90多个国

90 countries.

In order to further promote the dissemination of traditional Chinese medicine in the world, *A Newly Compiled Practical English-Chinese Library of Traditional Chinese Medicine*, compiled by Nanjing University of TCM with Professor Zuo Yanfu as the general compiler-in-chief and published by the Publishing House of Shanghai University of TCM, aims at systematic, accurate and concise expounding of traditional Chinese medical theory and introducing clinical therapeutic methods of traditional medicine according to modern medical nomenclature of diseases. Undoubtedly, this series of books will be the practical textbooks for the beginners with certain English level and the international enthusiasts with certain level of Chinese to study traditional Chinese medicine. Besides, this series of books can also serve as reference books for WHO to internationally standardize the nomenclature of acupuncture and moxibustion.

The scientific, safe and effective use of traditional medicine will certainly further promote the development of traditional medicine and traditional medicine will undoubtedly make more and more contributions to human health in the 21st century.

Zhang Xiaorui

WHO Coordination Officer

December, 2000

家和地区的留学生。

在南京中医药大学左言富教授主持下编纂的、由上海中医药大学出版社出版的《(英汉对照)新编实用中医文库》，旨在全面、系统、准确、简要地阐述中医基础理论，并结合西医病名介绍中医临床治疗方法。因此，这套文库可望成为具有一定英语水平的初学中医者和具有一定中文水平的外国中医爱好者学习基础中医学的系列教材。这套文库也可供世界卫生组织在编写国际针灸标准术语时参考。

传统医学的科学、安全、有效使用必将进一步推动传统医学的发展。传统医学一定会在 21 世纪为人类健康做出更大的贡献。

张小瑞

世界卫生组织传统医学协调官员

2000 年 12 月

Preface

The Publishing House of Shanghai University of TCM published *A Practical English-Chinese Library of Traditional Chinese Medicine* in 1990. The Library has been well-known in the world ever since and has made great contributions to the dissemination of traditional Chinese medicine in the world. In view of the fact that 10 years has passed since its publication and that there are certain errors in the explanation of traditional Chinese medicine in the Library, the Publishing House has invited Nanjing University of TCM and Shanghai University of TCM to organize experts to recompile and translate the Library.

Nanjing University of TCM and Shanghai University of TCM are well-known for their advantages in higher education of traditional Chinese medicine and compilation of traditional Chinese medical textbooks. The compilation of *A Newly Compiled Practical English-Chinese Library of Traditional Chinese Medicine* has absorbed the rich experience accumulated by Nanjing University of Traditional Chinese Medicine in training international students of traditional Chinese medicine. Compared with the previous Library, the Newly Compiled Library has made great improvements in many aspects，fully demonstrating the academic system of traditional Chinese medicine. The whole series of books has systematically introduced the basic theory and thera-

前　言

上海中医药大学出版社于 1990 年出版了一套《(英汉对照)实用中医文库》,发行 10 年来,在海内外产生了较大影响,对推动中医学走向世界起了积极作用。考虑到该套丛书发行已久,对中医学术体系的介绍还有一些欠妥之处,因此,上海中医药大学出版社特邀南京中医药大学主编、上海中医药大学主译,组织全国有关专家编译出版《(英汉对照)新编实用中医文库》。

《(英汉对照)新编实用中医文库》的编纂,充分发挥了南京中医药大学和上海中医药大学在高等中医药教育教学和教材编写方面的优势,吸收了作为 WHO 传统医学合作中心之一的两校,多年来从事中医药学国际培训和留学生学历教育的经验,对原《(英汉对照)实用中医文库》整体结构作了大幅度调整,以突出中医学术主体内容。全套丛书系统介绍了中医基础理论和中医辨证论治方法,讲解了中药学和方剂学的基本理论,详细介绍了 236 味中药、152 首常用方剂和 100 种常用中成药;详述

peutic methods based on syndrome differentiation, expounding traditional Chinese pharmacy and prescriptions; explaining 236 herbs, 152 prescriptions and 100 commonly-used patent drugs; elucidating 264 methods for differentiating syndromes and treating commonly-encountered and frequently-encountered diseases in internal medicine, surgery, gynecology, pediatrics, traumatology and orthopedics, ophthalmology and otorhinolaryngology; introducing the basic methods and theory of acupuncture and moxibustion, massage (tuina), life cultivation and rehabilitation, including 70 kinds of diseases suitable for acupuncture and moxibustion, 38 kinds of diseases for massage, examples of life cultivation and over 20 kinds of commonly encountered diseases treated by rehabilitation therapies in traditional Chinese medicine. For better understanding of traditional Chinese medicine, the books are neatly illustrated. There are 296 line graphs and 30 colored pictures in the Library with necessary indexes, making it more comprehensive, accurate and systematic in disseminating traditional Chinese medicine in the countries and regions where English is the official language.

This Library is characterized by following features:

1. Scientific　Based on the development of TCM in education and research in the past 10 years, efforts have been made in the compilation to highlight the gist of TCM through accurate theoretical exposition and clinical practice, aiming at introducing authentic theory and practice to the world.

2. Systematic　This Library contains 14 sepa-

264 种临床内、外、妇、儿、骨伤、眼、耳鼻喉各科常见病与多发病的中医辨证论治方法；系统论述针灸、推拿、中医养生康复的基本理论和基本技能，介绍针灸治疗病种 70 种、推拿治疗病种 38 种、各类养生实例及 20 余种常见病证的中医康复实例。为了更加直观地介绍中医药学术，全书选用线图 296 幅、彩图 30 幅，并附有必要的索引，从而更加全面、系统、准确地向使用英语的国家和地区传播中医学术，推进中医学走向世界，造福全人类。

本丛书主要具有以下特色：
(1) 科学性：在充分吸收近 10 余年来中医教学和科学研究最新进展的基础上，坚持突出中医学术精华，理论阐述准确，临床切合实用，向世界各国介绍"原汁原味"的中医药学术；(2) 系统性：本套丛书包括《中医基础理论》、《中医诊断学》、《中药学》、《方剂学》、《中医内

rate fascicles, i. e. *Basic Theory of Traditional Chinese Medicine*, *Diagnostics of Traditional Chinese Medicine*, *Science of Chinese Materia Medica*, *Science of Prescriptions*, *Internal Medicine of Traditional Chinese Medicine*, *Surgery of Traditional Chinese Medicine*, *Gynecology of Traditional Chinese Medicine*, *Pediatrics of Traditional Chinese Medicine*, *Traumatology and Orthopedics of Traditional Chinese Medicine*, *Ophthalmology of Traditional Chinese Medicine*, *Otorhinolaryngology of Traditional Chinese Medicine*, *Chinese Acupuncture and Moxibustion*, *Chinese Tuina (Massage)*, *and Life Cultivation and Rehabilitation of Traditional Chinese Medicine*.

3. Practical　Compared with the previous Library, the Newly Compiled Library has made great improvements and supplements, systematically introducing therapeutic methods for treating over 200 kinds of commonly and frequently encountered diseases, focusing on training basic clinical skills in acupuncture and moxibustion, tuina therapy, life cultivation and rehabilitation with clinical case reports.

4. Standard　This Library is reasonable in structure, distinct in categorization, standard in terminology and accurate in translation with full consideration of habitual expressions used in countries and regions with English language as the mother tongue.

This series of books is not only practical for the beginners with certain competence of English to study TCM, but also can serve as authentic textbooks for international students in universities and colleges of TCM in China to study and practice TCM. For those from TCM field who are going to go

科学》、《中医外科学》、《中医妇科学》、《中医儿科学》、《中医骨伤科学》、《中医眼科学》、《中医耳鼻喉科学》、《中国针灸》、《中国推拿》、《中医养生康复学》14个分册,系统反映了中医各学科建设与发展的最新成果;(3)实用性:临床各科由原来的上下两册,根据学科的发展进行大幅度的调整和增补,比较详细地介绍了200多种各科常见病、多发病的中医治疗方法,重点突出了针灸、推拿、养生康复等临床基本技能训练,并附有部分临证实例;(4)规范性:全书结构合理,层次清晰,对中医各学科名词术语表述规范,对中医英语翻译执行了更为严格的标准化方案,同时又充分考虑到使用英语国家和地区人们的语言习惯和表达方式。

本丛书不仅能满足具有一定英语水平的初学中医者系统学习中医之用,而且也为中医院校外国留学生教育及国内外开展中医双语教学提供了目前最具权威的系列教材,同时也是中医出国人员进

abroad to do academic exchange, this series of books will provide them with unexpected convenience.

Professor Xiang Ping, President of Nanjing University of TCM, is the director of the Compilation Board. Professor Zuo Yanfu from Nanjing University of TCM, General Compiler-in-Chief, is in charge of the compilation. Zhang Wenkang, Minister of Health Ministry, is invited to be the honorary director of the Editorial Board. Li Zhenji, Vice-Director of the State Administrative Bureau of TCM, is invited to be the director of the Approval Committee. Chen Keji, academician of China Academy, is invited to be the General Advisor. International advisors invited are Mr. M. S. Khan, Chairman of Ireland Acupuncture and Moxibustion Fund; Miss Alessandra Gulí, Chairman of "Nanjing Association" in Rome, Italy; Doctor Secondo Scarsella, Chief Editor of YI DAO ZA ZHI; President Raymond K. Carroll from Australian Oriental Touching Therapy College; Ms. Shulan Tang, Academic Executive of ATCM in Britain; Mr. Glovanni Maciocia from Britain; Mr. David, Chairman of American Association of TCM; Mr. Tzu Kuo Shih, director of Chinese Medical Technique Center in Connecticut, America; Mr. Helmut Ziegler, director of TCM Center in Germany; and Mr. Isigami Hiroshi from Japan. Chen Ken, official of WHO responsible for the Western Pacific Region, has greatly encouraged the compilers in compiling this series of books. After the accomplishment of the compilation, Professor Zhu Qingsheng, Vice-Minister of Health Ministry and Director of the State Administrative Bureau of TCM, has set a high value on the books in his fore-

行中医药国际交流的重要工具书。

全书由南京中医药大学校长项平教授担任编委会主任、左言富教授任总主编，主持全书的编写。中华人民共和国卫生部张文康部长担任本丛书编委会名誉主任，国家中医药管理局李振吉副局长担任审定委员会主任，陈可冀院士欣然担任本丛书总顾问指导全书的编纂。爱尔兰针灸基金会主席萨利姆先生、意大利罗马"南京协会"主席亚历山大·古丽女士、意大利《医道》杂志主编卡塞拉·塞肯多博士、澳大利亚东方触觉疗法学院雷蒙特·凯·卡罗院长、英国中医药学会学术部长汤淑兰女士、英国马万里先生、美国中医师公会主席大卫先生、美国康州中华医疗技术中心主任施祖谷先生、德国中医中心主任赫尔木特先生、日本石上博先生担任本丛书特邀外籍顾问。世界卫生组织西太平洋地区官员陈恩先生对本丛书的编写给予了热情鼓励。全书完成后，卫生部副部长兼国家中医药管理局局长朱庆生教授给予了高度评价，并欣然为本书作序；WHO 传统医学协调官员张小瑞对于本丛书的编写给予高度关注，百忙中也专为本书作序。我国驻外教育机构，特别是中国驻英国曼彻斯特领事张益群先生、中国驻美国休斯敦领事严美华

word for the Library. Zhang Xiaorui, an official from WHO's Traditional Medicine Program, has paid great attention to the compilation and written a foreword for the Library. The officials from the educational organizations of China in other countries have provided us with some useful materials in our compilation. They are Mr. Zhang Yiqun, China Consul to Manchester in Britain; Miss Yan Meihua, Consul to Houston in America; Mr. Wang Jiping, First Secretary in the Educational Department in the Embassy of China to France; and Mr. Gu Shengying, the Second Secretary in the Educational Department in the Embassy of China to Germany. We are grateful to them all.

The Compilers
December, 2000

女士、中国驻法国使馆教育处一秘王季平先生、中国驻德国使馆教育处二秘郭胜英先生在与我们工作联系中,间接提供了不少有益资料。在此一并致以衷心感谢!

编 者
2000 年 12 月

Note for compilation

Chinese Tuina is one important component of Chinese traditional medicine, and it is also an important clinical subject of TCM. Sticking to the distinctive features of TCM, this book comprehensively introduces the basic theories, manipulations, clinical application of Chinese tuina therapy, which are expounded in five chapters in an orderly way and step by step, and illustrated with 101 figures.

Chapter One, Basic Knowledge of Tuina, gives a brief review of the development of Chinese Tuina, its acting principles and research. In the part of acting principles, the relationship between tuina therapy and the theories of yin-yang, five elements, zang and fu, qi, blood, etc. is briefly discussed. Meridians and collaterals, commonly-used acupoints, approaches of tuina liangong, diagnosis, reinforcing and reducing therapies, indications and contraindications of tuina are also introduced in this part. In the second chapter, commonly-used manipulations for adults and infants are chiefly discussed, including the main points of manipulations, clinical applications, and methods and steps of manipulation practice. In the third chapter, commonly-used auxiliary tuina therapies such as ointment for massage (Gaomo), medicated hot compress are described so as to expand its clinical application range and strengthen its clinical therapeutic effects. Chapter Four mainly presents clinical therapies of 38 common adult and infant diseases with tuina. Each disease is concisely interpre-

编写说明

中国推拿是中国传统医学的重要组成部分,亦是中医的一门重要临床学科,本书坚持中医特色,全方位地介绍了中国推拿疗法的基础、手法和临床应用等知识,以循序渐进的形式,分五大章节进行了叙述,并附图 101 幅。

第一章推拿基础中简略地介绍了中国推拿发展简史、作用原理和研究进展,并在作用原理中简略说明阴阳五行、脏腑、气血等与推拿疗法的关系,扼要介绍了经络和常用穴位、推拿练功方法及诊断、补泻、适应证和禁忌证等。第二章着重介绍了成人及小儿推拿的常用手法,从动作要领、临床应用等方面作了详细讲解,并介绍了手法练习的方法和步骤。第三章介绍中国推拿常用的辅助方法,诸如膏摩、热敷等,以扩大推拿临床的应用范围和加强推拿临床的治疗效果。第四章着重介绍了成人和小儿推拿临床 38 个常见疾病的治疗,每个病证都简略地从中医和现代医学的病因、病理方面进行了概述,明确了诊断要点、基本治法和随症加减。第五章则从分部与对证两部分介绍了一些操作简便、行

ted from the view of etiology and pathology of TCM and modern medicine，and all the diagnostic points, basic therapeutic manipulations and modified manipulations with syndrome differentiation are made clear. Chapter Five elucidates some easily-operated，effective self-tuina methods with syndrome differentiation for all the parts of the body，which can be used to treat and prevent diseases in zang and fu organs and other parts.

Many thanks are to Ding Xiaohong, Liu Xue, Zhao Mei and Wu Yunchuan for their work in the course of compilation of this book.

The Compiler
December，2000

之有效的自我推拿方法，用以防治人体各相关部位和脏腑的病证。

本书编写过程中，丁晓红、刘雪、赵玫、吴云川等参加了具体工作，在此一并表示感谢。

编　者
2000 年 12 月

CONTENTS

目 录

1 Basic Knowledge

1.1 An Outline

Chinese Tuina was called massage or Mosuo in ancient times. The term Tuina was first seen in the Ming Dynasty. Chinese Tuina is a therapeutic approach guided by the theory of traditional Chinese medicine (TCM) and used to treat diseases through massage manipulations or by means of some massage tools applied to certain parts or points on the human body surface. It belongs to the category of external treatment in TCM. Tuina is an important component of Chinese medicine, which is very effective in curing and preventing diseases and has made great contributions to thriving and prosperity of the Chinese nation.

1.1.1 Brief Account of Development of Chinese Tuina

Tuina originated from labor, and labor was the first essentials for the survival of the human beings. In the prehistoric age the human beings hunted and opened up wastelands to fill their belly, broke branches and piled up stones to build their shelters, sewed leather and made clothes to keep themselves warm and trudged very far to look for living stuff. While doing so, injuries such as fractures, contusions and strains happened to them constantly. In this case man would instinctively press with hands to stop bleeding and rub to eliminate swelling and pains. After long-term accumulation, the ancient people gradual-

第一章 基础知识

第一节 概述

中国推拿,古称按摩、摩挲。推拿一名最早见于明代。推拿是以中医理论为指导,医生运用推拿手法或借助于一定的推拿工具作用于患者体表的特定部位或穴位来治疗疾病的一种治疗方法,属于中医外治法范畴。推拿是中医学的重要组成部分,防病治病,卓有成效,为中华民族的繁衍昌盛作出了巨大的贡献。

一、中国推拿发展简史

推拿起源于劳动。劳动是人类生存的第一要素。史前时代,人类打猎开荒以充口腹,折技垒石以筑巢居,缝革连衣以暖躯体,跋涉劳顿以寻生资。所有这些都会造成跌仆折骨之类的损伤,因之人类本能地用手按以止血,摩以消肿止痛。经过漫长的日积月累,终于领悟和总结出一些原始的推拿方法,并成为人们治

ly understood and summed up some primitive Tuina methods, which later became one of the commonly used techniques in treating diseases.

The period from the Xia, Shang and Zhou dynasties to the time when Qin Shihuang (the first emperor of the Qin Dynasty) united China is called the prior-Qin period in Chinese history. It was recorded in the literatures that in this period there had been a lot of medicinal books circulating among the people. Unfortunately all the books were lost later in wars. Of the great many treatises on medicine compiled by hundreds of scholars, only very a few had been kept down. Therefore the knowledge of the achievements in tuina of this period is mainly from the two important archaeological discoveries: the unearthed oracle inscriptions on bones or tortoise shells of the Yin-Shang Dynasty and the records of the medical books from the tombs of the Han Dynasty in Mawangdui, Changsha. The people of the Yin-Shang Dynasty were superstitious and they chiefly used prayer and sacrifice to eliminate illnesses and misfortunes when they were ill. So although there were a lot of records about diseases in the oracle inscriptions on bones or tortoise shells, only very few on treatment with medicines could be seen. Yet in these inscriptions there were many words about tuina therapy, which showed that besides sacrifice, the people of the Yin-Shang Dynasty mainly used tuina to treat diseases. Tuina was their creation and they were very skillful in applying it. Among the medical books written on silk unearthed in Mawangdui, the book *Wushi'er Bingfang* (*Fifty Two Medical Prescriptions*) mostly involved treatment of diseases with tuina. Tuina therapy in this book had two striking characteristics. One was the record about medicated tuina and ointment tuina, which were the earliest methods in the development of tuina in spite of being simple in making.

疗疾病的常用方法之一。

自夏商周以来,至秦始皇统一中国,史称先秦时期。据文献记载,此间曾有不少医书流传于世,后因兵燹战火,率皆亡佚。诸子百家对医药之论也只是一鳞半爪。因而对这一时期的推拿成就的了解,主要来自于 20 世纪考古学的两项重大发现,即殷墟甲骨卜辞和长沙马王堆汉墓医书的记载。殷人迷信鬼神,患病时以祷告祭祀为消灾祛病的主要方法。因而甲骨卜辞中记载的疾病虽多,用医药治疗之事却甚少。在甲骨卜辞中,有许多字与推拿治疗有关。这说明除祭祀之外,殷人的主要治病手段是推拿,推拿是殷人发明并擅长的。马王堆帛简医书中以《五十二病方》涉及推拿治病最多。该书中的推拿疗法有下列两个显著特点:一是记载了推拿发展史上制作虽然简单,但系最早的药摩和膏摩方法。二是记载了推拿时运用的许多富有特色的工具,如治疗疝气的木椎,治疗小儿惊风用的钱匕,最富特色的是一种"药巾",用以治疗某些性功能障碍或进行养生保健,这应该是推拿保健史上

The other was the record of plenty of tuina tools with distinguished features. For example, the taper wood tool used for treating hernia, the copper coin for infantile convulsion and the most characteristic medicated towel. The towel was used to treat certain sexual disorders and for health preservation, which could be counted as a great invention in the history of tuina. In fact, the earliest and most primitive tuina tool was Bianshi (a kind of prepared stone), which had many kinds, and each kind had its own functions. Therefore, it could be concluded that Bianshi was not only used for acupuncture, but also for tuina. The utilization of tuina tools made tuina therapy more effective.

The Qin and Han Dynasties were an important period in the development of tuina. It was recorded in the book, *Hanshu-Yiwenzhi-Fangjilüe* (*Han Book*, *Literature and Arts*, *Methods and Skills*) that *Huangdi Qibo Anmo Shijuan* (*Ten Volumes on Tuina of Huangdi and Qibo*) and *Huangdi Neijing* (*Huangdi's Canon of Medicine*), short for Neijing, came out at the same time. The former was the first monograph on massage in Chinese Tuina history, and the latter was the earliest great TCM works in existence. In classification, *Huangdi Qibo Anmo Shijuan* must have mainly concentrated on tuina, and by medical origin it was surely one branch of the same source with *Huangdi Neijing*, which was the other branch. *Huangdi Neijing* mainly recorded the theories of TCM and acupuncture, while *Huangdi Qibo Anmo Shijuan* was chiefly about tuina and health care. It was a pity that the great works of ten volumes on Tuina was unable to survive wars so that nowadays we could not have an all-round understanding of the development of tuina in the time before the Western Han Dynasty. Little to our relief, there were some literatures on tuina in *Huangdi's*

的一大发明。其实推拿最早最原始的工具是砭石。砭石有很多种类,不同的砭石其功用也不同,故砭石并非仅用于针刺。推拿工具的使用,使推拿治疗效果更为显著。

秦汉时期是推拿历史发展的重要阶段。据《汉书·艺文志·方技略》记载,我国推拿史上第一部推拿专著《黄帝岐伯按摩十卷》与中医学中现存最早的渊薮巨著《黄帝内经》同时问世。从分类来看,此书以记载保健按摩为主;从医学源流来看,此书与《黄帝内经》应是一源两歧。《黄帝内经》载述的是以中医理论、针灸为主,而《黄帝岐伯按摩十卷》则是主要涵括了推拿按摩、养生保健的内容。令人惋惜的是,这部篇幅长达 10 卷的推拿学巨著,未能幸免于战火,早已亡佚,致使我们无法窥视西汉以前推拿学发展的全貌。然而,在《黄帝内经》中还记载了大量的推拿文献,这多少让我们得到一点慰藉。

Canon of Medicine. It could be seen through a comprehensive view of *Neijing* that the unique therapeutic system of tuina had been formed in the Qin and Han period. Many paragraphs in the book were the theoretical summarization of tuina treatment from the Yin-Shang Dynasty. It was pointed out in *Neijing* that Chinese Tuina originated from and formed in the central region, equivalent to today's Luoyang area of Henan Province, which was the border of the Yin-Shang people at that time. That tallied with the contents of tuina described in the oracle inscriptions on bones or tortoise shells of the Yin-Shang Dynasty. Inspection, listening and smelling, interrogation and palpation diagnoses are the most important diagnostic methods of tuina. In *Neijing* there were many parts about the application of tuina manipulations to palpation diagnosis, which improved the accuracy of diagnosing diseases. *Neijing* fully affirmed the therapeutic effect of tuina and held that tuina had the function of promoting qi to activate blood, eliminating cold to stop pain, dredging the meridians and reducing fever to tranquilize the mind. The book also pointed out that attention should be paid to reinforcement and reduction of tuina and its coordination with acumox, medication and other therapeutic methods. In addition, there were a great many records about tuina manipulations in *Neijing*: pressing, rubbing, cutting, palpating, feeling, clapping, flicking, grasping, pushing, weighing down, flexing, stretching, rocking and so on, among which pressing and rubbing manipulations were most commonly used. That was why tuina was also called Anmo (pressing and rubbing) at that time. It was mentioned in *Neijing* that round needle and Di needle of the nine kinds of acupuncture needles might also be used as tuina tools, and the round one was used for reduction and the Di needle for reinforcement. Discussion and summary

综观《内经》全书,可以看出,秦汉时期推拿独特的治疗体系已经形成,这部巨著中许多条文是对殷商以来推拿疗法的理论总结。《内经》指出了我国推拿发源形成在我国中央地区,相当于现今河南洛阳一带,这正是殷、商人的疆界,与甲骨卜辞中有关推拿内容是吻合的。望、闻、问、切诊是推拿学中最重要的诊断方法,将推拿手法运用到切诊中,以加强疾病诊断的准确性,在《内经》中比比皆是。《内经》充分肯定了推拿的治疗作用,认为推拿具有行气活血、散寒止痛、疏经通络、退热宁神等作用,同时提出推拿要注意补泻,注重与针灸、药物等其他方法的协同配合。另外,《内经》中记载的推拿手法也很丰富,有按、摩、切、扪、循、拊、弹、抓、推、压、屈、伸、摇等多种方法,这些方法中以按、摩二法运用最多,故而当时以按摩作为这种治疗方法的名称。《内经》中述及针灸九针中的圆针和鍉针可作为按摩推拿的工具,圆针用于泻法,鍉针用于补法。总之,《内经》对推拿学的总结和论述,远远不止以上这些。重要的在于《内经》奠定了中医基本理论的同时,其中的主要内容,如脏腑

about tuina were certainly much more than the above in *Neijing*. *Neijing* established the basic theory of TCM, its main theories were also the most important guiding principles of tuina, which included the theories of zang-fu, meridians, yin-yang, five elements, qi, blood and body fluids and diagnostic methods and therapeutic principles as well.

The prominent doctor of the Han Dynasty, Zhang Zhongjing, listed the ointment tuina as one of the methods of health care for the first time in his book *Jingui Yaolüe* (*Synopsis of Golden Chamber*). He also introduced a massage powder for treating Toufeng (headache due to wind) with tuina, the prescription only contained Fuzi (Radix Aconiti Praeparata) and salt. Modinggao (an ointment for massage on the head) and its similar kinds that appeared in later time, all derived from it. In the same book Zhang also carefully recorded a tuina technique for saving persons who hanged themselves, which was generally acknowledged as the earliest scientific method recorded for rescuing the hanged by the medical world and a proud achievement in the history of tuina. Another famous doctor, Hua Tuo promoted the frolics of five animals, which led daoyin (physical and breathing exercises) and tuina close to bionics, and provided a set of effective means of health care for the later generations. He was good at applying ointment massage and the first person to employ the ointment massage extensively in clinic.

In a word, from instinctive pressing and rubbing behavior, through long time of accumulation, up to the summaries made in *Huangdi Qibo Anmo* and *Huangdi Neijing*, tuina finally developed into a clinical subject with its own unique therapeutic system. It was not only summarized and improved theoretically, but also became clinically mature and extensive with its own unique feature through the introduction and application of that time's

经络学说, 阴阳五行、气血津液学说, 诊断方法, 治疗原则等, 也都成为推拿学中最重要的指导原则。

汉代名医张仲景所著《金匮要略》中, 首次将膏摩疗法列为预防保健方法之一, 还介绍了一首用于推拿治疗头风的"摩散", 方仅附子与盐两味, 但后世"摩顶膏"之类, 皆由此衍化而出。在该书中, 张仲景还详细记载了推拿救治自缢的方法, 此法为医学界公认为世界上最早的救治缢死的科学记载, 是推拿史上值得骄傲的杰出成就。另一名医华佗倡导"五禽戏", 使导引按摩向仿生学靠拢, 为后世提供了一套行之有效的保健方法。其治病善用膏摩, 是第一位将膏摩广泛用于临床的医家。

总之, 推拿自本能按摩行为, 经历漫长岁月的不断积累, 至《黄帝岐伯按摩》和《内经》的总结, 终于发展成为一门具有独特治疗体系的临床学科, 不仅在理论上得到总结和提高, 而且经当时名医扁鹊、张仲景、华佗等倡

famous doctors Bian Que, Zhang Zhongjing, Hua Tuo, etc. Therefore the Qin and Han Dynasties were both the period of formation of the specific therapeutic system and the flourishing age of tuina, which linked the past and future in its history of development.

In the Jin and Tang Dynasties the rulers gradually valued tuina therapy. In the Office of Imperial Health of the Sui Dynasty, the title of massage doctor was authorized for the first time. On the basis of the Sui's office, Emperor Tang Taizong set up an Imperial Health Administration with larger scale and better facilities, in which there was a tuina department. Three academic titles were given to masseurs, i. e. massage academicians, massagists and massage workers. Assisted by the massagists and massage workers, the academicians taught the massage apprentices Daoyin methods (a self-tuina exercise) to take away diseases and rectify injuries. Tunia teaching came to be organized. Self-tuina was also laid stress on in this period. Many records about methods of self-tuina such as tuina method of ancient India and Laozi Tuina could be found in Ge Hong's *Zhouhou Beijifang* (*Handbook of Prescriptions for Emergencies*) and Sun Simiao's *Qianjinfang* (*Valuable Prescriptions*). In each chapter of *Zhubing Yuanhoulun* (*General Treatise on the Causes and Symptoms of Diseases*), Chao Yuanfang included daoyin method for health preservation. He especially valued the technique of abdominal tuina for that purpose. The extensive use of self-tuina indicated that massotherapy began to be used for health care and prevention of diseases and for exertion of patients's subjective initiative in fighting against diseases. The complementing effect of medication and tuina manipulations greatly promoted the development of massotherapy. Ge Hong took application

导和运用，在临床也更成熟和广泛，而且富有特色。因此秦汉时期既是推拿独特治疗体系的形成时期，也是推拿发展史上第一个承前启后的鼎盛时期。

晋唐之际，封建君主逐渐重视推拿疗法。隋太医署中首次设有按摩博士的职衔。唐太宗则在隋代已有的基础上，建立了规模更大、设置更加完备的太医署，并专门设立了按摩科，将推拿医生正式确定为按摩博士、按摩师和按摩工三个等级。按摩博士在按摩师和按摩工的协助下，教按摩生"导引之法以除疾，损伤折跌者正之"，开始了有组织的推拿教学。自我推拿在这一时期也得到了广泛的重视，在葛洪《肘后备急方》、孙思邈《千金方》中记载了许多自我推拿的方法，如天竺国按摩法、老子按摩法等。巢元方在《诸病源候论》的每一章节，均附有养生导引法，尤其重视摩腹养生之术。自我推拿的广泛开展，说明推拿疗法开始注重预防保健，注意发挥病人与疾病作斗争的主观能动性。药物与手法相得益彰的作用，更促使按摩疗法有了很大发展。葛洪十分重视膏摩的运用，是第一位系统论述膏摩方

of ointment tuina seriously and was the first specialist to expound it systematically and make it perfect in syndrome, therapeutic principle, prescription and medication. He said that illnesses occurring newly or in the past needed different therapies; ailments in the superficial parts of the body responded well to ointment and tuina. He also stressed that a quick result could be obtained by rubbing forcefully until heat produced and that when a patient was placed close to fire and rubbed with hand twice or three times a day, good effects would be gained after hundreds of times of operation. In his above-mentioned book Ge Hong recorded eight medical formulae of ointment tuina, which were mostly from the celebrities at that time. In addition to the ccyodinic recipe with ointment tuina in *Liujuanzi Guiyifang* (*Liu Juanzi's Magic Prescriptions*), two other ccyodinic tuina skills with salt and decoction were added in *Waitai Miyao* (*Medical Secrets of an Official*), in which many famous prescriptions of ointment tuina with their sources were listed too. The therapeutic indications of tuina were also gradually expanded in this period. For instance, in *Tangliudian* (*Six Classics of the Tang Dynasty*) there were records about eight kinds of diseases caused by pathogenic wind, cold, heat, dampness, hunger, overeating, overwork and lack of exercise, which could be treated with tuina. In *Waitai Miyao* a record about tuina used for EFD (exogenous febrile disease) could be seen, which said when EFD was first caught with headache and stiffness in the back, tuina could be applied with satisfactory results. It was in this period that tuina techniques were introduced into Korea, Japan, India, Europe and some Arabic countries.

In the Song, Jin and Yuan Dynasties, massotherapy gained more extensive use and the doctors attached more importance to the analysis of tuina manipulations. In

法,使膏摩证、法、方、药齐备的医家。他认为"病有新旧,疗法不同,邪在毫毛,宜服膏及摩之";强调"摩时宜极力,令作热,乃速效","向火以手摩","日两三度","数百遍佳"等。《肘后方》记载的葛洪常备膏摩方有8首,这些膏方多出自当时名医之手。《外台秘要》在《刘涓子鬼遗方》膏摩催产的基础上,又增添了盐摩与汤摩两种催产方法。该书罗列了诸多膏摩名方,且多有出处。这一时期推拿治疗范围也逐渐扩大,如《唐六典》中记载:推拿可除八疾,即风、寒、暑、湿、饥、饱、劳、逸。《外台秘要》记载:"如初得伤寒一日,若头痛背强,宜摩之佳。"推拿也正是这一时期传入朝鲜、日本、印度、阿拉伯及欧洲。

宋金元时期,推拿运用范围更加广泛,而且更为注重对手法的分析。《圣济总录》首

Shengji Zonglu（*General Collection for Holy Relief*）a professional treatise on tuina was listed in the first place, in which summaries and induction of massotherapy were made. It was the earliest and most complete tuina works in existence. In the book the author first made some explanation of the implications of pressing and rubbing and their distinction："Pressing and rubbing are sometimes used in combination, in this case they are generally called pressing-rubbing or Anmo. But pressing is not rubbing, and rubbing is not pressing, for pressing is done only by hand while rubbing can also be administrated with the aid of medication. Which to be used, pressing or rubbing, just depends upon their suitability to cases." The writer also believed that massage should be distinguished from daoyin. He pointed out that there existed a tendency not to differentiate the former from the latter in explanation and to confuse them in use, which showed lack of sufficient reflection. Next the author made an incisive summary of the mechanism of massotherapy："Generally speaking, the purpose of tuina therapy completely lies in removal and inhibition. Removal means eliminating or dispersing the obstruction, while inhibition is to have the hyperaction under control." His inference was considered an incisive summarization of the function of tuina and greatly valued by the later generations. Afterwards, on the basis of the original of *Neijing* the author elaborated on the applicable indications of massotherapy, and pointed out under what conditions pressing manipulation can stop pain, not be effective, make pain severe and gain a comfortable sensation. This differentiation was very significant in guiding the clinical application of tuina. Though the treatise on tuina in *Shengji Zonglu of Medicine* was not long, it made thorough analyses of the important problems in tuina therapy and drew precise conclusions,

列"按摩"专论,对按摩疗法进行总结和归纳,是现存最早最完整的推拿专论。首先,作者就按摩的含义及按与摩的区别进行了解释:"可按可摩,时兼而用,通谓之按摩。按之弗摩,摩之弗按,按止以手,摩或兼以药,曰按曰摩,适所用也。"其次,作者认为应当将按摩与导引分别开来:"世之论按摩,不知析而治之,乃合导引而解之,益见其不思也。"接着,作者对按摩治疗的机制进行了精辟的概括:"大抵按摩法,每以开达抑遏为义。开达则壅敝者以之发散,抑遏则慓悍者有所归宿。"这一论断,被认为是对按摩作用机制的经典概括,为后世医家所重视。而后,作者以《内经》原文为基础,对推拿疗法的应用范围详加阐发,指出在何种情况下,"按之痛止,按之无益,按之痛甚,按之快然"。这一区分,对于推拿疗法的临床运用,有很大的指导意义。《圣济总录》中这篇推拿专论文字虽不长,但就推拿疗法中的几个重要问题分析透彻,结论准确,对推拿疗法的发展作出了重要的理论贡献。这一时期,膏摩疗法又有了新的发展。《太平圣惠方》记载了六首治疗目疾的摩顶膏方,为膏摩治疗眼病

so it made great contributions to the development of massotherapy theoretically. In this period ointment tuina was also developed further. In *Taiping Shenghuifang* (*Imperial Health-benefiting Prescriptions*) there were six recorded ointment formulae about treating eye diseases by rubbing the top of the head, which were the earliest records in this problem. The book also recorded for the first time some ointment recipes of rubbing the lower back, and it was a medical book recording the most prescriptions of ointment tunia of a kind from every dynasty and most greatly influencing the development of ointment tuina of the later generations. Among the four medical celebrities of the Jin and Yuan Dynasties, Zhang Congzheng was the one who introduced the most about tuina. In his book *Rumen Shiqin* (*Essential Affairs in the Confucianists*) he classified pressing and rubbing as Hanfa (diaphoretic therapy), which could really be a distinctive view surpassing his predecessors. The method for correcting dislocation of shoulder joints by sitting on a stool or supporting a ladder, reduction of dislocated hip joints by downward hanging and reduction of fracture of spine by suspension recorded in *Shiyi Dexiaofang* (*Curative Prescriptions for Doctors in the World*) could be used to replace traction manipulation. That was an important invention in the history of tuina and set up a new remedy to cure bone diseases with instrumental traction in Chinese medical history.

The Ming and Qing Dynasties witnessed another flourishing age in the history of tuina development. In the field of infantile tuina professional works were published in succession. *Xiao'er Tuina Fangmai Huoying Mizhi Quanshu* (*Imperial Physician's Complete Classic of the Secret Principles of Tuina to Bring Infants Back to Life*), also called *Complete Classic of Infantile Tuina*,

的最早记载,该书还首次记载了摩腰膏方,是历代医书中记载膏摩方最多的医书,对后世膏摩发展影响巨大。金元四大家中,对推拿介绍最多的,首推张从正。他在《儒门事亲》中将按摩列为汗法之一,这不能不说是一种超越前人的独特见解。《世医得效方》中所载肩关节脱位的坐凳架梯法、髋关节脱位的倒吊复位法和脊椎骨折的悬吊复位法等都可以替代拔伸手法,是推拿史上的重大发明,开辟了中国医学史上以器械牵引治疗骨科疾病的新篇章。

明清时期,是推拿发展史上的又一个鼎盛时期。在小儿推拿方面,推拿专著纷纷面世。太医龚云林的《小儿推拿方脉活婴秘旨全书》(又称《小儿推拿全书》),属单行本流行最早者;周于蕃的《小儿推拿

was the earliest published book in separate edition. *Xiao'er Tuina Mijue* (*the Secret of Infant Tuina Therapy*) written by Zhou Yufan most vividly described eight manipulations. Xiong Yingxiong's *Xiao'er Tuina Guangyi* (*Elucidations of Tuina for Infants*) had attached remedies commonly used for children, which was considered the perfect book in the Qing Dynasty. Xia Yuzhu's *Youke Tiejing* (*the Iron Mirror of Pediatrics*) showed ingenuity and had many more differences from other books. He also wrote *Tuina Daiyao Fu* (*the Prose of Tuina Used for Replacing Medication*), which made people find everything fresh and new. *Youke Tuina Mishu* (*Secrets of Tuina of Pediatric Speciality*), written by Luo Rulong, was the most minute and incisive book with clear presentation, and a shortcut of learning infantile tuina. *Tuina Sanzijing* (*the Three-character Classics on Tuina*), written by Xu Qianguang, is read smooth and rhythmic. If it is learned by heart, you can employ them with high proficiency in treatment. In his *Lizheng Anmo Yaoshu* (*Revised Synopsis of Tuina*), Zhang Zhenjun absorbed the strong points of many scholars and put forward for the first time eight manipulations of infantile tuina: pressing, rubbing, nipping, kneading, pushing, arc-pushing, palm-twisting and rotating, which symbolized the formation of independent therapeutic system of infantile tuina. Meanwhile, adult tuina was further developed. It presented a situation of hundreds of flowers blossoming and decades of schools coming into being, such as bone-setting tunia, point-pressing tuina, one finger meditation tuina, eye tuina, surgery tuina, internal exercise tuina, keep-fit tuina, too numerous to enumerate. In a word, the Ming and Qing Dynasties were an important period of overall development, summarization and creation in the history of tuina.

秘诀》，描述小儿推拿八法最为精彩；熊应雄的《小儿推拿广意》附录儿科常用方药，被誉为清代最善之本；夏禹铸《幼科铁镜》匠心独运，与诸书存异处甚多，更作"推拿代药赋"，令人耳目一新。骆如龙《幼科推拿秘书》，最为详晰，条理清楚，是小儿推拿之入门捷径；徐谦光的《推拿三字经》朗朗上口，烂熟于胸必临证应手；张振鋆的《厘正按摩要术》博采众家之长，首次提出小儿推拿八法，即"按、摩、掐、揉、推、运、搓、摇"。这些标志着小儿推拿独特治疗体系的形成。成人推拿也得到了更大发展，可谓百花齐放，流派纷呈，诸如正骨推拿、点穴推拿、一指禅推拿、眼科推拿、外科推拿、内功推拿、保健推拿，真是举不胜举。因此，明清时期是推拿发展史上一个较为全面发展、总结、创造的重要时期。

The Republic of China constituted the key period of linking up the preceding and the following and forming schools in the history of tuina. These schools included one-finger manipulation tuina, meridian and visceral tuina, point-pressing tuina, abdominal diagnosis tuina, internal exercise tuina, rolling tuina, gastropathy tuina, etc. Yet owing to some historical limitations the academic schools of tuina were developed only among the people, inherited and taught in the master-apprentice mode and passed on through oral instruction and learned by heart. It was a pity that they could not be sorted out systematically and fostered and enhanced.

1.1.2　Research and Advance of Chinese Tuina

Ever since the founding of the People's Republic of China, tuina medicine has entered an overall new developing period. The main achievements of tuina study and advance in this period were embodied in the following five aspects:

Firstly, ancient books on tuina were excavated and sorted out, and a lot of new works on tuina were published. Besides the ancient books sorted out and published again, which were mostly specialized treatises on infantile tuina, in this period there were restricted publications *Erzhi Dingchan* (*Fixed Two-finger Meditation*), *Yizhi Yangchun* (*One-finger Spring Season*), etc., which made contributions to the excavation of ancient medical tuina books. New works on tuina included the following kinds: ① Popular literatures which are of combination of basic theories with clinical knowledge. ② Books in the form of clinical specialities. ③ Books which are of characteristic of schools or unique experience. ④ Specific treatises on manipulations or exercises. ⑤ Great complete

民国时期,是推拿发展史上承上启下,形成流派的关键时期,这些流派包括一指禅推拿、经络脏腑推拿、点穴推拿、腹诊推拿、内功推拿、滚法推拿、胃病推拿等。但由于历史原因的限制,这些推拿学术流派的发展多是在民间流传,并限于"以师带徒,口授心传"的方式继承和传授,惜未能系统整理和发扬光大。

二、中国推拿的研究和进展

中华人民共和国成立后至今,推拿学的发展进入了一个全新时期。这一时期推拿的研究和进展的主要成就集中表现在下列五个方面。

第一,推拿古籍得到全面的发掘和整理,并出版了大量推拿新著。这一阶段整理再版的推拿古籍除多部小儿推拿专著外,有内部刊物《二指定禅》、《一指阳春》等,为古代推拿医籍的发掘作出了贡献。推拿新著有以基础理论与临证知识相结合的通俗著作,有以临证专科形式出现,有以流派和独到的经验见长,有专论手法、功法者,也有集大成之类的巨著,如《中国按摩大全》、《中国推拿》、《中华推拿

works. Among them were *Zhongguo Anmo Daquan* (*the Complete works of Chinese Anmo*), *Zhongguo Tuina* (*Chinese Tuina*), *Zhonghua Tuina Dacheng* (*the Great Collection of Chinese Tuina*), and *Tuina Dacheng* (*the Great Collection of Tuina*), etc. A general survey showed that all the works had the common features of the enhancement of science and logic of tuina, the breakthrough in tuina principle, the increase of proofs of modern researches and the combination of treatment of diseases with diagnostic and anatomic knowledge of Western medicine.

Secondly, the practice and summarization of clinical experience of tuina became more scientific day by day. The progress of science and culture and the development of health and medicine made tuina practice more scientific. The accumulated rich experience in practice and the education of modern medical knowledge raised the quality of massagists greatly. For example, diagnosis of tuina was no longer confined to the traditional four diagnostic methods. Many massagists have commanded modern medical techniques such as X-ray examination, ultrasonic scanning, electromyographic examination, CT examination and nuclear magnetic resonance. In treatment sectarian bias were gradually thrown away. Massagists have mastered a set of theories of treatment based on syndrome differentiation. They are able to select and employ the best ones from the principles, methods, prescriptions and techniques. Thousands of theses on tuina have been published in many sorts of periodicals of China, which summed up tuina therapy from all respects scientifically and offered an important guide to tuina clinic.

Thirdly, the teaching system of tuina has been improving day by day. Since Shanghai Health School started a tuina training class in October, 1956, tuina teaching has

大成》、《推拿大成》等。综观这些著作,其共同特点是推拿理论的科学性和逻辑性增强,在推拿原理方面有所突破,增加了现代研究的佐证,在疾病的治疗方面多结合西医学的诊断和解剖知识。

第二,推拿实践及临床经验的总结日趋科学化。科学文化的进步,医药卫生事业的发展,使推拿实践也日趋科学化。医疗实践方面丰富经验的积累和现代医学知识的教育使推拿医师整体素质大大提高。如在诊断方法上,已不再仅局限于中医传统四诊,现代医学的 X 线诊断、超声波检查、肌电图、CT 检查、核磁共振等已为广大推拿医师所掌握。在治疗方面,门户之见逐渐消除,推拿医师已掌握了一整套辨证论治的理论,理、法、方、术,择善而从之。全国各类期刊发表了数以千计的推拿论文,对推拿各方面进行了科学总结,对推拿临床起到了重要的指导作用。

第三,推拿教学体系日趋完善。自 1956 年 10 月上海卫生学校开办了推拿训练班起,

gone out of the old master-apprentice mode and has been on the way of formal education. Since the late 1970s, and early 1980s, all the TCM colleges in China have organized tuina speciality one after another and consummated the educational system of tuina subject including professional training, undergraduate, postgraduate, doctorate and international education, which have trained quite a lot of advanced specialists on tuina. Tuina teaching activities have been carried out at all TCM colleges of China and the foreign exchanges has greatly increased. Textbooks of tuina have also possessed different styles and different levels. With the development of tuina subject, tuina teaching has divided into different courses: basic tuina, tuina therapy, tuina manipulation, tuina exercise training, and infantile tuina, etc.

Fourthly, scientific researches into tuina has been advancing rapidly. Since the 1950s scientific researchers on tuina have conducted extensive clinical and experimental studies of the functional mechanism of tuina by means of modern scientific and medical knowledge and made exciting progress. For instance, the gate control theory in neurophysiology was employed to successfully explain the analgesic principle of tuina. It was deduced that the distinct changes of circulating speed of blood and lymph-vascular fluid before and after tuina manipulations might be one of action principles of eliminating swelling and blood stasis with tuina. It was also demonstrated that lowering blood pressure by tuina had a stable effect, the contents of 5-HT in the blood increased after tuina treatment and the therapy of nipping the spine apparently promoted the absorption of the small intestine.

Finally, many new tuina therapies have been summed

推拿教学就从过去师带徒形式走上了正规教育的途径。20世纪70年代末、80年代初以来，全国各中医院校相继成立推拿专业，完善了推拿专业专科、本科、硕士研究生、博士研究生和外国留学生教育体系，为中医推拿培养了大量的高级人才。推拿教学活动在全国各中医院校全面展开，而且对外交流也日益加强，推拿教材方面也具备了各种不同体例、不同层次的教材。并随着推拿学科的发展，推拿教学逐渐分为推拿学基础、推拿治疗学、推拿手法学、推拿练功学、小儿推拿学等课程。

第四，推拿科研发展迅速。从20世纪50年代起，推拿科研人员运用现代科学和现代医学知识对推拿作用机制进行了广泛的临床和实验研究，取得了令人振奋的进展。如运用神经生理学中闸门控制学说能够较为完满地解释了推拿镇痛原理；推拿前后血液及淋巴管液循环速度差异明显，可能是推拿消肿化瘀的作用原理之一；推拿降血压，效果恒定，推拿后血液中5-HT含量增加；捏脊疗法明显促进小肠的吸收功能等。

第五，总结和创造出许多

up and created such as ear point tuina, foot point tuina, the second metacarpal bone tuina, sports tuina and anaesthesia by tuina. In a word, today's China is in the unprecedented golden age in the history of tuina. There appears a flourishing situation in tuina practice, teaching, scientific research, publication of works and periodicals and the construction of tuina practitioners.

1.1.3　How to Learn Chinese Tuina

Chinese Tuina is a clinical subject of TCM with intensive theory and practice. Tuina doctors should not only have the basic knowledge of Chinese and Western medicine, understand the methods of diagnosis and treatment based on syndrome differentiation, have specialized in theoretical knowledge of tuina, but also possess a good physical constitution and proficient manipulation techniques for clinical practice. So in addition to the study of elementary theories of Chinese and Western medicine, the students of tuina speciality must systematically study tuina courses and carry out strict constitutional physical exercise and technical training in manipulation.

In respect of medical elementary theories, the study of TCM theories of yin-yang, five elements, zang-fu organs, meridians, wei, qi, ying, and blood, cause and mechanism of diseases, four diagnostic methods and eight principles, differentiating syndrome to decide treatment and the study of anatomy, physiology, pathophysiology, pathoanatomy and physical diagnosis of Western medicine should be put at the first place. Anatomic structure of the human body, athletic physiology, neural segments, circu-

新的推拿疗法,如耳穴推拿、足穴推拿、第二掌骨推拿法、运动推拿、推拿麻醉等。总之,现今的中国是推拿史上前所未有的黄金时期,中国推拿的临床、教学、科研以及推拿著作和刊物的出版、推拿队伍的建设和发展,都出现了空前的繁荣。

三、怎样学习中国推拿

推拿学是一门理论性和实践性都比较强的中医临床学科。推拿医生不仅要通晓中西医基础知识、诊断及辨证论治方法、推拿专业理论知识,而且还要具备能适应推拿临床工作的身体素质和熟练的手法操作技能。所以,推拿学生,除了学习中西医基础理论课程外,还要系统学习专业课,并且要进行严格的身体素质锻炼和手法操作的技能训练。

在医学基础理论方面,要特别强调中医的阴阳五行、脏腑经络、营卫气血、病因病机、四诊八纲、辨证论治和西医的解剖、生理、病理生理、病理解剖、物理诊断等内容的学习。尤其要熟知人体的解剖结构、运动生理、神经节段和十四经络的循环、常用穴的位置、作

lation of the fourteen meridians, location and function of commonly used points have great practical value in tuina practice. Students should especially master them.

In professional technical training students should first do the common exercises hard with the methods introduced in the section of Tuina Liangong of this book step by step. During the exercise both the training of physical constitution including strength, endurance, pliability and toughness and the cultivation of psychological quality should be devoted to. That means while building up one's physique, one should develop indomitable willpower and quality to bear hardships and stand strenuous work so as to lay a good foundation for the long-term tuina practice in future. Next, under the guidance of teachers, one should seriously learn and practice all kinds of manipulations introduced in this book, fully and strictly accomplish the training in the three elementary stages, which refer to training on a sand sack, training on the human body and training of manipulations in treating commonly encountered diseases. Furthermore, one should study carefully the parts of tuina therapy in this book and combine them with frequent clinical practice so as to improve the result of study.

Generally speaking, after a period of conscientious training, for those with some knowledge of medical science, it is not too hard to cross the threshold of tuina within a short period of time. But it is difficult to come up to professional standards, particularly hard to gain a perfect command and serviceable application of some technically difficult manipulations such as pushing manipulation with one-finger meditation, rolling manipulation in clinic. So a long period of special training is the only approach to

用等,这些在推拿临床极有实用价值。

在专业技能方面,首先要根据本书"练功"卷所介绍的常用功法及其练习方法,按步骤进行认真练功。在练功过程中,不仅要注意力量、耐力、柔韧性等身体素质的锻炼,而且还要加强心理素质的培养。即在锻炼身体素质的同时,培养自己吃苦耐劳、坚韧不拔的精神,为将来长期从事推拿工作打下良好的基础。其次,在老师的指导下,认真学习和练习本教材手法篇中所介绍的各种手法。严格按照动作要求循序渐进、持之以恒地完成沙袋练习、人体练习与常见病操作练习三个基本阶段的训练。第三,认真学习本书有关推拿治疗的内容,并坚持勤于临床实践,这样理论与实践相结合将大大提高学习效果。

总之,掌握了一定医学基础知识的人,经过一段时间的认真训练,推拿是不难在短期内入门的,但是要达到推拿专业医师的水平,特别是要熟练掌握一指禅推法、滚法等技术难度较高的手法并能得心应手地运用于临床,则必须经过长时间的专业训练,才能达到

reach the realm——once in clinic, while you massage the exterior of the body, effect can produce in the interior. Your hands manipulate along with the mind's meditation and curative therapy comes out of your excellent manipulations, as stated in *Yizongjinjian* (*Golden Mirror of Medicine*).

1.2   Acting Principles of Tuina

Tuina attains the purpose of preventing and treating diseases by means of applying therapeutic manipulations to certain points or superficial parts of the human body to regulate the physiological and pathological conditions. So its curative action depends upon the property and quantity of the applied manipulations, the special nature of the locations being treated and the selected points. The acting principles of tuina include balancing yin and yang, regulating the zang-fu organs, dredging the meridians and promoting circulation of qi to activate blood.

1.2.1   Balancing Yin and Yang

Yin-yang is a concept of ancient Chinese philosophy. The initial meaning of yin and yang was very simple, just referring to side facing or opposing the sunlight, i. e. the side facing it being yang while the side opposing it yin. Later on, this meaning was extended to mean warmth and cold in climate, up and down, left and right, internal and external in location, excitement and inhibition of motion state, etc. The ancient thinkers observed that everything in the universe comprised two opposing aspects. Yin and yang were the summarization of the two opposing aspects of related things and phenomena in the nature. The occurrence, development and change of everything in the universe

《医宗金鉴》所说"一旦临证，机触于外，巧生于内，手随心转，法从手出"的境界。

第二节　推拿作用原理

推拿是通过手法作用于人体体表的特定穴位或部位，来调节机体的生理病理状态，达到防治疾病的目的。因此，推拿疗效的产生取决于手法的性质和量、治疗部位或穴位的特异性。推拿作用原理可概括为平衡阴阳、调和脏腑、疏通经络、行气活血等。

一、平衡阴阳

阴阳是中国古代的一个哲学概念。阴阳的最初涵义是很朴素的，是指日光的向背，向日为阳，背日为阴。后来引申为气候的寒暖，方位的上下、左右、内外，运动状态的躁动和宁静等。古代思想家看到自然界万事万物都有正反两个方面，阴阳是对自然界相互关联的某些事物和现象对立双方的概括，宇宙间一切事物的发生、发展和变化，都

were the outcome of motion of yin and yang in opposition and unity of two aspects in one contradiction. It is said in *Plain Questions*, *the Treatise on the Correspondence between Man and the Universe* that yin and yang are the law of the universe, the great outlines of everything, the parents of all changes, the origin of birth and death and the source of mental activities. Over two thousand years ago, the yin-yang theory had been introduced into TCM and became an important component of its basic theory, used to explain the organic structure, the physiological functions and the pathological changes of the human body as well as guide clinical diagnosis and treatment.

The yin-yang theory holds that the human body is composed of two opposite but unified aspects: materials and functions, i.e. yin and yang. In terms of the parts of the human body, the exterior is yang and the interior is yin; the upper part is yang and the lower part is yin; the back is yang and the abdomen is yin. As for the zang-fu organs, the six fu-organs are yang and the five zang-organs are yin. As for qi and blood, qi is yang and blood is yin. In terms of function and material, function is yang and material is yin. As far as functional state is concerned, excitement is yang and inhibition is yin; activity is yang and static condition is yin; growth is yang and decline is yin. When it comes to functional activity of qi, upward is yang while downward is yin; outward is yang and inward is yin and so on. When yin and yang are in dynamic equilibrium, life activity of the body will remain in a healthy state known as "yin and yang in equilibrium". But if the relative balance between yin and yang is upset by the six pathogenic factors, seven emotions and traumatic injuries, there may appear a series of pathological changes due to imbalance between yin and yang. For example, excess of yang causes heat, while excess of yin leads to

是阴阳对立统一矛盾运动的结果。所以《素问·阴阳应象大论》说:"阴阳者,天地之道也,万物之纲纪,变化之父母,生杀之本始,神明之府也。"早在两千多年前,阴阳学说就被引用到中医学中,成为中医基本理论的一个重要组成部分。中医用阴阳学说来解释人体的组织结构、生理功能、病理变化等,并指导着临床诊断和治疗。

阴阳学说认为,人体是由两种既对立又统一的物质与功能,即阴和阳构成的。就人体部位而言,体表为阳,体内为阴;上部为阳,下部为阴;背部为阳,腹部为阴。就人体脏腑而言,六腑为阳,五脏为阴。就人体气血而言,气为阳,血为阴。就功能与物质而言,功能为阳,物质为阴。就功能活动的状态而言,兴奋为阳,抑制为阴,活动为阳,静止为阴,增长为阳,减退为阴。就气机运行而言,上升为阳,下降为阴,向外为阳,向内为阴等。当阴阳双方处于相对动态平衡状态时,人体的生命活动便处于"阴平阳秘"的健康状态。如因六淫、七情或跌仆损伤等因素的作用使人体阴阳的相对平衡状态遭到破坏时,就会导致一系列阴阳失调的病理

cold; excess of yin results in disorders of yang, excess of yang results in disorders of yin; deficiency of yang produces exterior cold, deficiency of yin brings about interior heat, etc. Clinically syndromes of different degrees and properties such as yin, yang, exterior, interior, cold, heat, deficiency and excess may be present. It is clear that all physiological and pathological changes in the human body can be summarized with yin and yang, which correspond to asthenia or sthenia of zang-fu organs, disharmony between qi and blood, obstruction of the meridians, irregulation of the ying and wei systems. They are all due to predominance or decline of yin and yang or imbalance between yin and yang, which is the root cause of the occurrence of diseases and presents in the whole process of the occurrence and development of diseases. It is said in the book *Jingyue Quanshu—Chuanzhonglu* that though they are complex, medical tenets can still be summed up in one word: yin and yang.

Tuina treatment follows the principle "examining the conditions of yin and yang carefully so as to get them in relative balance" described in *Huangdi Neijing*. According to syndrome differentiation, massagists employ different manipulations with different stimulations clinically to change pathological conditions of the body caused by imbalance of yin-yang, restore their relative equilibrium and remove pathogenic factors. Manipulations may be light or heavy, slow or rapid, forceful or gentle. They can be used to treat asthenic syndrome with reinforcing method, sthenic syndrome by reduction, heat syndrome by cooling, cold syndrome by warming, stasis or stagnation by removing and dispersing, exopathogens in the exterior of the body by diaphoresis and half-exterior and half-interior syndrome by expelling and regulating therapy. The purpose of regulating yin and yang is accomplished mainly

变化,如阳盛则热,阴盛则寒;阴盛则阳病,阳盛则阴病;阳虚生外寒,阴虚生内热等。临床可表现为阴、阳、表、里、寒、热、虚、实等多种不同层次、不同性质的病证。可见,人体内部的一切生理病理变化均可以阴阳概括,脏腑虚实、气血不和、经络不畅、营卫失调等病理变化,不外乎阴阳的偏盛或偏衰,均属于阴阳失调的范畴。阴阳失调是疾病产生的根本原因,贯穿于一切疾病发生、发展的始终。《景岳全书·传忠录》说,"医道虽繁,可一言以蔽之,阴阳而已。"

推拿治病遵循《黄帝内经》"谨察阴阳所在而调之,以平为期"的原则,根据辨证分型,推拿医生采用或轻、或重、或缓、或急、或刚、或柔等不同刺激量的手法,使虚者补之,实者泻之,热者寒之,寒者热之,壅滞者通之,结聚者散之,邪在皮毛者汗而发之,病在半表半里者和而解之,以改变人体内部阴阳失调的病理状态,从而达到恢复阴阳的相对平衡、邪去正复之目的。这种调整阴阳的功能,主要是通过经络、气血而起作用的。推拿手法作用于局部,在局部通经

through the meridians, qi and blood. That is, tuina manipulations act on the local areas to dredge the meridians, promote circulation of qi and blood and nourish the bones and muscles and through them further affect the corresponding viscera and other parts. For instance, proper manipulations applied to cases with hyperperistalsis of the intestine at the Back-Shu and Front-Mu acupoints can inhibit its hyperactivity and make it back to a normal condition; on the contrary, hypoperistalsis of the intestine can also be improved to the healthy condition with tuina manipulations. Some researchers observed the peristalsis of the stomach by massaging Pishu (BL 20), Weishu (BL 21) and Zusanli (ST 36). They found that massaging Pishu (BL 20) and Weishu (BL 21) quickened its movement, while massaging Zusanli (ST 36) and other points inhibited it. Further studies showed that when the movement of the stomach is enhanced, tuina can make it decrease, however, when its movement decreases, tuina can enhance it.

1.2.2 Regulating Zang and Fu Organs

The visceral manifestation theory is an extremely important part of the theoretical system of traditional Chinese medicine, which has the universal significance in expounding the physiology and pathology of the human body and guiding clinical practice. Zang-fu organ is a general term of the internal organs. According to their physiological functional characteristics these internal organs can be divided into three categories i. e. zang-organ, fu-organ and extraordinary fu-organ. Zang-organ refers to the heart, lung, spleen, liver and kidney, together known as the five zang-organs. Fu-organ includes the gallbladder, stomach, small intestine, large intestine, urinary bladder and triple energizer, collectively called the six fu-organs.

络、行气血、濡筋骨,并通过气血、经络影响相应的脏器与相关部位。如对肠蠕动亢进者,在背部和腹部的俞募穴上使用适当的手法,可使其亢进状态受到抑制而恢复正常。反之,肠蠕动功能减退者,亦可通过手法加快其蠕动而恢复正常。有人通过穴位推拿观察胃的运动,对两侧脾俞、胃俞、足三里等穴位进行推拿的结果表明:脾俞、胃俞在推拿后引起胃运动增强,足三里则引起胃运动抑制。进一步研究发现,在胃运动增强时,推拿后往往胃的运动减弱,而在胃运动减弱时,推拿后往往使胃的运动增强。

二、调和脏腑

藏象学说在中医学理论体系中占有极其重要的地位,对阐明人体的生理和病理,指导临床实践具有普遍的指导意义。脏腑,是内脏的总称。按照脏腑的生理功能特点,可分为脏、腑、奇恒之腑三类。脏,即心、肺、脾、肝、肾,合称为五脏;腑,即胆、胃、小肠、大肠、膀胱、三焦,合称六腑;奇恒之腑,即脑、髓、骨、脉、胆、女子胞(子宫)。五脏的共同生理特点,是化生和贮藏精

And the brain, marrow, bones, vessels, gallbladder and uterus belong to the category of the extraordinary fu-organs. The common physiological function of the five zang-organs is to produce and store the vital essence or essential qi, while that of the six fu-organs is to receive, digest, transport and transform foodstuff. And the extraordinary fu-organs refer to a kind of fu-organs, which are different from the six fu-organs physiologically and morphologically. They do not directly contact water and foodstuff and are relatively enclosed organs. But like the five zang-organs functionally, they have the property of storing essential qi. That's why they are termed as the extraordinary fu-organs. It is said in *Plain Questions*, *Special Classics on the Five Zang-Organs* that the five Zang-organs store essential qi, but do not excrete, so they can be full, but can't be over stuffed; while the six fu-organs transport and transform foodstuff, but do not store, so they can be stuffed, but can't be full. The reason is that when foodstuff is taken in, it makes the stomach full, but the intestine is still empty; when the foodstuff is transported and transformed from the stomach into the intestines, the former is empty, while the latter is full. So there is the so-called "stuffed but not full, and full but not stuffed". Wang Bing once said, "Essential qi is to be full, and water and food are to be stuffed. The five zang-organs only store essential qi, so they are full, but not stuffed; the six fu-organs do not store essential qi, but receive water and food, so they are stuffed, but not full." This difference between zang and fu organs not only indicates their physiological functional features, but also is helpful in guidance of clinical practice. Disorders of the zang-organs are mostly of asthenic syndrome, diseases of the fu-organs are sthenic. So when a zang-organ is excessive, purging its corresponding fu-organ will be effective

气;六腑的共同生理特点,是受盛和传化水谷;奇恒之腑,即是指这一类腑的形态及生理功能均有异于"六腑",不与水谷直接接触,而是一个相对密闭的组织器官,并还具有类似于脏的贮藏精气的作用,因而称为奇恒之腑。所以,《素问·五藏别论》说:"所谓五藏者,藏精气而不泻也,故满而不能实。六府者,传化物而不藏,故实而不能满也。所以然者,水谷入口,则胃实而肠虚;食下,则肠实而胃虚。故曰,实而不满,满而不实也。"王冰说:"精气为满,水谷为实。五脏但藏精气,故满而不实;六腑则不藏精气,但受水谷,故实而不能满也。"脏与腑的这些区别,并不仅仅是说明其生理上的功能特点,而且也具有指导临床实践的意义。如脏病多虚,腑病多实;脏实者可泻其腑,腑虚者可补其脏等,至今仍不失为指导临床的准则。

and vice versa, if a fu-organ is deficient, the approach to tonifying its related zang-organ can be used. This principle is still guiding clinical practice.

Regulating zang and fu organs with tuina is accomplished mainly through manipulations applied to a certain part of the body. Through the connection of the meridians tuina manipulations bring about some physiological changes in the corresponding zang or fu organs, reinforce asthenia and reduce sthenia to treat diseases. Modern physiological researches demonstrate that for some tissues, weak stimulations can activate and excite their physiological functions, whereas strong stimulations can inhibit them. In clinic, patients with splenogastric asthenia respond well to the treatment of long-term rhythmic stimulations of mild pushing manipulation with one finger on the points of Pishu (BL 20), Weishu (BL 21), Zhongwan (CV 12), Qihai (CV 6) and so on. For the cases of gastroenterospasm, performing pressing and digital-pressing manipulations with short-time powerful stimulations on the corresponding Back-Shu acupoints can relieve spasm. The treatment of hypertension is the same. Hypertension caused by hyperactivity of liver yang can be relieved by applying pushing, pressing, kneading, grasping manipulations to the point qiaogong with very strong stimulations to calm the liver to suppress hyperactive liver yang. And hypertension due to retention of phlegmatic dampness can be lowered by performing pressing and rubbing manipulations at Pishu (BL 20) and Shenshu (BL 23) on the back and abdomen with long-time gentle stimulations to invigorate the spleen to eliminate dampness. From the above examples it can be seen that though it does not have any tonic or purgative into the body, through manipulations to stimulate certain superficial parts of the body, tuina is able to promote visceral functions or inhibit their hyperac-

推拿调和脏腑的作用,主要是运用手法作用于人体某一部位,通过经络的联系,使体内相应的脏腑产生相应的生理变化,补虚泻实,以达到治疗的目的。现代生理研究表明:对某一组织来说,弱刺激能活跃、兴奋其生理功能,强刺激能抑制其生理功能。在临床上,对脾胃虚的患者,治疗时,在脾俞、胃俞、中脘、气海等穴用轻柔的一指禅推法进行较长时间的有节律的刺激,可取得好的疗效;胃肠痉挛患者,则在其背部相应的俞穴,用点、按等较强的手法作短时间刺激,痉挛即可缓解。对高血压病的治疗也是如此,由于肝阳上亢而致的高血压病,可在桥弓穴用推、按、揉、拿等手法作重刺激,平肝潜阳,从而降低血压;由于痰湿内阻而致的高血压病,则可在腹部及背部脾俞、肾俞用推摩等手法,作较长时间的轻刺激,健脾化湿,从而降低血压。从以上例子可以看出,推拿虽无直接补、泻物质进入体内,但从本质上看依靠手法在体表一定的部位刺激,可起到促进脏腑功能或抑制其亢进的

tivities. Of course, the light or heavy degrees of manipulations should vary according to individual physique, location of receiving manipulations and the threshold value of stimulation, which are measured by aching or distending sensations obtained by the patients in clinic. Manipulations inducing a strong aching and distending sensation are heavy manipulations, and those producing a mild sensation are light ones.

In tuina therapy frequency and direction of manipulations are also very important in regulating the functions of the viscera. The variety of frequency of manipulations in certain limits is only the change of quantity, but the variety beyond the limits will be a leap from the quantitative change to the qualitative change. For instance, the common frequency of pushing manipulation with one finger meditation only has the function of dredging the meridians and regulating ying and wei systems. But the high frequency of this manipulation has the action of activating blood circulation to eliminate swelling and the action of pus-draining and toxin-expelling, which is often used clinically to treat carbuncle and boil, because they are able to permeate tissues effectively and produce an effect of clearing away, resolving and draining toxins with less energy diffused. This kind of effect is called reduction or purging, the opposite is reinforcement or tonifying. Directions of manipulations have different reinforcing or reducing actions at specific treated areas, too. For example, while rubbing the abdomen, if the direction of manipulations and the moving direction of the area being treated are both clockwise, the manipulations will have a noticeable reducing effect. If the direction of the manipulation is counterclockwise and the moving direction of the part being treated is clockwise, the manipulation will have a reinforcing effect of promoting the digestive function of

作用。当然手法的轻重,因各人的体质、接受手法的部位,接受刺激的阈值而异,在临床上则从患者的酸胀感来衡量,产生较强烈的酸胀感为重手法,轻微的酸胀感为轻手法。

在推拿治疗中,手法的频率和方向对调和脏腑功能亦起着重要的作用,手法的频率在一定范围内变化,仅是量的变化,但超过一定范围的变化,则出现了从量变到质变的飞跃。如一般频率的一指禅推法,仅具有舒通经络、调和营卫的作用,但高频率的一指禅推法则具有活血消肿、托脓排毒的作用,临床上常用来治疗痈疖等疾病。因高频率的手法,能量扩散少,能有效地深透于组织中起到"清、消、托"等作用,称之为泻,反之则为补。手法的方向在特定的治疗部位有不同的补泻作用,如在腹部摩腹,手法操作方向与治疗部位移动的方向为顺时针时,有明显的泻下作用,若手法的操作方向为逆时针,而治疗部位的移动方向为顺时针时,则有增加肠胃的消化功能,起到补的作用。在沿经络的推拿中,一般顺经推拿为补,逆经推拿为泻。

the stomach and intestine. In tuina along the meridians, manipulations along the circulating direction of the meridians produce reinforcement and manipulation against their direction has reducing effect.

1.2.3   Dredging Meridians and Collaterals

Jingluo (the meridian system) is the passages of circulating qi and blood throughout the whole body, interconnecting the zang and fu organs with the extremities and linking up the lower part with the upper, and the interior with the exterior of the body. Jingluo is a collective term for the meridians and the collaterals. The meridians are the main trunks, and the collaterals are branches derived from the meridians. The meridians mostly go in the deep parts of the body and have their definite routes. The collaterals are widely and superficially distributed throughout the body like an interlacing network linking the zang and fu organs, body orifices as well as the skin, muscles, tendons, bones and other tissues into an organic integral whole. So the meridian theory is also an important component of TCM, which can not only be used to explain the physiological functions of the body, but more importantly, to expound the pathological changes and guide diagnosis and treatment of diseases.

The meridian system consists of the meridians and collaterals. The meridians include the twelve regular meridians, the eight extraordinary vessels and the divergences of twelve meridians, the tendons of twelve meridians and the twelve skin divisions, which are subordinate to the twelve regular meridians. The collaterals comprise the fifteen collaterals, the superficial collaterals and the minute collaterals, etc. The twelve regular meridians refer to the lung meridian of hand-taiyin, the pericardium meridian of hand-jueyin, the heart meridian of hand-shaoyin, the large intestine meridian of hand-yangming,

三、疏通经络

经络是运行全身气血,联络脏腑肢节,沟通上下内外的通路。经络,是经脉和络脉的总称。经脉是主干,络脉是分支。经脉大多循行于深部,络脉循行于较浅的部位。经脉有一定的循行径路,而络脉则纵横交错,网络全身,把人体所有的脏腑、器官、孔窍以及皮肉筋骨等组织联结成一个统一的有机整体。可见,经络学说是中医学的一个十分重要的组成部分。它不仅可以用来解释人体的生理功能,而且更重要的是它还可用来阐述人体的病理变化,指导疾病的诊断和治疗。

经络系统是由经脉和络脉组成的。其中经脉包括十二经脉和奇经八脉,以及附属于十二经脉的十二经别、十二经筋、十二皮部。络脉有十五络、浮络、孙络等。十二经脉即手太阴肺经、手厥阴心包经、手少阴心经、手阳明大肠经、手少阳三焦经、手太阳小肠经、足阳明胃经、足少阳胆经、足太阳膀胱经、足太阴脾

the triple energizer meridian of hand-shaoyang, the small intestine meridian of hand-taiyang, the stomach meridian of foot-yangming, the gallbladder meridian of foot-shaoyang, the bladder meridian of foot-taiyang, the spleen meridian of foot-taiyin, the liver meridian of foot-jueyin and the kidney meridian of foot-shaoyin. They are the main part of the meridian system, therefore, also called Zhengjing (regular meridians). Here are the distributions of the twelve regular meridians on the body surface. They are symmetrically distributed in the head, face, trunk and extremities and going longitudinally through the whole body. The six yin meridians are distributed in the chest, the abdomen and the medial aspect of the limbs. Among them the three hand yin meridians are in the medial aspect of the upper limbs, and the three foot yin meridians in the medial aspect of the lower limbs. The six yang meridians are distributed in the head, face, trunk and the lateral aspect of the limbs, among which the three hand yang meridians are in the lateral aspect of the upper limbs and the three foot yang meridians in the lateral aspect of the lower extremities. The interior-exterior, pertaining-linking relations of the twelve regular meridians are as follows. Internally, the twelve regular meridians pertain to the zang and fu organs, which have interiorly-exteriorly linking up relations. And the yin and yang meridians also have interior-exterior relations. The yin meridians pertain to zang-organs and connect fu-organs, while the yang meridians pertain to fu-organs and link with zang-organs. The mutually interior-exterior meridians are physiologically connected to each other closely, pathologically affect each other and able to be mutually used in treatment. The circulating courses of the twelve regular meridians are as follows : the three yin meridians of hand travel from the chest to the hands; the three yang meridians of hand go

经、足厥阴肝经和足少阴肾经的总称。它们是经络系统的主体,故又称为"正经"。十二经脉在体表的分布规律:它们左右对称地分布于头面、躯干和四肢,纵贯全身。六条阴经分布于四肢的内侧和胸腹,其中上肢的内侧是手三阴经,下肢的内侧是足三阴经;六条阳经分布于四肢的外侧和头面躯干,其中上肢的外侧是手三阳经,下肢的外侧是足三阳经。十二经脉的表里属络关系:十二经脉内属脏腑,脏与腑有表里相合的关系,阴经与阳经有表里络属的关系。阴经属脏络腑,阳经属腑络脏。互为表里的经脉在生理上密切联系,病变时相互影响,治疗时相互为用。十二经脉的循行走向是:手三阴经从胸走手,手三阳经从手走头,足三阳经从头走足,足三阴经从足走腹(胸)。十二经脉的交接规律是:阴经和阳经多在四肢部衔接,阳经与阳经(指同名经)在头面部相接,阴经与阴经(即手足三阴经)在胸部交接。由于十二经脉通过手足阴阳表里经的连接而逐经相传,所以就构成了一个周而复始、如环无端的传注系统,气血通过经脉,内到脏腑器官,外达肌表,营养全身。奇经八

from the hand to the head; the three yang meridians of foot run from the head to the foot and the three yin meridians of foot pass from foot to the abdomen or chest. The connective law of the twelve regular meridians is as follows: the yin and yang meridians connect to each other at the extremities; the yang meridians of hand and foot join at the head and face, and the yin meridians of hand or foot are connected to each other in the chest. By means of the connection of the yin and yang, interior and exterior meridians, the twelve regular meridians connect and form a circulatory endless ring-like conductive system. Through the meridians, qi and blood internally get to the viscera, and externally to the muscles on the surface to nourish the whole body. The eight extraordinary vessels are a collective term for the governor vessel, conception vessel, thoroughfare vessel, belt vessel, yinwei vessel, yangwei vessel, yinqiao vessel and yangqiao vessel, which are different from the twelve regular meridians. They are neither directly connected with the zang and fu organs, nor interiorly-exteriorly related to each other. They go along other paths different from the regular meridians, so are called extraordinary meridians. The eight extraordinary vessels are crossward distributed among the twelve regular meridians, and perform the function of strengthening the ties among the twelve regular meridians, participating in regulation of the storage and permeation of qi and blood within the twelve regular meridians. The five zang and six fu organs, four limbs, five sense organs, skin, muscles, tendons and bones make up the human body. Although each of them has their own specific physiological function, it is through the connecting and linking role of the meridians that the human body is kept in a coordinative state of the upper and lower, interior and exterior, and constituted as an organic whole . The meridian system has the

脉是督脉、任脉、冲脉、带脉、阴维脉、阳维脉、阴跷脉、阳跷脉的总称。它们与十二正经不同,既不直属脏腑,又无表里配合的关系,"别道奇行",故称奇经。奇经八脉交错的循行分布于十二经之间,沟通了十二经脉之间的联系,并参与调节十二经脉气血的蓄积和渗灌。人体的五脏六腑、四肢百骸、五官九窍、皮肉筋骨等组织器官,虽各有不同的功能,但依靠经络系统的联络沟通作用,使机体内外上下保持协调一致,构成一个有机的整体。经络具有运行气血、濡养周身、抗御外邪、保卫机体等作用。在正虚邪盛的情况下,经络又是病邪传注的途径。当体表受到病邪侵袭时,可通过经络由表及里,由浅入深;脏腑之间、脏腑与体表组织器官之间病变也可通过经络相互影响;内脏病变又可由经络反应到体表组织器官。在推拿治疗中,经络是手法刺激信息到达相应脏腑、组织器官的传导通路。推拿治疗通过按揉腧穴,以疏通经络,恢复调节人体脏腑气血的功能,从而达到治疗的目的。

function of circulating qi and blood, nourishing the body, resisting exogenous pathogenic factors and protecting the body. But under the condition of weakened vital qi and excessive pathogenic factors, the meridians may become the passages of transmitting diseases. When the superficial part of the body is attacked by pathogenic factors, they may be conveyed from the exterior into the interior, from the superficial portion into the deep part. Diseases of the viscera or the superficial tissues and organs can affect each other through the meridians. Diseases of the viscera may also be reflected in the superficial tissues and organs through the meridians. In tuina treatment, the meridians are conductive paths of information of manipulative stimulations to corresponding viscera, tissues and organs. By pressing and kneading the points, tuina therapy dredges the meridians, restores the function of regulating the visceral qi and blood of the human body and achieves the purpose of treating diseases.

TCM holds that the injury of the human tissues and organs such as the joints, tendons and muscles may cause blood to stray out of the vessels, which will obstruct the vessels and meridians resulting in stagnation of qi and blood. Obstruction gives rise to pain. So stagnation of qi and blood in circulation may cause some clinical syndromes with pain as the cardinal symptom. The key point of tuina therapy is to restore the smooth flow of qi and blood, for the pain will subside when obstruction is removed. The purpose to remove obstruction is to dredge the meridians and make qi and blood circulate smoothly so as to remove pain. Dredging the meridians by tuina is accomplished through the following three ways.

中医学认为人体的关节、筋络、肌肉等组织器官受到损伤后,由于血离经脉,经脉受阻,气血流行不通,不通则痛,从而出现以疼痛为主症的临床病证。推拿治疗的关键在于"通",通则不痛。通的目的是疏通经络,使气血运行畅通,消除疼痛。推拿疏通经络是通过下列三个途径实现的。

1.2.3.1 Relaxing Muscles and Tendons and Activating the Meridians

After tissues are injured, the injured site may send

(一) 舒筋活络

在组织损伤后,损伤部位

out some painful stimuli, which cause muscles to contract and the involved tissues to be in an alert state through the nerve reflex and transmission of transmitter. Tension or even spasm of muscles is the manifestation of this state, the effect of which is to reduce the activities of the body to avoid pain and another injury due to traction of the injured portion by too many movements. If at this time a timely treatment is not given or the treatment is not thorough or muscular tension and spasm can not be relieved, the spasmodic muscles will compress the blood vessels going among them, leading to a marked decrease of blood supplies to the muscles. Since spasmodic muscles need much more blood than relaxed ones, the accumulation of lots of metabolic products will result in inflammatory pains. Long-term chronic ischemia and hypoxia may bring about different degrees of connective tissue proliferation, even adhesion, fibrosis or cicatrization in the injured tissues with harmful stimulations sent out, which will aggravate pain, muscular tension and spasm and form a vicious cycle. Where there is pain, there must be muscular tension, and vice versa. Pain and muscular tension have become two aspects of mutual causality. Tuina therapy should aim at treatment of pain and muscular tension so as to break up the vicious cycle, speed up renovation and recovery of the affected tissues. Clinical practice shows that if the focus of pain is removed, muscular tension will be relaxed. And on the contrary, when muscular tension is removed, pain will be apparently relieved or disappear. Tuina can not only directly relax muscles, but also get rid of the factors causing muscular tension. The mechanism of directly relaxing muscles by tuina includes three aspects. Firstly, tuina enhances local circulation and raises the temperature of local areas. Secondly, the threshold value of pain is increased through proper manipulation stimulations . Thirdly , tuina is to lengthen the tense and

可以发出疼痛刺激,通过人体神经、介质的反射与传递,该刺激可以使机体有关组织处于警觉状态,肌肉收缩、紧张直至痉挛是这一状态的表现,其目的是为了减少肢体的活动,防止过度的运动而牵拉受损处,从而引起疼痛或再损伤。此时如不及时治疗或治疗不彻底,肌肉紧张、痉挛不能得到较好的缓解,痉挛的肌肉压迫穿行于其间的血管,致使肌肉的供血量明显减少,而痉挛状态的肌肉所需的供血量远较松弛状态的肌肉为高,因此,代谢产物大量堆积,引起炎性疼痛;肌肉的长期的、慢性的缺血、缺氧,使损伤组织形成不同程度的结缔组织增生,以至粘连、纤维化或瘢痕化,长期发出有害刺激,从而加重疼痛及肌肉的紧张、痉挛,形成恶性循环。凡有疼痛则肌肉必紧张,凡有肌紧张又势必疼痛,它们成为互为因果的两个方面。推拿治疗的目标应针对疼痛和肌紧张这两个主要环节,打破恶性循环,加速损伤组织的修复和恢复。临床治疗表明,消除了疼痛病灶,肌紧张也就解除;如果使紧张的肌肉松弛,则疼痛也就明显减轻或消失。推拿不但可以直接放松肌肉,而且能解除引起肌紧张的原因。

spasmodic muscles, which will help to remove muscular tension and spasm and eliminate pain. The principle of removing muscular tension by tuina is to promote blood circulation in the injured tissues, accelerate their renovation, increase absorption of edema and hematoma in the local injured site and relax and strip off the adhesion in the adhesive soft tissues. In tuina therapy the first thing is to pinpoint the exact location of the primary tender point. The position of most tender points is usually the injured area and also the cardinal portion to be treated. Generally, the most sensitive tender points are often located at the starting and ending points of anadesma and muscle, on the border of two muscles or their crisscrossing areas. By curing tender points, the pathological base of muscular tension is eliminated, which creates good conditions for restoring the normal function of the body. Relaxing tendons and activating the meridians is able to have the tense and spasmodic muscles relaxed and qi and blood of the meridians flow smoothly so as to get rid of pains.

1.2.3.2　Treating and Restoring Injured Soft Tissues and Promoting Their Recovery and Renovation

Many kinds of diseases caused by various agents leading to anatomic abnormal position of the tissues can be rectified by direct external force exerted by tuina manipulations, which can also smooth the circulation of qi and blood in the meridians. For cases with joint dislocation, the joint can be restored to its normal anatomic position by

推拿直接放松肌肉的机理有三个方面:一是加强局部循环,使局部组织温度升高;二是在适当的刺激下,提高了局部组织的痛阈;三是将紧张或痉挛的肌肉充分拉长,从而解除其紧张痉挛,以消除疼痛。推拿可以消除肌紧张的原理是:加强损伤组织的循环,促进损伤组织的修复;促进损伤局部水肿、血肿的吸收;对软组织有粘连者,可以松解粘连。在推拿治疗中,抓住原发性压痛点是关键。大多数压痛点是损伤的部位,也就是推拿治疗的关键部位。一般来说,最敏感的压痛点往往在筋膜、肌肉的起止点,两肌交界或相互交错的部位。通过对压痛点的治疗,消除了肌紧张的病理基础,为恢复肢体的正常功能创造了良好的条件。舒筋活络,可使紧张痉挛的筋肉放松,经络气血得以畅通,消除病痛。

(二) 理筋整复

因各种原因造成的有关组织解剖位置异常的一系列疾病,都可以通过手法外力的直接作用得到纠正,使经络气血运行流畅。推拿对关节脱位者,可以通过运动关节类手

applying manipulations of moving it. Take dislocation of the shoulder joint for example, tell the patient to be in a sitting position, apply pulling and stretching manipulations to the shoulder joint, that will get it normal. In cases with half dislocation of sacro-iliac joint, pain may appear due to incarceration and squeezing of the articular synovium and the dragging of local soft tissues. Applying techniques of obliquely pulling, flexing-extending the hip and knee joints and other passive movements can rectify the dislocation, and pain will be lessened or disappear. In patients with posterior articular disturbance syndrome of the vertebrae, the spinous processes are askew to one side and the joint capsules and ligaments surrounding them are injured due to being pulled and dragged, which can also be rectified with obliquely pulling manipulation. Another example is the case of protrusion of lumbar intervertebral disc, which is commonly seen in clinic. The projections compress the nerve roots inducing pain in the lumbar region and radiating pain in the lower limbs. Tuina manipulations such as lifting the straight leg with force, obliquely pulling, traction can change the position of the projection or the nerve root and remove the compression of the projections to the nerve roots so as to relieve pain.

For cases of malposition of the soft tissues, tuina can also make it restore to its normal state through the action of external force of manipulations. For example, in the case of slipped tendon, a streaky projection can be felt in the slipped site and there is a severe disturbance of joint activities. In tuina therapy, plucking manipulation or pushing-pulling manipulation may be used to restore it to the normal condition. For cases with complete laceration of the tendon or ligament, a suture is needed to reconstruct them, while for partial laceration, a proper manipulation of regulating the tendon may first smooth out the

法使关节回复到正常的解剖位置,如肩关节的脱位,可嘱患者取坐位,作跨肩关节的拔伸,即可令肩关节回复正常。骶髂关节半脱位者,因关节滑膜的嵌顿挤压和局部软组织的牵拉而出现疼痛,可通过斜扳、伸屈髋膝等被动运动,将脱位整复,疼痛亦随之减轻、消失。脊柱后关节紊乱患者,棘突偏向一侧,关节囊及邻近的韧带因受牵拉损伤,也能用斜扳法进行纠正。又如临床上常见的腰椎间盘突出症患者,由于突出物对神经根的压迫而引起腰部疼痛及下肢的放射痛,应用强迫直腿抬高、斜扳、牵引等手法,可以改变突出物与神经根的位置,从而解除突出物对神经根的压迫,消除疼痛。

对软组织错位者,推拿也可以通过手法外力作用使之回复正常。如肌腱滑脱者,在滑脱部位可以摸到条索样隆起,关节活动严重障碍,推拿中可使用弹拨或推扳手法使其回复正常。肌肉肌腱、韧带完全断裂者,必须用手术缝合才能重建,但对部分断裂者,可使用适当的理筋手法,使组织抚顺,然后加以固定。对关

tissues and then fix them. For cases with injury of intra-articular chrondral plate, locked joints, which often cause difficulty in limb activities, can be relieved through proper tuina manipulations. In a word, tuina can treat and restore injured soft tissues through the action of manipulations to make all the tissues in their normal place, joints smooth and qi and blood in the meridians flowing straightway so as to cure diseases.

1.2.3.3　Promoting Blood Circulation to Remove Blood Stasis

Motion is the characteristic of tuina therapy. In the course of tuina treatment, for the patient motion involves the following three aspects of implication: firstly to promote the activities of the tissues of the body, secondly to promote circulation of qi and blood of the meridians, and thirdly to make the joints do passive movements.

Tuina manipulations have the direct action of promoting and regulating functional activities of the soft viscera in the body cavity. For instance, applying proper manipulations on the abdomen can regulate the activities of the stomach and intestine, which has been confirmed by plenty of clinical practice. The effect on restoration of injured soft tissues produced by tuina manipulation can also be proved by experiments. For proper manipulations can regulate muscular contraction and stretching, which can further regulate the pressure among tissues. That will result in promotion of blood circulation around injured tissues and increasing perfusion flow of tissues so as to produce the effect of activating blood circulation to dissipate blood stasis or removing blood stasis to promote blood circulation. In addition, proper manipulations may also restore the mechanical balance among muscles. In recent years some people use the theory of compensatory regulation to explain the mechanism of soft tissue injury and believe that

节内软骨板损伤者，常因关节交锁而致使肢体活动困难，推拿可使用适当的手法，解除关节的交锁。总之，推拿可以通过手法作用进行理筋整复，使各种组织各守其位，关节通顺，经络气血畅通，从而起到治疗作用。

（三）活血祛瘀

"动"是推拿疗法的特点。在治疗过程中，对患者来说"动"包括三个方面：一是促进肢体组织的活动；二是促进经脉气血的流动；三是肢体关节的被动活动。

推拿手法对柔软体腔内的脏器有直接促进和调整其功能活动的作用，如在腹部施以适当的手法可调整胃肠的活动，早已被大量临床实践所证实。推拿对于加速软组织损伤恢复的影响也可在诸多实验研究中得到证明，如适当的手法可调节肌肉的收缩和舒张，使组织间压力得到调节，以促进损伤组织周围的血液循环，增加组织灌流量，从而起到"活血化瘀"、"祛瘀生新"的作用。不仅如此，适当的手法还可使肌肉间的力学平衡得到恢复。近年来，有人用补偿调节论来解释软组织损伤的机

once muscular spasm occurs, it will cause corresponding changes in the related muscles, which is called corresponding compensatory regulation. For example, lumbodorsal muscular tension may cause compensatory regulation of the abdominal muscles. And muscular tension of the left lumbar muscles may cause that of the right lumbar muscles. The muscular tension and spasm caused by corresponding regulation may also induce the injury reaction of soft tissues. In clinic, it is frequently seen that lingering lumbago on one side causes pain on both sides, and prolonged lumbago leads to pain on the back or buttock areas. Tuina can regulate the incoordinative mechanical relations among muscles and restore them to a normal state so as to alleviate or eliminate pain. Passive movement is an important component of tuina manipulations. For cases with adhesion and rigidity of joints, proper passive movements help relax and remove adhesion and smooth joints. For cases with degeneration of local soft tissues, passive movement has the effect of improving local nutrient supplies, promoting metabolism and increasing the extension of muscles so as to get degenerated tissues improved and recovered gradually.

1. 2. 4 Promoting Circulation of Qi and Activating Blood

Qi and blood are the fundamental substances constituting the human body. They are also the basis of the normal life activities, which are the outcome of change and motion of qi and blood. The elemental qi of the human body is the primordial qi, the formation of which depends on the integration of the essence qi in the kidney, cereal essence and the clear qi in the nature. The exertion of its physiological function depends upon smooth flow of functional

理,认为一旦肌肉痉挛,可引起对应肌肉的相应变化,称为对应补偿调节。如腰背肌紧张,可引起腹肌的补偿调节;而左侧腰肌紧张,又可引起右侧腰肌的补偿调节。对应调节所产生的肌紧张、痉挛,同样可引起软组织的损伤反应。临床不乏见到一侧腰痛日久不愈而引起对侧腰痛,腰痛日久又引起背痛或臀部痛的病例。推拿能使肌肉间不协调的力学关系得到改善或恢复,从而使疼痛减轻或消失。被动运动是推拿手法的一个重要组成部分。对关节粘连僵硬者,适当的被动活动则有助于松解粘连,滑利关节;对局部软组织变性者,则可改善局部营养供应,促进新陈代谢,增大肌肉的伸展性,从而使变性的组织逐渐得到改善或恢复。

四、行气活血

气血是构成人体的基本物质,是正常生命活动的基础,人的生命活动是气血运动变化的结果。人体中最基本的气是元气,它的生成有赖于肾中的精气、水谷精气和自然清气的结合,其生理功能的发挥有赖于气机的调畅。血是

qi. Blood is derived from cereal nutrients transformed by the spleen and stomach. Blood and nutritive qi circulate alongside in the vessels, flow to all parts of the body and have the function of nourishing the limbs, viscera and the whole body. Therefore it is clear that the formation of qi and blood needs abundant supplies of cereal nutrients, which further depends upon the receiving and digestive function of the stomach and the transporting and transforming function of the spleen. The function of spleen refers to digestion, absorption and distribution of essential substances and so on. Through invigorating the stomach and spleen, tuina improves the formation of qi and blood. And it also makes qi activities regular and smooth by dredging the meridians and reinforcing the liver's function of governing normal flow of qi, which, in turn, strengthens qi in its function of producing, circulating and controlling blood and promotes physiological circulation of the body, which result in abundant and smooth qi and blood in the body. As it is said in the ancient book *Lingshu* that regular and smooth circulation of blood is the guarantee of vigor and keen mind.

The function of promoting qi circulation to activate blood of tuina is accomplished by strengthening the spleen and stomach and soothing the liver to regulate qi and other means. In clinical practice, the method of rubbing the abdomen is often used to promote the descending function of the stomach. Kneading manipulation, pressing manipulation and pushing manipulation with one-finger meditation are also applied to Pishu (BL 20), Weishu (BL 21), Zusanli (ST 36), Zhongwan (CV 12) and other acupoints to improve the function of the spleen and stomach and promote the circulation of qi and blood. Up-and-down rubbing the governor vessel or transversely rubbing the splenogastric area on the left side of the back may also produce the

由脾胃运化的水谷精气化生而成,血与营气共行脉中,在心、肝、脾的作用下流注全身,起濡养全身肢体脏腑的作用。由此可见,气、血的生成都需水谷精微的充分供给,而这又有赖于胃的受纳腐熟功能及脾的运化功能。脾的运化功能包括消化、吸收及输布精微等方面。推拿通过健脾和胃,来促进人体气血的生成,同时通过疏通经络加强肝的疏泄功能来促进气机的调畅,这样又加强了气生血、行血、摄血的功能,促进或改善人体生理循环,使人体气血充盈而调畅。《灵枢》说:"血脉和利,精神乃居。"

推拿行气活血的作用是通过健脾和胃、疏肝理气等方法来体现的。临床治疗经常用摩腹来促进胃的通降功能;用一指禅推法、揉法、按法等作用于脾俞、胃俞、足三里、中脘等穴,或用直擦督脉及横擦左侧背部脾胃区域,以促进脾胃功能,加强气血的运行。推拿治疗时可用按揉章门、期门、肝俞等穴位来疏肝理气。在四肢和背部的搓、揉、搓或轻拿肩井可直接活血行气。

same effect as above. Pressing and kneading Zhangmen (LR 13), Qimen (LR 14), Ganshu (BL 18), etc. can disperse stagnated liver qi in tuina treatment. Rolling, kneading and palm-twisting the limbs and the back or grasping slightly Jianjing (GB 21) have the immediate effect of promoting qi circulation to activate blood. Blood stasis is a pathologic product formed by irregular circulation of blood resulting in the coagulation of blood in a certain area. This product can become the etiological factor of some diseases. Tuina can promote qi circulation and activate blood by applying appropriate manipulations with the result of eliminating blood stasis.

瘀血是因血行失度而使机体某一局部的血液凝聚而形成一种病理产物,而这一产物在机体内又会成为某些疾病的致病因素,推拿也可以通过适当的手法行气活血,而消除瘀血。

1.3 Practising Exercises for Tuina Therapy (Tuina Liangong)

第三节 推拿练功

1.3.1 Characteristics of Tuina Liangong

The work of a tuina doctor is to cure diseases by applying various manipulations to patients to help them conduct passive movements. For this purpose a tuina doctor needs an excellent constitution and necessary strength of the finger, arm, loin and leg, which requires a self-training process to obtain. In the long course of development, Chinese tuina has formed and summed up a set of training methods for practising exercises, including bare-handed liangong, liangong with apparatus, Wushu Liangong, Qigong Liangong and therapeutic liangong, among which bare-handed liangong mostly bears the traditional features. The characteristics of tuina liangong can be chiefly summarized as follows.

一、推拿练功的特点

推拿医生的工作,是其通过采用各种手法帮助病人进行被动运动来达到治病目的。为此,推拿医生必须具备良好的身体素质和指力、臂力及腰腿的力量,这也就需要一个自我锻炼的过程。中国推拿在漫长的发展过程中,逐渐形成了包括徒手练功、器械练功、武术练功、气功练功以及医疗练功等方法的练功学内容,而在这些内容的练功方法中,尤以徒手练功最具传统特色。中国推拿练功主要有以下几个特点。

1.3.1.1　Explicit Actions with Capacity of Comprehensive Training

Bare-handed liangong and liangong with apparatus selected in tuina liangongfa have very clear aim, and therefore is very effective in the cultivation of the human constitution and strength. In bare-handed liangong, for example, training of foot postures and stances are put at the first place. And an overall exercise of the muscles and ligaments of the lower limbs and the abdominal, lumbar and back muscles are required to be given through various kinds of flexing and up-and-down movements of the lower limbs. Through long-term exercises the muscles of the lower limbs can become thick and strong, which is just in conformity with the so-called theory "Building up the lower parts means strengthening the body constitution." The powerful lower limbs with great strength will lay a good foundation for tuina liangong.

In bare-handed liangong, many actions are chiefly based on movement of the palm. The palm emerges from the hypochondrium, rubbing and pushing. Both hands rise and fall with spiral strength. Flexion and extension and contraction of the muscles of every part and their confrontation with each other greatly train the muscles of the finger, palm and upper limbs.

1.3.1.2　Attaching Importance to Mind and Qi and Emphasizing Internal Strength

According to the theory of qi and blood in TCM, qi is the origin of life. The bones, arms, legs and the five zang and six fu organs all depend upon qi and blood conveyed by the meridians and vessels to nourish themselves and maintain their normal vital activities. Any human being with smooth and flourishing qi and blood will have a strong body with good health. The special property of clinical tuina requires tuina doctors to have a healthy physique

（一）动作明确，锻炼全面

推拿练功法中的徒手与器械练功方法对人体素质和力量锻炼很明显，练功中针对性很强。如徒手练功法中，首先强调步型、档势，要求通过下肢各种屈曲、起伏，使下肢肌肉、韧带以及腹肌、腰肌、背肌等都得到全面的锻炼，长期练习，可使下肢肌肉充实，力量大增，这就是中国练功家们所谓"筑其基，壮其体"之说。有了扎实而坚强的下肢力量，即是练功顺利进行的良好基础。

徒手练功法中还有许多动作都是以掌为主要动作基础，掌从胁肋下擦推而出，两手起落多有螺旋劲等，这样通过各部肌肉的伸展收缩，相互争衡，从而使指掌、上肢肌肉力量得到更大的锻炼。

（二）注重"意""气"，强调"内劲"

根据中医气血学说，"气"是生命之本，人体四肢百骸、五脏六腑无不有赖于经脉之气血运行以充养，这样才能维持正常生命活动，而气血畅旺者自然身体强盛。推拿临床工作的特殊性质，更要求推拿医务人员具有"阴平阳秘"的

with yin and yang in equilibrium. Tuina liangong stresses the restoration and nourishment of qi and replenishment of essence and blood. And in order to attain this physiological state, a long period of training process of every technique in tuina liangong is needed. During the training practice, the high devotion of thought activities can effectively promote the formation and transformation of essence, qi and blood in the human body, improve their function and quality and further attain the so-called status: mind (or thought) leading qi, and qi controlling strength. So an internal strength can be produced by that, which indicates the full exertion of human functional activities. This exertion benefits the vital functions of the tuina doctor himself as well as has an active recovery effect on patients receiving tuina therapy.

1.3.1.3　Combining Treatment with Practising Exercises to Improve Therapeutic Results

There is an old saying that wise doctors can prevent diseases from occurring, while poor doctors can only treat diseases. Following this saying, people pay attention not only to the treatment of diseases, but also to the prevention of their occurrence and development. This practice is also embodied in tuina liangongfa, among which some actions are fit for patients to practice and are helpful in eliminating diseases. They are also a good method of reinforcing the body resistance to eliminate pathogenic factors and mobilizing patient's initiative.

For example, in bare-handed liangong there are actions such as Qiantui Bapima (pushing eight horses forward) and Daola Jiutouniu (pulling nine oxen backward), in which the hands are pushed forward from both sides of the hypochondrium, which causes qi to circulate and come out from the middle energizer. So these actions can invigorate the spleen and stomach, improve gastrointestinal

健康状态。所以推拿练功法中强调蓄养气机,充实精血。要达到这种良好的生理状态,则需经过各种推拿练功法的锻炼过程。进行这种锻炼,由于高度的意念活动,可有效地促生、转化人体"精、气、血"类物质,提高其功能、质量,进而"以意领气,以气贯力",使人体产生所谓的"内劲"。这种"内劲"的产生,可以说是人体功能态的最好发挥,其不仅有益自身的生命机能,更可以在对他人实施推拿手法治疗时产生积极的康复作用。

(三) 医练结合,增强疗效

古人云:"上工治未病,下工治已病"。推拿临床工作中,正是恪遵了这一说法,不仅重视疾病的治疗,而且更加注意预防疾病的发生和发展,推拿练功法中亦有着良好的体现。推拿练功法中一些动作,很适合病患者练习,有利于消除疾病,是一种扶正祛邪和调动病员积极性的好方法。

如徒手练功法中前推八匹马、倒拉九头牛一类动作,两手自胁肋两侧向前推出,使气机蓄行出于中焦,故能健脾和胃,促进胃肠功能,使摄纳增加,化生有源,气血因此充沛。凤凰展翅一类动作,两臂

functions to increase the amount of food taken in, which offers a source for transformation of nutrients and makes qi and blood ample. In the movements of Fenghuang Zhanchi (phoenix spreading its wings), the two arms extend transversely sideward, which causes the chest to expand and qi of the upper energizer to be extended, resulting in alleviating depression to regulate qi and calming the liver to invigorate the lung. Due to the above effect, qi activity is regulated and the adverse liver yang descends. So these actions can be used to treat and prevent hypertension, vertigo and other diseases. In the movements such as Liangshou Tuotian (two hands supporting the heaven) and Bawang Juding (the overlord holding-up the tripod), two palms push upward to direct clear yang qi to go up to the head, which can be used in treating and preventing headache, insomnia, etc. Besides, in the course of tuina liangong, various exercises of bare-handed liangong and liangong with apparatus also lay emphasis on the actions of the lower limbs. They require the lower limbs to use hegemonic force, that is to say, to use enough strength, all the toes clutch at the ground, the heels stand fully, the legs straighten and the thighs exert force. These actions can invigorate qi activities, strengthen the spleen and waist and have therapeutic and preventive effect on diseases of the urogenital systems. Furthermore, there are some other liangong actions, including training and exercises of the joints of the neck, shoulder, loin, back and extremities, which improve muscular strength and functions of these areas as well as treat and prevent common diseases frequently encountered in these parts.

1. 3. 2　Approaches of Cultivating Shaolin Neigong (Shaolin Internal Cultivation Exercises)

Shaolin Neigong is the main practicing method of

横向两侧展开，使胸廓扩张，上焦气机得以舒展，可有宽胸利气、平肝健肺的作用，并因而调整了气机，使亢逆之肝阳下降，故能防治高血压、眩晕等疾病。两手托天、霸王举鼎之类动作，两掌向上推出，引清阳之气上行巅顶，故能防治头昏、失眠之类疾病。另外，推拿练功过程中，徒手及器械各种功法锻炼，都强调一定的下肢动作，要求下肢运用"霸力"（即用足力气，以五趾抓地，足跟踏实，下肢挺直，两股用力），使下焦气机畅旺，以健脾壮腰，故而对泌尿系统、生殖系统疾病有着防治作用。再有其他各种练功动作，都包含了对颈、肩、腰、背各关节、肢体的活动锻炼，既使这些部位功能、肌肉力量有所改善，又能防治这些部位的常见病、多发病。

二、少林内功练习方法

"少林内功"是徒手练功

bare-handed liangong. According to a legend, Shaolin Neigong was derived from Shaolin Martial Arts actions by Bodhidharma, the founder of Buddhism. It is a method of practicing exercises and can strengthen the body health as well as cure and prevent diseases. Because of its real and excellent effect in practising exercises, Shaolin Neigong was gradually introduced into tuina liangong as the traditional preserved exercises. In training practice Shaolin Neigong requires the lower limbs to exert hegemonic force. That is to say, it requires the lower limbs to use enough strength, all the toes to clutch at the ground, the heels to stand fully, the legs to straighten with the front part of the foot turned inward, the thighs to press forcefully inward and the trunk to straighten with the chest upright, the abdomen contracted and the lower jaw tucked in. While exercising the upper limbs, one should focus strength on the shoulder, arm, elbow, wrist and finger. Respiration should not be held, but be conducted naturally, and coordinative with actions, keeping a state of tightness outside and relaxation inside. During practicing exercises, strength should reach the extremities, back and waist, and get qi going with it and infusing into the meridians and vessels so as to make qi and blood circulate smoothly and able to nourish the whole body. It is through this persistent repeated practice that the human body is kept in a healthy state with qi and blood flourishing and yin and yang in equilibrium and diseases are kept away. There are mainly five basic stances and ten basic actions in the practicing methods of Shaolin Neigong.

1.3.2.1 The Basic Stances

1.3.2.1.1 The Upright Standing Stance
ACTIONS

(1) Stand erect. The left foot takes a step leftward with a distance between the feet wider than the shoulder.

法中主要的锻炼方法。它相传是佛教达摩祖师根据中国少林武术动作衍化而成的强身健体并能防治疾病的练功方法。以其有良好而切实的练功效果,遂逐渐被引用为推拿练功的传统保留功法。"少林内功"在锻炼中,要求下肢运用"霸力",也就是用足力气,以五趾抓地,足跟踏实,下肢挺直,脚尖内收,两股用力内夹,躯干挺拔,做到挺胸、收腹、含颏。上肢在进行锻炼时,要求凝劲于肩、臂、肘、腕、指。呼吸要自然,不可屏气,并与动作相协调,保持"外紧内松"。练功时,要力贯于四肢、腰背,气随力行,注于经脉,使气血循行畅通,荣灌四肢百骸、五脏六腑。也就是在这种经常性的练功重复过程中,人体才能气血充盈,阴阳平衡,进而更能强身健体,祛除病邪。"少林内功"练功方法主要有 5 种裆势和 10 种基本动作。

(一)基本裆势

1. 站裆势
【动作】

(1)立正,左足向左平跨一步,约相当于肩宽,足尖略

The toe tips turn in to form inward splayfeet. All the toes touch the ground, and strength is directed from the top to the feet with hegemonic force.

（2）The chest squares slightly, the buttock being tucked in. The hands stretch backward with the elbow and wrist straightened. The shoulder and armpit tighten. The four fingers are put close alongside with the thumbs parting outward. The eyes look straight ahead. The head should not turn round. And the mind concentrates with voluntary breath（Fig. 1）.

收成内八字,五趾着地,运用霸力,劲由上贯下注足。

（2）前胸微挺,后臀要蓄,两手后伸,挺肘伸腕,肩腋莫松,四指并拢,拇指外分,两目平视,头勿左右盼顾,精神贯注,呼吸随意(图1)。

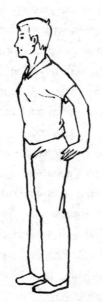

Fig. 1 The Upright Standing Stance
图1 站裆势

ESSENTIALS Three straightnesses and four levelnesses. Three straightnesses refer to straightnesses of the buttock, loin and legs, while four levelnesses include levelnesses of the head, shoulders, palms and feet. The foot tips turn in with hegemonic force. Press the scapulae inward, straighten the elbow, extend the wrist, turn the palm to get the fingers upright. And square the chest,

【要领】 三直四平。三直:臀、腰、腿。四平:头、肩、掌、脚,两脚内扣,运用霸力。夹肩、挺肘、伸腕、翻掌、立指。挺胸收腹,舌抵上腭,呼吸自然,两目平视。

contract the abdomen, get the tongue to touch the palate, the eye look straight ahead and breathe naturally.

1.3.2.1.2　The Horse-riding Stance

ACTIONS

(1) Stand upright. The left foot takes a step leftward. And bend the knees and squat with the foot heels apart wider than the shoulder. The knees and foot tips turn slightly inward and the heels turn outward to form inward splayfeet.

(2) Extend the hands backward with the elbow straightening and wrist stretching, the thumb apart and the four fingers close together. Or both the hands rest on the hips horizontally with Hukou (the part between the thumb and index finger) facing inward. The trunk leans slightly forward with the chest stuck out and the abdomen held in. The body weight center is kept between the legs. The head feels as if supporting an object. The eyes look straight ahead with voluntary breath (Fig. 2).

2. 马裆势

【动作】

(1) 立正，左足向左平开一步，屈膝下蹲，足跟距离较肩为宽，两膝和脚尖微向内扣，两脚跟微向外蹬，足尖成内八字形。

(2) 两手后伸，肘直腕伸，拇指分开，四指并拢，或两手平放两胯处，虎口朝内。上身挺胸，收腹微微前倾，重心放在两腿之间，头如顶物，目须平视，呼吸随意（图2）。

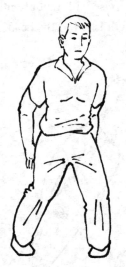

Fig. 2　The Horse-riding Stance
图2　马裆势

ESSENTIALS　Sinking the lower back and bending the knees, sticking out the chest and holding in the abdo-

【要领】　沉腰屈膝，挺胸收腹，两目平视，呼吸自然。

men, looking forward and breathing naturally.

1.3.2.1.3 The Bow-step Stance
ACTIONS

(1) Stand upright. The body rotates rightward. The right foot takes a big step rightward and forward to have a proper distance between the feet according to the body height. The front right leg bends the knee and half squats to keep the knee and the toes in a vertical line and the foot tips turn slightly inward. The left leg is at the rear with its knee straight, the foot turning out slightly and the heel on the ground to form a posture of bow-shaped front leg and arrow-shaped rear leg.

(2) The upper body leans slightly forward. The body weight center sinks and the buttock holds in slightly. The arms extend backward, the elbow straightens and the wrist extends with strength gathering on the palmar root. Or the hands rest on the hips with Hukou facing inward. Store up energy to get ready for exercise with rapt attention. The neck is relaxed and strength is led to the head. Breathe naturally (Fig. 3).

3. 弓箭裆势
【动作】

（1）立正，身向右旋，右足向右前方跨出一大步，距离可根据自己身体高矮取其自然；在前之右腿屈膝半蹲，膝与足成垂直线，足尖微向内扣；左腿在后，膝部挺直，足略向外撤，脚跟必须着地，成前弓后箭之势。

（2）上身略向前俯，重心下沉，臀须微收，两臂后伸，挺肘伸腕，掌根蓄劲（或两手叉腰），虎口朝内，蓄势待发，全神贯注，虚领顶劲，呼吸随意（图3）。

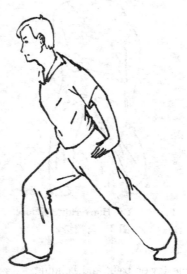

Fig. 3   The Bow-step Stance
图3   弓箭裆势

ESSENTIALS The front leg is bow-shaped and the back leg is arrow-shaped. The body weight center sinks. The chest squares and the abdomen contracts with natural breath.

1.3.2.1.4 The Opposite Foot Tips Stance
ACTIONS

(1) Stand upright. The foot heels move outward as much as possible and the foot tips get opposite to each other. The toes clutch at the ground with even force.

(2) The arms stretch slightly backward with the elbows and wrists straight, the palms facing downward, the fingers close together and the thumb apart. The eyes look straight ahead (Fig 4).

ESSENTIALS The same as that in the Standing Stance.

1.3.2.1.5 The Wide-apart-feet Standing Stance
ACTIONS

(1) The left foot takes a big step leftward and the knees straighten and the feet stand firmly.

(2) The arms stretch backward with Hukou opposite to each other, the fingers close together and the elbows and wrists stretching (Fig. 5).

【要领】 前弓后箭,重心下沉,挺胸收腹,呼吸自然。

4. 并裆势
【动作】

(1) 立正,两足跟尽力向外蹬,足尖相对,五趾着实,用力宜匀。

(2) 两手挺肘伸腕,微向后伸,掌心朝下,四指并拢,拇指外分,目须平视(图4)。

【要领】 同站裆势。

5. 大裆势
【动作】

(1) 左足向左分开一大步,膝直足实。

(2) 两手后伸,虎口相对,四指并拢,肘直腕伸(图5)。

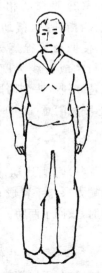

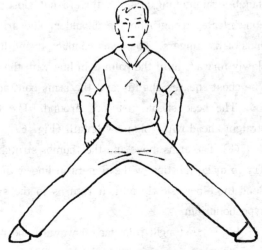

Fig. 4 **The Opposite Foot Tips Stance**
图 4 并裆势

Fig. 5 **The Wide-apart-feet Standing Stance**
图 5 大裆势

ESSENTIALS The same as that in the Standing Stance.

COMMENTS The above five basic stances are also the main basic standing-posture exercises of Shaolin Neigong. Since all the exercises need exertion of hegemonic force through the lower limbs as well as focusing strength on the back and waist, the practice of these exercises will have the effect of strengthening the kidney and the loin and cultivating primordial qi to consolidate the body resistance. If combined with basic actions, the exercises will have a good supportive action in the treatment of various diseases.

1.3.2.2 The Sets of Basic Actions

1.3.2.2.1 Qiantui Bapima（Pushing Eight Horses Forward）

PREPARATORY POSTURE Keep a standing stance or a given stance.

ACTIONS

（1）Bend the elbows and rest the straight hand on the hypochondrium.

（2）Have the palms facing to each other with the thumb straightening and the fingers put close together. Concentrate strength on the shoulder, the arm and the ends of the fingers. The arms conduct strength and push slowly forward until the palm is in line with the shoulder. The chest squares slightly and the arms contract slightly too. The head should not look around. The eyes look straight ahead with voluntary breath (Fig. 6).

（3）The arms move and the thumbs stretch upward. Try to make the tips of the fingers in line with the arm. Bend the elbow slowly until it returns to the side of the hypochondrium.

（4）The straight palm face downward and press. The arms stretch backward and then reduce to the starting stance.

【要领】 同站裆势。

【按语】 以上 5 种基本裆势也是少林内功的主要基本站桩功,由于均要求下肢运用霸力,蓄劲于腰背,因此练习这些裆势还可以健肾强腰,培元固本,再配合各种基本动作,可对各种疾病起到很好的辅助防治作用。

（二）基本动作

1. 前推八匹马

【预备】 站好站裆或指定的裆势。

【动作】

（1）两手屈肘,直掌于两胁。

（2）两掌心相对,拇指伸直,四指并拢,蓄劲于肩臂指端,使两臂徐徐运力前推,以肩与掌成直线为度。胸须微挺,臂略收,头勿盼顾,两目平视,呼吸随意(图 6)。

（3）手臂运动,拇指上翘,指端力求与手臂成直线,慢慢屈肘,收回于两胁。

（4）由直掌化俯掌下按,两臂后伸,回原裆势。

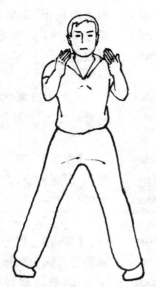

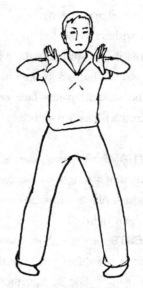

Fig. 6 Pushing Eight Horses Forward
图 6 前推八匹马

Fig. 7 Pulling Nine Oxen Backward
图 7 倒拉九头牛

ESSENTIALS Concentrating strength on the fingers and arms，erecting the fingers，directing qi and pushing slowly，looking straight ahead and breathing naturally.

1.3.2.2.2 Daola Jiutouniu（Pulling Nine Oxen Backward）

PREPARATORY POSTURE Keep a standing stance or a given stance.

ACTIONS

(1) Bend the elbows and place the extending hand beside the hypochondrium.

(2) The hands push forward along the hypochondria. Meanwhile，the forearms turn gradually inward until they are completely straightened with Hukou downward. The fingers are close together and the thumbs separate as much as possible with wrists and elbows straight to the same level of the shoulders (Fig. 7).

(3) Flex the five fingers inward and change a palm into a fist just like holding an object. Direct strength to

【要领】 指臂蓄力，立指运气慢推，两目平视，呼吸自然。

2. 倒拉九头牛

【预备】 站好站裆或指定的裆势。

【动作】

（1）两手屈肘，直掌于两胁。

（2）两掌沿两胁前推，边推边将前臂渐渐内旋，手臂完全伸直时，虎口正好朝下。四指并拢，拇指用力外分，腕、肘伸直，力求与肩平（图7）。

（3）五指向内屈收，由掌化拳如握物状，劲注拳心，旋

the fist center. Turn the wrist to get the fist hole upward. Then withdraw the fist to the hypochondrium and change the fist into a straight palm. The trunk leans a little forward and the buttock tucked in slightly.

(4) The straight palms face downward and press. The arms stretch backward and then reduce to the preparatory posture.

ESSENTIALS Turning the straight palms while pushing, directing strength to the fist center, straightening the wrist and elbow to the same level of the shoulder and pulling them tightly backward.

COMMENTS In the above two sets of actions, the hands are both pushed forward from the hypochondriac areas to get qi to circulate in the middle energizer, which therefore has an effect of strengthening the spleen and stomach, improving the gastrointestinal function and increasing food intake with the result of obtainment of a source of transformation of plenty of qi and blood. The actions have good therapeutic effect on indigestion, belching, distending pain in the epigastric area and borborygmus, etc. caused by dysfunction of the stomach, intestine, liver and gallbladder.

1.3.2.2.3　Danzhang Lajinhuan（Pulling Gold Ring with One Hand）

PREPARATORY POSTURE Keep a standing stance or a given stance.

ACTIONS

(1) Bend the elbows and put the straight palm beside the hypochondrium.

(2) Push the right hand forward, meanwhile turn the forearm inward to get Hukou facing downward and the palm center outward. The fingers are close together and the thumb is outward apart. Concentrate strength on the arm and exert force on the side of the palm. Straighten

腕拳眼朝上，紧紧内收，化直掌于两胁，身微前倾，臀部微收。

（4）由直掌化俯掌下按，两臂后伸，恢复原裆势。

【要领】　直掌旋推，劲注拳心，肘腕伸直，力求肩平，紧紧后拉。

【按语】　以上两节，两手自胁肋两侧向前推出，使气行于中焦，故能健脾和胃，促进胃肠功能，使人体摄纳增加，化生有源，气血充沛，对于因胃、肠、肝、胆导致的消化不良、嗳气、胃脘胀痛、肠鸣等病证有较好的防治作用。

3. 单掌拉金环

【预备】　站好站裆或指定的裆势。

【动作】

（1）两手屈肘，直掌于两胁。

（2）右手前推，边推边将前臂内旋，虎口朝下，掌心朝外，四指并拢，拇指外分，臂欲蓄劲，掌侧着力，肘腕伸直，松肩，身体正直，两目平视，呼吸

the elbow and wrist, relax the shoulders, keep the body upright and the eyes looking straight ahead. Breathe naturally (Fig. 8).

随意（图 8）。

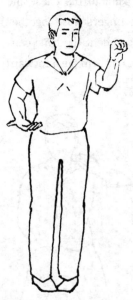

Fig. 8   Pulling Gold Ring with One Hand
图 8   单掌拉金环

（3）Clench the knuckles into a fist and direct strength to the fist center. Turn the wrist to get the fist hole facing upward. Change the fists into the straight palms and withdraw them closely to the hypochondria to protect them. Movements of the left hand are the same as the right one.

（3）五指内收握拳，使劲注掌心，旋腕，拳眼朝上，紧紧内收，化直掌护肋。左手动作与右手相同。

（4）The straight palm faces downward and presses. The arm stretches backward and then reduces to the preparatory posture.

（4）由直掌化俯掌下按，两臂后伸，恢复原档势。

ESSENTIALS   The same as that in Daola Jiutouniu.

1.3.2.2.4   Xianren Zhilu (the Celestial Pointing the Way)

PREPARATORY POSTURE   Keep a standing stance or a given stance.

【要领】   同倒拉九头牛。

4. 仙人指路

【预备】   站好站档或指定的档势。

ACTIONS

（1）Bend the elbows and rest the up-facing palm beside the waist.

（2）Raise the up-facing right palm to the chest and get it out in a vertical palm. Put the fingers close together with the thumb stretching straight and dent the hand center into a concave shape. The elbow and arm push forward in a vertical palm with even force (Fig. 9).

【动作】

（1）两手屈肘，仰掌于腰部。

（2）右仰掌上提至胸前立掌而出，四指并拢，拇指伸直，手心内凹成瓦楞状，肘臂运动立掌向前推出，力要均匀（图9）。

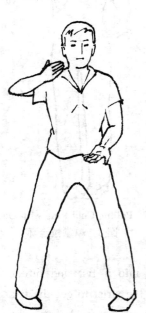

Fig. 9   The Celestial Pointing the Way
图9   仙人指路

（3）Flex the wrist and erect the palm after pushing them straight. Withdraw the arms inward with force, in the meantime, turn the forearm outward and change the upright palms into the up-facing palms and rest them at the waist.

（4）Turn the up-facing palm into the down-facing palm and have them press downward. Stretch the arms backward just as the starting stance.

（3）推直后屈腕立掌，蓄劲内收，边收边外旋前臂，仰掌于腰部。

（4）由仰掌化俯掌下按，两臂后伸，同原裆势。

(5) Alternate the left hand with the right hand and make the same movements with it as the right hand has done.

ESSENTIALS　Raising the up-facing palm, placing the upright palm in front of the chest, denting the palm center in a concave shape, pushing the arm and hand forcefully forward, and turning the wrist and pulling the arm backward.

COMMENTS　In the above two sets of actions, Strength is concentrated on the shoulder, arm, elbow, wrist and fingers. The wrist turns and pushes forward, and the palm turns and does grasping actions. All the actions can excite qi in the twelve meridians and have the effect of invigorating the brain to clear the mind, promoting qi circulation to activate blood and dredging the meridians. They also have good therapeutic and preventive action on neurosis, numbness of the extremities, stiffness of muscles and joints, over-strained injury of joints in the neck, shoulder, palm and fingers and pain caused by wounds.

1.3.2.2.5　Fenghuang Zhanchi (Phoenix Spreading Its Wings)

PREPARATORY POSTURE　Stand in a bow-step stance or a given stance.

ACTIONS

(1) The elbows bend, the hands go upward to the superior chest and cross.

(2) The upright palms turn into the down-facing palms, then part slowly and forcefully to the right and left sides respectively, the arms extend as straight as possible like stretching wings. The fingers are put close together and slightly raised up and the thumbs separate outward. The head looks like supporting an object. The eyes look forward. The torso bends slightly forward, but the shoulders should not be raised. Breathe naturally (Fig. 10).

（5）左右交换，左掌动作与右掌动作相同。

【要领】　仰掌上提，立掌胸前，手心内凹，如同瓦楞，臂指用力前推，旋腕后拉。

【按语】　以上两节，凝劲于肩、臂、肘、腕、指，旋腕前推，翻掌空抓，可以激发十二经脉经气，有健脑开窍、行气活血、疏通经脉的作用，对神经衰弱，肢体麻木，筋骨不利以及颈、肩、掌、指各关节的劳损、伤痛有良好的防治作用。

5. 凤凰展翅

【预备】站好弓箭裆或指定的裆势。

【动作】

（1）两手屈肘上行，徐徐至上胸成立掌交叉。

（2）由立掌化为俯掌，缓缓用力向左右外分，两臂尽力伸直，形如展翅，四指并拢，拇指外分，指欲上翘，头如顶物，两目平视，上身微倾，切勿抬肩，呼吸随意（图10）。

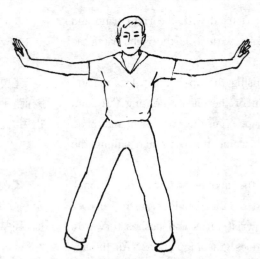

Fig. 10 Phoenix Spreading Its Wings
图 10 凤凰展翅

(3) Rotate the wrists. Flex and withdraw the elbows inward. Concentrate and exert strength on both sides. Pull the arms slowly inward with force until both palms gradually face to each other and cross them in front of the chest in upright position.

(4) Change the upright palms in front of the chest into the down-facing palms and press them downward. The arms extend backward and reduce back to the starting stance.

ESSENTIALS   Erecting the palms and crossing them. Extending the arms outward with force. Exerting force like pulling a bow. Straightening the shoulder，elbow and wrist. Withdrawing the arms inward with concentrated strength.

1.3.2.2.6   Fengbai Heye (Wind Swaying Lotus Leaf)

PREPARATORY POSTURE   Stand in the bow-step stance or in a given stance.

ACTIONS

(1) Bend the elbow and put the hands at the side of the waist with the palm facing upward.

（3）两掌旋腕，屈肘内收，两侧蓄劲着力，徐徐收回，使掌心逐渐相对，处于胸前交叉立掌。

（4）由上胸之立掌化俯掌下按，两臂后伸，恢复原裆势。

【要领】 立掌交叉，用力外展，劲如开弓，肩肘腕平，蓄劲内收。

6. 风摆荷叶

【预备】 站如弓箭裆或指定的裆势。

【动作】

（1）两手屈肘，仰掌于腰部。

（2）Push the arm upward-forward to the front of the chest with the palm facing upward, the four fingers close together and the thumb stretched straight, then overlap the left hand on the right one. Move and push the feet forward, then separate them slowly toward both sides with force. The shoulder, elbow and palm should be straight in line. Concentrate strength on the lateral side of the thumbs and keep both hands in a horizontal position. The head seems to be in a pose of supporting an object and the eyes look straight ahead. Breathe naturally (Fig. 11).

（2）掌心向上，四指并拢，拇指伸直，向前上方推出，至胸部左掌在右掌上相叠，运动向前推足，然后缓缓用力向左右外分，肩肘掌须平成直线形，拇指外侧着力含蓄，使两手托成水平线，头如顶物，两目平视，呼吸自然（图 11）。

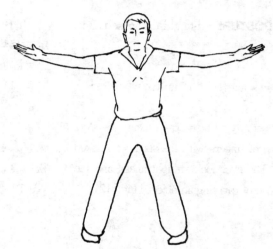

Fig. 11   Wind Swaying Lotus Leaf
图 11   风摆荷叶

（3）Both up-facing palms move slowly toward each other from both sides of the body, cross and overlap them with the left palm above the right one, then withdraw them back to the waist.

（4）Turn the up-facing palms into the down-facing palms and press them downward, stretch the arms backward, then reduce them to the starting stance.

ESSENTIALS   Crossing the up-facing palms and pushing them forward, turning the elbows outward and pulling them apart and keeping the shoulder, elbow, wrist

（3）两仰掌用力从两侧向内慢慢合拢，右下左上交叉相叠，再收于腰部。

（4）由仰掌化俯掌下按，两臂后伸，回原裆势。

【要领】 仰掌交叉前推，外旋双肘拉开，肩、肘、腕掌平齐。

and palm straight in line.

COMMENTS The above two sets of actions extend forward and stretch outward the upper arms, which expand the chest so as to extend the qi in the upper energizer. That has the function of alleviating depression to regulate qi, strengthening the heart and dispersing the lung and regulating qi activities. The actions are also very effective in treating and preventing diseases of the heart and lung such as coronary heart disease, atelectasis, etc.

1.3.2.2.7 Liangshou Tuotian (Both Hands Supporting the Sky)

PREPARATORY POSTURE Stand in a horse-riding stance or a given stance.

ACTIONS

(1) Bend the elbows and set the up-facing palms at the side of the loin.

(2) Raise the hands slowly with the palm facing the sky. Exert strength at the end of fingers with the shoulder relaxed and the elbow straight. The eyes look straight ahead and the head seems to be in a pose of carrying an object (Fig. 12).

【按语】 以上两势,上臂运动前伸、外展,使胸廓尽量张开,上焦气机得以舒展,起到宽胸理气,强心宣肺的作用,因而调整气机,对心肺疾患,诸如冠心病、肺不张等有良好的防治作用。

7. 两手托天

【预备】 站好马裆或指定的裆势。

【动作】

(1) 两手屈肘,仰掌于腰部。

(2) 两仰掌上托,掌心朝天,缓缓上举。指端着力,肩松肘直,两目平视,头如顶物。(图12)。

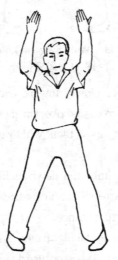

Fig. 12 Both Hands Supporting the Sky
图12 两手托天

(3) Turn the palmar bases outward, part them leftward and rightward with four fingers close together, concentrate strength and slowly drop them down to the chest and change them into the up-facing palms by rotating the wrists, and withdraw them to the waist.

(4) Change the up-facing palms into the down-facing palms and press them downward. Stretch the arms backward and reduce them to the starting stance.

ESSENTIALS　Raising the palms with them facing the sky. Exerting strength with the end of the fingers, relaxing the shoulders and straightening the elbows. The eyes look straight ahead.

1.3.2.2.8　Bawang Juding (the Overlord Lifting up the Tripod)

PREPARATORY POSTURE　Stand in a bow-step stance or a given stance.

ACTIONS

(1) Bend the elbows and set the hands at the loin with the palms facing upward.

(2) Slowly hold up the hands with the palms facing the sky until they are over the shoulders. Turn the palmar bases outward and rotate the fingertips inward from the left and right sides to make the two Hukou opposite to each other to set a posture just like holding a heavy object. Raise the arms slowly up. Straighten the elbows with the tips of the fingers opposite to each other, the fingers close together and the thumb parting outward. The eyes look straight ahead. And breathe naturally (Fig. 13).

(3) Rotate the wrists and turn the palms to get the tips of the fingers pointing upward and the sides of the palms opposite to each other and the thumbs apart outward. Concentrate strength and lower the arms gradually and withdraw the palms beside the loin.

（3）掌根外旋，四指并拢分向左右，蓄力徐徐而下，至胸部旋腕变仰掌收回护腰。

（4）由仰掌化俯掌下按，两臂后伸，同原裆势。

【要领】　仰掌上托，掌心朝天，指端运劲，松肩挺肘，两目平视。

8.　霸王举鼎

【预备】　站好弓箭裆势或指定的裆势。

【动作】

（1）两手屈肘仰掌于腰部。

（2）仰掌缓缓上托，掌心朝天，过于肩部掌根外展，指端由左右向内旋转，虎口相对，犹托重物，徐徐上举，肘部要挺，指端相对，四指并拢，拇指外分，两目平视，呼吸自然（图 13）。

（3）旋腕翻掌，指端朝上，掌侧相对，拇指外分，蓄力而下，渐渐收回腰部。

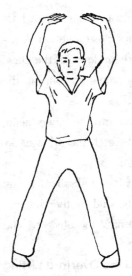

Fig. 13 The Overlord Lifting up the Tripod
图13 霸王举鼎

(4) Change the up-facing palms into the down-facing ones and press them downward, stretch the arms backward and reduce them to the original stance.

ESSENTIALS Supporting upward with the up-facing palms over the shoulder, rotating the wrists and turning the palms, getting the tips of the fingers opposite to each other. Stretching the elbows and holding them up. Rotating the wrists, turning the palms and withdrawing the arms. Having the tips of the fingers pointing upward and the sides of the palms opposite to each other.

COMMENTS In the above two sets of actions, the arms and the palms push slowly upward, which leads clear yang qi to go upward around the vertex and nourish the brain marrow. They also exert force upward, vibrating the muscles, tendons, superficies, zang and fu organs. Therefore these actions are very effective in treating and preventing general weakness, dizziness, insomnia, gastroptosia, nephroptosia and other visceral ptosis.

（4）在腰部之仰掌化俯掌下按，两臂后伸同原裆势。

【要领】 仰掌上托,过肩旋腕翻掌,指端相对,挺肘上举,回收旋腕翻掌直下,指端朝上,掌侧相对。

【按语】 以上两节,掌臂徐缓向上推动,引清阳之气上行于巅顶,营养脑髓。同时发力向上,振动肌肉、筋腱、体表、脏腑,故对体虚头晕,失眠以及胃、肾等各种内脏下垂疾患,均有良好的防治作用。

1. 3. 2. 2. 9   Dingtian Baodi（Sustaining the Heaven and Holding the Earth）

PREPARATORY POSTURE   Stand in a wide-apart-feet stance or a given stance.

ACTIONS

（1）Bend the elbows and set the up-facing palms beside the loin.

（2）Hold up the up-facing palms until over the shoulder. Rotate the wrists and turn the palms with the palmar bases extending outward and the fingertips turning inward to be opposite to each other. Raise the hands upward slowly to the most extent, then rotate the wrists and turn the palms again. Separate the arms to the right and left sides and insert the hands downward, at the same time bend the torso forward. Close both palms gradually together with the thumbs apart outward and overlap the hands with the right one on the above. Make the dorsum of the hand close to the ground as much as possible and get ready for the next posture（Fig. 14）.

9. 顶天抱地

【预备】　站好大裆或指定的裆势。

【动作】

（1）两手屈肘，仰掌于腰部。

（2）仰掌上托，过于肩部旋腕翻掌，掌根外展，指端内旋相对，徐徐上举，待推足后，旋腕翻掌，慢慢向左右外分下抄，同时身向前俯，两掌逐渐合拢，拇指外分，两掌相叠（右掌在上）。掌背尽量靠底待发（图14）。

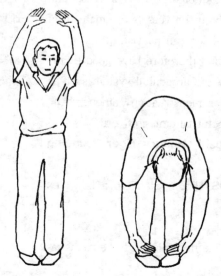

Fig. 14   Sustaining the Heaven and Holding the Earth
图 14　顶天抱地

(3) Lift the palms slowly to the chest just like carrying a heavy object and have the palms facing up and protecting the waist, in the meantime, straighten the torso and look straight ahead.

(4) Change the up-facing palms into the down-facing palms and press downward. Stretch the arms backward and reduce to the original stance.

ESSENTIALS　Support the up-facing palms upward. Rotate the wrists and turn the palms to get them facing up and the fingertips opposite to each other after the arms rise over the shoulders. Separate the turned palms right and left, and insert them downward with the upper body leaning forward. Close the palms with one palm overlapping another and lift them in a posture of carrying an object.

COMMENTS　This set of actions concentrates strength on the lumbus and the back. On the basis, separate the hands and insert them downward and hold them together. Bend the upper body forward and backward. All those movements can excite qi of the governor vessel and the conception vessel, as both the vessels originate from the lower abdomen. The action can nourish qi and blood and regulate yin and yang and therefore have good therapeutic effect on diseases of the urogenital system such as general weakness, irregular menstruation, amenorrhea, leukorrhea, impotence, nocturnal emission, etc.

1.3.2.2.10　Ehu Pushi (Hungry Tiger Pouncing on Its Prey)

PREPARATORY POSTURE　Stand in a bow-step stance.

ACTIONS

(1) Set the hands beside the waist with the palms facing upward.

(2) Change the up-facing palms into straight palms

（3）两掌如抬重物缓缓提到胸部成仰掌护腰，上身随势而直，目须平视。

（4）两仰掌化俯掌下按，两臂后伸，同原裆势。

【要领】　仰掌上托，过肩旋腕翻掌，掌心朝上，指端相对，两翻掌外分下抄，身向前俯，两掌合拢相叠，如抱物上提。

【按语】　本节动作，蓄劲于腰背，在此基础上，分掌抄抱，仰俯曲身，此均可以激发任、督两脉经气。皆因任督脉俱起于胞中，故能益养气血，通调阴阳，对于体虚衰弱、月经不调、闭经、带下及阳痿、遗精等泌尿生殖系统疾病都有较好的防治作用。

10. 饿虎扑食

【预备】　弓箭裆势。

【动作】

（1）两手仰掌护腰。

（2）两仰掌化直掌前推，

and push forward. Meanwhile rotate the forearms inward. The wrists stretch backward and the two Hukou face downward. Following that, the lumbus leans forward. The front leg is kept in the position and the back leg exerts force without relaxation (Fig. 15).

同时两前臂内旋,两腕背伸,虎口朝下,腰随势前俯,前腿得势后腿使劲勿松(图 15)。

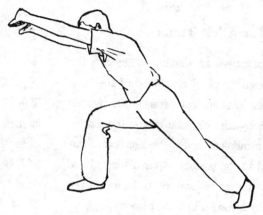

Fig. 15　Hungry Tiger Pouncing on Its Prey
图 15　饿虎扑食

(3) Flex the five knuckles and clench a fist. Rotate the wrist with the fist hole upward. Bend the elbow and withdraw it closely to the waist with the palm facing upward.

(4) Change the up-facing palm into the down-facing palm and press it downward. Stretch the arms backward and reduce them to the original stance.

ESSENTIALS　Push spirally with the palm facing up. The lumbus leans forward. Concentrate strength on the fist center, bend the elbow and withdraw it tightly.

COMMENTS　In this set, a bow-step stance is adopted with intention to take a posture of the bow-step front leg and the arrow-step back leg so as to exert strength of the whole body. In combination with leaning the back forward and stretching the arms and pushing them forcefully, the will, qi and strength can be merged and coordinated. Persistent practice of this set of actions will produce a good therapeutic and

　(3) 五指内收握拳,旋腕,拳眼朝天,屈肘紧收,成仰掌护腰。

　(4) 由仰掌化俯掌下按,两臂后伸,同原裆势。

【要领】　仰掌旋推,腰向前俯,劲注拳心,屈肘紧收。

【按语】　本节多采取弓箭裆势,意取前弓后箭,尽全身之力,配合腰背前俯,伸臂劲推,使意、气、力相融一致,久练此势可对全身伤痛、关节屈伸不利以及各种慢性疾病都有较好的防治效果。

preventive effect on general pain and injury, stiff joints and various kinds of chronic diseases.

1.4 Commonly Used Acupoints in Tuina

1.4.1 Acupoints for Adult Tuina

Acupoints are also known as shuxue. They are the specific locations, through which qi and blood of the zang and fu organs and the meridians and collaterals are transfused and transported to the body surface. Shu means transportation, transfusion and transmission, and xue means hole. Acupoints are closely related to the passage of circulating qi and blood of the body, i.e. the meridians and collaterals. The 361 acupoints traditionally recorded in TCM respectively pertain to the 14 main meridians, so they are also called jingxue (meridian point). Since each meridian pertains to and connects with a certain visceral organ of the body, an indivisible physiological and pathological relationship between acupoints and the meridians and the viscera is formed.

Accurately locating acupoints is very important in prevention and treatment of diseases with tuina. There are several ways to locate acupoints, but the most commonly used is the proportional measurement, in which the bone segments are converted as measurement standards of equal portions to measure the width and length of various portions of the body. The bone-length measurement is applicable to all patients regardless of sex and age, height and physique (See Fig. 16). Now the commonly used bone-length measurement and the main acupoints listed in this book and some other acupoints which do not pertain to the 14 main meridians but called extraordinary acupoints, and their locations and functions are shown in the following:

第四节 常用穴位

一、成人穴位

穴位又叫腧穴,是人体脏腑、经络气血输注于体表的特定部位。腧有转输的含义,穴即孔隙的意思。穴位与人体运行气血的通路——经络紧密关联。中医传统记载的 361 个穴位分别归属于人体主要的 14 条经脉,因此这些穴位又叫做经穴。由于经脉隶属联络着人体的各个脏腑器官,这样就形成了穴位—经络—脏腑在人体生理、病理上不可分割的关系。

推拿防治疾病过程中,准确地选择穴位非常重要,取穴有许多方法,最常用的是骨度分寸法,即将人体多部的骨骼尺寸折算成一定的等分,不论男女老少,高矮胖瘦均按这一标准度量(图 16)。兹将骨度分寸和本书中所涉及的主要经穴以及一些不在十四经所属,称之为经外奇穴的穴位的定位、功用等介绍如下。

The Commonly Used Bone-length Measurement (Fig. 16)

Portion of Body	Beginning and Ending	Size of Bone-length Measurement	Method	Explanation
Head & Face	From the anterior hairline to the posterior hairline	12 cun	Longitudinal measurement	If the anterior and posterior hairlines are not clear, the distance from the ophryon to Dazhui (GV 14) is taken as 18 cun; to the anterior hairline, 3 cun; from Dazhui to the posterior hairline, 3 cun
	Between the two mastoid processes	9 cun	Horizontal measurement	Equal to the distance between the two Touwei (ST 8) acupoints on the forehead, used to measure the head and face transversely
Neck & Nape	From the posterior hairline to Dazhui (GV 14)	2.5 cun	Longitudinal measurement	Taken as 3 cun in acupoint-locating measurement
	From Adam apple to Tiantu (CV 22) (the center of the suprasternal fossa)	4 cun	Longitudinal measurement	i. e. from the larynx to the suprasternal notch
Chest, Abdomen and Hypochondrium	From Tiantu (CV 22) to the xiphosternal synchondrosis	9 cun	Longitudinal measurement	i. e. from the suprasternal notch to the xiphosternal synchondrosis. Acupoint-location in the chest and hypochondrium is also determined by ribs i. e. a rib or the intercostal space is counted as 1. 6 cun
	From the xiphosternal synchondrosis to the centre of the umbilicus	8 cun	Longitudinal measurement	Used for acupoint-location on the upper abdomen
	Between the centre of the umbilicus and the upper margin of pubic bone	5 cun	Longitudinal measurement	Used for acupoint-location on the lower abdomen
	Between the two nipples	8 cun	Horizontal measurement	Used for transverse measurement of the chest and abdomen. In females the distance between the two acupoints Quepen (ST 12) instead
	From the area below the axilla to the lower border of the hypochondriac region	12 cun	Longitudinal measurement	The lower border of hypochondrium refers to the tip of the 11th rib
	From the 11th rib to the uppermost part of the lateral aspect of the thigh (the prominence of the greater trochanter)	9 cun	Longitudinal measurement	i. e. from the tip of the 11th rib to greater trochanter

(**Following table**)

Portion of Body	Beginning and Ending	Size of Bone-length Measurement	Method	Explanation
Back and Lumbus	From Dazhui (GV 14) to the coccyx	21 vertebrae in all	Longitudinal measurement	Location of the Back-Shu acupoints is determined by the vertebrae. The two inferior angles of the scapula are at the same level with the spinous process of the 7th thoracic vertebra, and the two iliac crests are at the same level with the spinous process of the 4th lumbar vertebra
	The distance between the vertebral margins of the scapula	6 cun	Horizontal measurement	
Upper limb	Between the end of the anterior axillary fold and the transverse cubital crease	9 cun	Longitudinal measurement	Used for location of the acupoints on the three hand yin and yang meridians
	Between the transverse cubital crease and the transverse wrist crease	12 cun		
Lower limb	From the level of the upper margin of the pubic bone to the upper margin of the internal condyle of femur	18 cun	Longitudinal measurement	Used for the location of acupoints on the three foot yin meridians
	From the lower margin of the internal condyle of femur (the lower margin of the medial condyle of tibia) to the tip of the medial malleolus	13 cun		
	From the prominence of the greater trochanter to the middle of knee	19 cun		Used for the location of acupoints on the three foot yang meridians. The height of the middle of knee levels with Dubi (ST 35) anteriorly and to Weizhong (BL 40) posteriorly
	From the transverse gluteal crease to the middle of knee	14 cun		
	Between the middle of knee and the tip of the lateral malleolus	16 cun		
	From the tip of the lateral malleolus to the lateral border of the sole	3 cun		

常用骨度分寸表(见图16)

分 部	部 位 起 止 点	度 数	度量法	说 明
头 面	前发际至后发际	12寸	直寸	如前后发际不明从眉心量至大椎18寸,眉心至前发际3寸,大椎至后发际3寸
	两耳后完骨(乳突)之间	9寸	横寸	与额部左右头维穴间距相当;用以度量头面部横寸
颈 项	后发际至大椎	2.5寸	直寸	取穴法作3寸
	喉结至天突穴	4寸	直寸	即喉头至胸骨上切迹
胸腹肋	天突穴至歧骨	9寸	直寸	即胸骨上切迹至胸剑联合;胸肋部取穴度量,一般根据肋骨计算,每一肋骨或上下两肋间折作1寸6分
	歧骨至脐中	8寸	直寸	用于上腹部定穴
	脐中至横骨上廉(耻骨联合上缘)	5寸	直寸	用于下腹部定穴
	两乳头之间	8寸	横寸	用于胸腹部横量;女性以两缺盆穴间距代替
	腋以下至季胁	12寸	直寸	季胁指11肋端
	季胁以下至髀枢	9寸	直寸	即11肋端至股骨大转子上
背 腰	大椎以下至尾椎	21椎	直量	背部腧穴根据脊椎定位;两肩胛骨下角平第7胸椎棘突,两髂嵴平第4腰椎棘突
	两肩胛骨脊柱缘之间	6寸	横寸	
上肢部	腋前纹头至肘横纹	9寸	直寸	用于手三阴、手三阳经的取穴定位
	肘横纹至腕横纹	12寸		
下肢部	横骨上廉至内辅骨上廉(股骨内髁上缘)	18寸	直寸	用于足三阴经的取穴定位
	内辅骨下廉(胫骨内髁下缘)至内踝高点	13寸		
	髀枢至膝中	19寸		用于足三阳经的取穴定位;膝中的水平:前面相当于犊鼻穴,后面相当于委中穴
	臀横纹至膝中	14寸		
	膝中至外踝高点	16寸		
	外踝高点至足底	3寸		

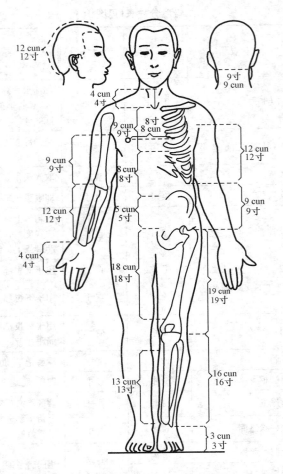

Fig. 16 The Commonly Used Proportional Measurement of
Acupoint Selection on the Human Body
图 16 人体取穴常用骨度分寸

1.4.1.1 Acupoints on the Head and Face

1.4.1.1.1 Yingxiang (LI 20)

LOCATION 0.5 cun lateral to the midpoint of the lateral border of ala nasi, in the nasolabial groove.

INDICATIONS Nasal obstruction, epistaxis, facial distortion, itching of the face and biliary colic.

MERIDIAN The Large Intestine Meridian of Hand-*Yangming*.

（一）头面部穴位

1. 迎香

【定位】 鼻翼外缘中点，旁开 0.5 寸，当鼻唇沟中。

【主治】 鼻塞，鼻出血，口眼歪斜，面痒，胆绞痛。

【归经】 手阳明大肠经。

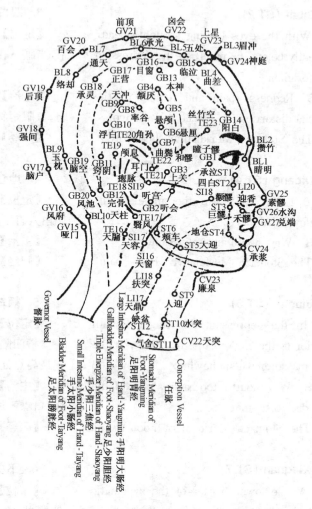

Fig. 17 - 1 Acupoints on the Head, Face and Neck
图 17 - 1 头面颈部穴位

1.4.1.1.2 Chengqi（ST 1）

LOCATION With the eyes looking straight ahead, the acupoint is directly below the pupil, between the infraorbital margin and the eyeball.

INDICATIONS Redness, swelling and pain of the eyes, lacrimation, night blindness and facial distortion.

MERIDIAN The Stomach Meridian of Foot-*Yangming*.

2. 承泣

【定位】 目正视,瞳孔直下,当眶下缘与眼球之间。

【主治】 目赤肿痛,流泪,夜盲,口眼歪斜。

【归经】 足阳明胃经。

1.4.1.1.3　Sibai (ST 2)

LOCATION　With the eyes looking straight ahead, the acupoint is directly below the pupil, in the depression at the infraorbital foramen.

INDICATIONS　Redness, pain and itching of the eyes, cataract, facial distortion, headache and vertigo.

MERIDIAN　The Stomach Meridian of Foot-*Yangming*.

1.4.1.1.4　Dicang (ST 4)

LOCATION　0.4 cun lateral to the angle of the mouth, directly below Sibai (ST 2).

INDICATIONS　Wry mouth and salivation.

MERIDIAN　The Stomach Meridian of Foot-*Yangming*.

1.4.1.1.5　Jiache (ST 6)

LOCATION　In the depression one finger-breadth anterior and superior to the angle of the mandible, at the prominence of m. masseter when chewing.

INDICATIONS　Wry mouth, toothache, pain of the cheek and aphasia due to trismus.

MERIDIAN　The Stomach Meridian of Foot-*Yangming*.

1.4.1.1.6　Xiaguan (ST 7)

LOCATION　At the lower border of the zygomatic arch, in the depression between the anterior part to the condyloid process of the mandible and the notch. The acupoint is located when the mouth is closed.

INDICATIONS　Deafness, tinnitus, toothache, trismus and facial paralysis.

MERIDIAN　The Stomach Meridian of Foot-*Yangming*.

1.4.1.1.7　Touwei (ST 8)

LOCATION　0.5 cun directly above the hairline at the corner of the forehead.

3. 四白

【定位】　目正视，瞳孔直下，当眶下孔凹陷中。

【主治】　目赤肿痛，目翳，口眼歪斜，头痛眩晕。

【归经】　足阳明胃经。

4. 地仓

【定位】　口角旁 0.4 寸。四白穴直下取之。

【主治】　口㖞，流涎。

【归经】　足阳明胃经。

5. 颊车

【定位】　下颌角前上方一横指凹陷中，咀嚼时咬肌隆起最高点处。

【主治】　口歪，齿痛，颊痛，口噤不语。

【归经】　足阳明胃经。

6. 下关

【定位】　颧弓下缘，下颌骨髁状突之前方的凹陷中。合口有孔，张口即闭。

【主治】　耳聋，耳鸣，齿痛，口噤，口眼歪斜。

【归经】　足阳明胃经。

7. 头维

【定位】　额角发际直上 0.5 寸。

INDICATIONS Headache, vertigo, pain of the mouth and lacrimation.

MERIDIAN The Stomach Meridian of Foot-*Yangming*.

1.4.1.1.8 Quanliao (SI 18)

LOCATION Directly below the outer canthus, in the depression on the lower border of the zygoma.

INDICATIONS Facial distortion, toothache and swelling in the cheek.

MERIDIAN The Small Intestine Meridian of Hand-*Taiyang*.

1.4.1.1.9 Tinggong (SI 19)

LOCATION Anterior to the tragus and posterior to the condyloid process of the mandible, in the depression formed when the mouth is open.

INDICATIONS Tinnitus, deafness, toothache, and depressive and maniac psychosis.

MERIDIAN The Small Intestine Meridian of Hand-*Taiyang*.

1.4.1.1.10 Jingming (BL 1)

LOCATION 0.1 cun lateral to the inner canthus.

INDICATIONS Conjunctival congestion with swelling and pain, lacrimation, blurred vision, dizziness, myopia, night blindness and color blindness.

MERIDIAN The Bladder Meridian of Foot-*Taiyang*.

1.4.1.1.11 Cuanzhu (BL 2)

LOCATION In the depression on the medial end of the eyebrow.

INDICATIONS Headache, facial paralysis, blurred vision, lacrimation, redness, swelling and pain of eyes, pain in the supraorbital region and blepharoptosis.

MERIDIAN The Bladder Meridian of Foot-*Taiyang*.

1.4.1.1.12 Tianzhu (BL 10)

LOCATION 0.5 cun directly above and 1.3 cun

【主治】 头痛,目眩,口痛,流泪。

【归经】 足阳明胃经。

8. 颧髎

【定位】 目外眦直下,颧骨下缘凹陷中。

【主治】 口眼歪斜,齿痛,颊肿。

【归经】 手太阳小肠经。

9. 听宫

【定位】 耳屏前,下颌骨髁状突的后缘,张口呈凹陷处。

【主治】 耳鸣,耳聋,齿痛,癫狂病。

【归经】 手太阳小肠经。

10. 睛明

【定位】 目内眦旁0.1寸。

【主治】 目赤肿痛,流泪,视物不明,目眩,近视,夜盲,色盲。

【归经】 足太阳膀胱经。

11. 攒竹

【定位】 眉头凹陷中。

【主治】 头痛,口眼歪斜,目视不明,流泪,目赤肿痛,眉棱骨痛,眼睑下垂。

【归经】 足太阳膀胱经。

12. 天柱

【定位】 后发际正中直

lateral to the midpoint of the posterior hairline, in the depression on the lateral margin of m. trapezius.

INDICATIONS Headache, neck rigidity, nasal obstruction, epilepsy, depressive and maniac psychosis, pain in the shoulder and back, and febrile diseases.

MERIDIAN The Bladder Meridian of Foot-*Taiyang*.

1.4.1.1.13 Yifeng (TE 17)

LOCATION Anterior-inferior to the mastoid process, in the depression posterior to the inferior border of the lobule of the ear.

INDICATIONS Tinnitus, deafness, facial paralysis, lockjaw, toothache, swelling of the cheek and scrofula.

MERIDIAN The Triple Energizer Meridian of Hand-*Shaoyang*.

1.4.1.1.14 Ermen (TE 21)

LOCATION In front of the superior notch of the tragus, in the depression on the posterior border of the mandibular condyloid process.

INDICATIONS Tinnitus, deafness and toothache.

MERIDIAN The Triple Energizer Meridian of Hand-*Shaoyang*.

1.4.1.1.15 Sizhukong (TE 23)

LOCATION In the depression at the lateral end of the eyebrow.

INDICATIONS Headache, conjunctival congestion with swelling and pain, toothache, depressive and maniac psychosis and epilepsy.

MERIDIAN The Triple Energizer Meridian of Hand-*Shaoyang*.

1.4.1.1.16 Tongziliao (GB 1)

LOCATION 0.5 cun lateral to the outer canthus, in the depression on the lateral edge of the orbit.

INDICATIONS Headache, redness, swelling and

上 0.5 寸,旁开 1.3 寸,当斜方肌外缘凹陷中。

【主治】 头痛,项强,鼻塞,癫狂痫,肩背痛,热病。

【归经】 足太阳膀胱经。

13. 翳风

【定位】 乳突前下方,平耳垂后下缘的凹陷中。

【主治】 耳鸣,耳聋,口眼歪斜,牙关紧闭,齿痛,颊肿,瘰疬。

【归经】 手少阳三焦经。

14. 耳门

【定位】 耳屏上切迹前,下颌骨髁状突后缘凹陷中。

【主治】 耳鸣,耳聋,齿痛。

【归经】 手少阳三焦经。

15. 丝竹空

【定位】 眉梢的凹陷中。

【主治】 头痛,目赤肿痛,齿痛,癫狂痫。

【归经】 手少阳三焦经。

16. 瞳子髎

【定位】 目外眦旁 0.5寸,眶骨外缘凹陷中。

【主治】 头痛,目赤痛,

pain of the eye, cataract and glaucoma.

MERIDIAN The Gallbladder Meridian of Foot-*Shaoyang*.

1.4.1.1.17 Tinghui (GB 2)

LOCATION Anterior to the intertragic notch, at the posterior border of the condyloid process of the mandible. The acupoint is located when the mouth is open.

INDICATIONS Deafness, tinnitus, toothache and wry mouth.

MERIDIAN The Gallbladder Meridian of Foot-*Shaoyang*.

1.4.1.1.18 Shangguan (GB 3)

LOCATION Directly above Xiaguan (ST 7), on the upper border of the zygomatic arch.

INDICATIONS Migraine, tinnitus, deafness, facial distortion, toothache and trismus.

MERIDIAN The Gallbladder Meridian of Foot-*Shaoyang*.

1.4.1.1.19 Yangbai (GB 14)

LOCATION With the eyes looking straight forward, the acupoint is directly above the pupil, 1 cun superior to the eyebrow.

INDICATIONS Headache, pain of the eye, blurred vision and eyelids twitching.

MERIDIAN The Gallbladder Meridian of Foot-*Shaoyang*.

1.4.1.1.20 Baihui (GV 20)

LOCATION 7 cun directly above the midpoint of the posterior hairline. (Simple location way: Directly above the apex auricula, on the midline of the head.)

INDICATIONS Headache, vertigo, post-apoplectic aphasia, depressive and maniac psychosis, prolapse of the rectum, prolapse of uterus and insomnia.

MERIDIAN The Governor Vessel.

目翳,青盲。

【归经】 足少阳胆经。

17. 听会

【定位】 耳屏间切迹前,下颌骨髁状突的后缘,张口有孔。

【主治】 耳鸣,耳聋,齿痛,口㖞。

【归经】 足少阳胆经。

18. 上关

【定位】 下关穴直上,当颧弓的上缘。

【主治】 偏头痛,耳鸣,耳聋,口眼歪斜,齿痛,口噤。

【归经】 足少阳胆经。

19. 阳白

【定位】 目正视,瞳孔直上,眉上1寸。

【主治】 头痛,目痛,视物模糊,眼睑瞤动。

【归经】 足少阳胆经。

20. 百会

【定位】 后发际正中直上7寸。(简便定位:耳尖直上,头顶正中)

【主治】 头痛,眩晕,中风失语,癫狂,脱肛,阴挺,不寐。

【归经】 督脉。

1.4.1.1.21　Shenting (GV 24)

LOCATION　0.5 cun directly above the midpoint of the anterior hairline.

INDICATIONS　Headache, vertigo, insomnia, rhinorrhea and epilepsy.

MERIDIAN　The Governor Vessel.

1.4.1.1.22　Shuigou (Renzhong GV 26)

LOCATION　At the junction of the superior 1/3 and the middle 1/3 of the philtrum.

INDICATIONS　Depressive and maniac psychosis, infantile convulsion, coma, facial distortion, rigidity and pain along the spinal column.

MERIDIAN　The Governor Vessel.

1.4.1.1.23　Lianquan (CV 23)

LOCATION　At the midpoint of the upper border of the hyoid bone.

INDICATIONS　Swelling and pain of the subglossal region, salivation with flaccid tongue, aphasia due to stiff tongue and difficulty in swallowing.

MERIDIAN　The Conception Vessel.

1.4.1.1.24　Chengjiang (CV 24)

LOCATION　In the centre of the mentolabial groove.

INDICATIONS　Swelling and pain of the gums, salivation, depressive and maniac psychosis.

MERIDIAN　The Conception Vessel.

1.4.1.1.25　Sishencong (EX-HN 1)

LOCATION　1 cun respectively anterior, posterior and bilateral to Baihui (GV 20), 4 acupoints in all.

INDICATIONS　Headache, vertigo, insomnia, amnesia and epilepsy.

MERIDIAN　Extraordinary acupoints.

1.4.1.1.26　Yintang (EX-HN 3)

LOCATION　At the midpoint of the line between the

---

21. 神庭

【定位】　前发际正中直上 0.5 寸。

【主治】　头痛，眩晕，失眠，鼻渊，癫痫。

【归经】　督脉。

22. 水沟(人中)

【定位】　在人中沟的上 1/3 与中 1/3 交界处。

【主治】　癫狂病，小儿惊风，昏迷，口眼歪斜，腰脊强痛。

【归经】　督脉。

23. 廉泉

【定位】　舌骨体上缘的中点处。

【主治】　舌下肿痛，舌缓流涎，舌强不语，吞咽困难。

【归经】　任脉。

24. 承浆

【定位】　颏唇沟的中点。

【主治】　齿龈肿痛，流涎，癫狂。

【归经】　任脉。

25. 四神聪

【定位】　百会穴前后左右各 1 寸处。

【主治】　头痛，眩晕，失眠，健忘，癫痫。

【归经】　经外奇穴。

26. 印堂

【定位】　两眉头连线的

medial ends of the two eyebrows.

INDICATIONS Headache, vertigo, epistaxis, rhinorrhea, infantile convulsion and insomnia.

MERIDIAN Extraordinary acupoints.

1.4.1.1.27 Qianzheng (EX-HN)

LOCATION 0.5 to 1 cun anterior to the ear lobule.

INDICATIONS Wry mouth and orolingual ulcer.

MERIDIAN Extraordinary acupoints.

1.4.1.1.28 Yiming (EX-HN 14)

LOCATION 1 cun posterior to Yifeng (TE 17)

INDICATIONS Eye diseases, tinnitus and insomnia.

MERIDIAN Extraordinary acupoints.

1.4.1.1.29 Anmian (EX-HN)

LOCATION At the midpoint of the line between Yifeng (TE 17) and Fengchi (GB 20).

INDICATIONS Insomnia, headache, vertigo, palpitation, depressive and maniac psychosis.

MERIDIAN Extraordinary acupoints.

1.4.1.2 Acupoints on the Neck and the Shoulder

1.4.1.2.1 Zhongfu (LU 1)

LOCATION On the latero-superior aspect of the chest, 6 cun lateral to the anterior midline, level with the 1st intercostal space.

INDICATIONS Cough, asthma, fullness of the lung and pain in the chest, back and shoulder.

MERIDIAN The Lung Meridian of Hand-*Taiyin*.

1.4.1.2.2 Yunmen (LU 2)

LOCATION On the latero-superior aspect of the chest, 6 cun lateral to the anterior midline, in the infraclavicular fossa of its lateral end.

INDICATIONS Cough, asthma and pain in the chest, shoulder and back.

MERIDIAN The Lung Meridian of Hand-*Taiyin*.

中点。

【主治】 头痛，眩晕，鼻衄，鼻渊，小儿惊风，失眠。

【归经】 经外奇穴。

27. 牵正

【定位】 耳垂前0.5～1寸。

【主治】 口歪，口舌生疮。

【归经】 经外奇穴。

28. 翳明

【定位】 翳风穴后1寸。

【主治】 目疾，耳鸣，失眠。

【归经】 经外奇穴。

29. 安眠

【定位】 翳风穴与风池穴连线的中点。

【主治】 失眠，头痛，眩晕，心悸，癫狂。

【归经】 经外奇穴。

（二）颈肩部穴位

1. 中府

【定位】 胸前壁外上方，前正中线旁开6寸，平第1肋间隙处。

【主治】 咳嗽，气喘，肺胀满，胸痛，肩背痛。

【归经】 手太阴肺经。

2. 云门

【定位】 胸前壁外上方，距前正中线旁开6寸，当锁骨外端下缘凹陷中取穴。

【主治】 咳嗽，气喘，胸痛，肩痛。

【归经】 手太阴肺经。

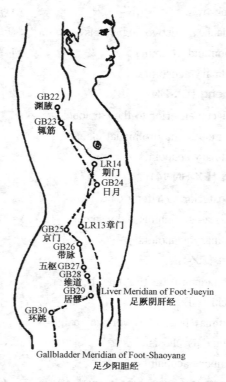

GB22
渊腋
GB23
辄筋
LR14
期门
GB24
日月
GB25
京门
LR13章门
GB26
带脉
五枢GB27
GB28
维道
GB29
居髎
GB30
环跳
Liver Meridian of Foot-Jueyin
足厥阴肝经
Gallbladder Meridian of Foot-Shaoyang
足少阳胆经

Fig. 17 - 2　Acupoints on the Armpit, Hypochondrium and Lateral Abdomen
图 17 - 2　腋胁侧腹部穴位

1.4.1.2.3　Jianyu (LI 15)

LOCATION　Inferior to the end of the acromion, between the acromion and the greater tuberosity of the humerus, and at the center of the lower portion of m. deltoideus. When the arm is abducted forward in level, there are two depressions on the shoulder. The acupoint is in the anterior depression.

INDICATIONS　Scrofula and spasmodic pain and paralysis in the shoulder and arm.

MERIDIAN　The Large Intestine Meridian of Hand-*Yangming*.

1.4.1.2.4　Renying (ST 9)

LOCATION　1.5 cun lateral to Adam's apple, just

3. 肩髃

【定位】　肩峰端下缘,当肩峰与肱骨大结节之间,三角肌下部中央。肩平举时,肩部出现两个凹陷,在前方的凹陷中。

【主治】　肩臂挛痛不遂,瘰疬。

【归经】　手阳明大肠经。

4. 人迎

【定位】　喉结旁1.5寸,

behind the common carotid artery, on the anterior border of m. sternocleidomastoideus.

INDICATIONS   Sore throat, asthma, scrofula, goiter and hypertension.

MERIDIAN   The Stomach Meridian of Foot-*Yangming*.

1.4.1.2.5   Jianliao (TE 14)

LOCATION   Posterior and inferior to the acromion, in the depression about 1 cun posterior to Jianyu (LI 15) when the arm is abducted outward.

INDICATIONS   Spasmodic pain and paralysis in the shoulder and arm.

MERIDIAN   The Triple Energizer Meridian of Hand-*Shaoyang*.

1.4.1.2.6   Fengchi (GB 20)

LOCATION   In the depression between m. sternocleidomastoideus and m. trapezius.

INDICATIONS   Headache, vertigo, conjunctival congestion with redness, swelling and pain, epistaxis, rhinorrhea, tinnitus, pain and stiffness of the neck, common cold, epilepsy, apoplexy, febrile diseases and malaria.

MERIDIAN   The Gallbladder Meridian of Foot-*Shaoyang*.

1.4.1.2.7   Jianjing (GB 21)

LOCATION   At the midpoint of the line joining Dazhui (GV 14) and the acromion.

INDICATIONS   Pain and rigidity of the head and neck, pain in the shoulder and back, motor impairment of the upper arm, dystocia, mastitis, alactation and scrofula.

MERIDIAN   The Gallbladder Meridian of Foot-*Shaoyang*.

1.4.1.2.8   Dazhui (GV 14)

LOCATION   Below the spinous process of the 7th

当颈动脉之后,胸锁乳突肌前缘。

【主治】 咽喉肿痛,气喘,瘰疬,瘿气,高血压。

【归经】 足阳明胃经。

5. 肩髎

【定位】 肩峰后下方,上臂外展,当肩髃穴后寸许的凹陷中。

【主治】 肩臂挛痛不遂。

【归经】 手少阳三焦经。

6. 风池

【定位】 胸锁乳突肌与斜方肌之间凹陷中。

【主治】 头痛,眩晕,目赤肿痛,鼻渊,衄血,耳鸣,颈项强痛,感冒,癫痫,中风,热病,疟疾。

【归经】 足少阳胆经。

7. 肩井

【定位】 大椎穴(督脉)与肩峰连线之中点。

【主治】 头项强痛,肩背疼痛,上肢不遂,难产,乳痈,乳汁不下,瘰疬。

【归经】 足少阳胆经。

8. 大椎

【定位】 第 7 颈椎棘突

cervical vertebra.

INDICATIONS　Febrile diseases, malaria, cough, dyspnea, hectic fever accompanied with night sweating, epilepsy, headache, rigidity of the neck and rubella.

MERIDIAN　The Governor Vessel.

1.4.1.2.9　Yamen (GV 15)

LOCATION　0.5 cun directly above the midpoint of the posterior hairline.

INDICATIONS　Sudden aphonia, aphasia due to stiffness of the tongue, depressive and maniac psychosis, epilepsy, headache and neck rigidity.

MERIDIAN　The Governor Vessel.

1.4.1.2.10　Fengfu (GV 16)

LOCATION　1 cun directly above the midpoint of the posterior hairline.

INDICATIONS　Headache, stiff neck, vertigo, sore throat, aphonia, depressive and maniac psychosis and apoplexy.

MERIDIAN　The Governor Vessel.

1.4.1.2.11　Tiantu (CV 22)

LOCATION　In the center of the suprasternal fossa.

INDICATIONS　Cough, asthma, pain in the chest, sore throat, sudden aphonia, goiter, globus hystericus and dysphagia.

MERIDIAN　The Conception Vessel.

1.4.1.3　Acupoints on the Chest and Abdomen

1.4.1.3.1　Rugen (ST 18)

LOCATION　In the 5th intercostal space, directly below the nipple.

INDICATIONS　Cough, short breath, hiccup, chest pain, mastitis and insufficient lactation.

MERIDIAN　The Stomach Meridian of Foot-*Yangming*.

下。

【主治】　热病，疟疾，咳嗽，气喘，骨蒸盗汗，癫痫，头痛项强，风疹。

【归经】　督脉。

9. 哑门

【定位】　后发际正中直上0.5寸。

【主治】　暴喑，舌强不语，癫狂痫，头痛项强。

【归经】　督脉。

10. 风府

【定位】　后发际正中直上1寸。

【主治】　头痛，项强，眩晕，咽喉肿痛，失音，癫狂，中风。

【归经】　督脉。

11. 天突

【定位】　胸骨上窝正中。

【主治】　咳嗽，气喘，胸痛，咽喉肿痛，暴喑，瘿气，梅核气，噎膈。

【归经】　任脉。

（三）胸腹部穴位

1. 乳根

【定位】　第5肋间隙，乳头直下。

【主治】　咳嗽，气喘，呃逆，胸痛，乳痛，乳汁少。

【归经】　足阳明胃经。

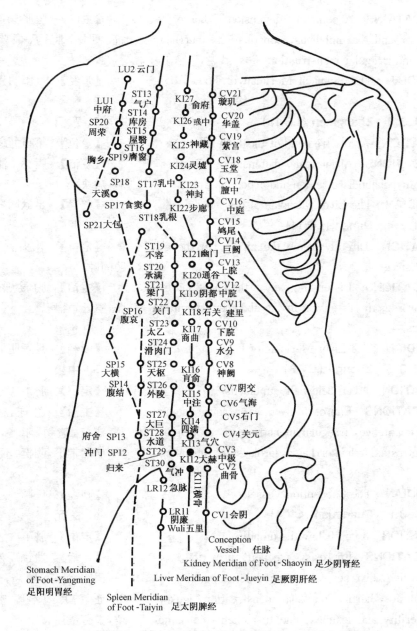

Fig. 17‑3 Acupoints on the Chest, Hypochondrium and Abdomen

图 17‑3   胸膺胁腹部穴位

1.4.1.3.2 Tianshu (ST 25)   **2. 天枢**

LOCATION 2 cun lateral to the umbilicus.   【定位】 脐旁 2 寸。

INDICATIONS Abdominal distension, borborygmus, pain around the umbilicus, constipation, diarrhea, dysentery and irregular menstruation.

MERIDIAN The Stomach Meridian of Foot-*Yangming*.

1.4.1.3.3　Zhangmen (LR 13)

LOCATION At the free end of the 11th rib.

INDICATIONS Abdominal distension, diarrhea, pain in the hypochondriac region and abdominal mass.

MERIDIAN The Liver Meridian of Foot-*Jueyin*.

1.4.1.3.4　Qimen (LR 14)

LOCATION Directly below the nipple, in the 6th intercostal space.

INDICATIONS Distending pain in the chest and hypochondriac region, distension in the abdomen, vomiting and mastitis.

MERIDIAN The Liver Meridian of Foot-*Jueyin*.

1.4.1.3.5　Zhongji (CV 3)

LOCATION 4 cun below the umbilicus.

INDICATIONS Enuresis, dysuria, hernia, seminal emission, impotence, irregular menstruation, metrorrhagia and metrostaxis, leukorrhagia, prolapse of uterus and sterility.

MERIDIAN The Conception Vessel.

1.4.1.3.6　Guanyuan (CV 4)

LOCATION 3 cun below the umbilicus.

INDICATIONS Enuresis, frequent urination, retention of urine, diarrhea, abdominal pain, seminal emission, impotence, hernia, irregular menstruation, leukorrhagia, sterility and leanness due to asthenia consumption.

MERIDIAN The Conception Vessel.

1.4.1.3.7　Qihai (CV 6)

LOCATION 1.5 cun below the umbilicus.

【主治】 腹胀肠鸣,绕脐痛,便秘,泄泻,痢疾,月经不调。

【归经】 足阳明胃经。

3. 章门

【定位】 第11肋端。

【主治】 腹胀,泄泻,胁痛,痞块。

【归经】 足厥阴肝经。

4. 期门

【定位】 乳头直下,第6肋间隙。

【主治】 胸胁胀痛,腹胀,呕吐,乳痈。

【归经】 足厥阴肝经。

5. 中极

【定位】 脐下4寸。

【主治】 遗尿,小便不利,疝气,遗精,阳痿,月经不调,崩漏带下,阴挺,不孕。

【归经】 任脉。

6. 关元

【定位】 脐下3寸。

【主治】 遗尿,小便频数,尿闭,泄泻,腹痛,遗精,阳痿,疝气,月经不调,带下,不孕,虚劳羸瘦。

【归经】 任脉。

7. 气海

【定位】 脐下1.5寸。

INDICATIONS   Abdominal pain, diarrhea, constipation, enuresis, hernia, seminal emission, irregular menstruation, amenorrhea and collapse due to asthenia depletion.

MERIDIAN   The Conception Vessel.

1.4.1.3.8   Shenque（CV 8）

LOCATION   In the center of the umbilicus.

INDICATIONS   Abdominal pain, edema, hernia, irregular menstruation and leukorrhagia.

MERIDIAN   The Conception Vessel.

1.4.1.3.9   Zhongwan（CV 12）

LOCATION   4 cun above the umbilicus.

INDICATIONS   Gastric pain, vomiting, acid regurgitation, abdominal distension, diarrhea, jaundice, depressive and maniac psychosis.

MERIDIAN   The Conception Vessel.

1.4.1.3.10   Jiuwei（CV 15）

LOCATION   Below the xiphoid process, 7 cun above the umbilicus.

INDICATIONS   Chest pain, abdominal distension, depressive and maniac psychosis, epilepsy.

MERIDIAN   The Conception Vessel.

1.4.1.3.11   Danzhong（CV 17）

LOCATION   On the anterior midline, level with the 4th intercostal space.

INDICATIONS   Cough, dyspnea, chest pain, palpitation, insufficient lactation, vomiting and dysphagia.

MERIDIAN   The Conception Vessel.

1.4.1.3.12   Zigongxue（EX-CA 1）

LOCATION   3 cun lateral to Zhongji（CV 3）.

INDICATIONS   Prolapse of the uterus, hernia and abdominal pain.

MERIDIAN   Extraordinary acupoints.

【主治】 腹痛,泄泻,便秘,遗尿,疝气,遗精,月经不调,经闭,虚脱。

【归经】 任脉。

8. 神阙

【定位】 脐的中间。

【主治】 腹痛,水肿,疝气,月经不调,带下。

【归经】 任脉。

9. 中脘

【定位】 脐上 4 寸。

【主治】 胃痛,呕吐,吞酸,腹胀,泄泻,黄疸,癫狂。

【归经】 任脉。

10. 鸠尾

【定位】 剑突下,脐上 7 寸。

【主治】 胸痛,腹胀,癫狂痫。

【归经】 任脉。

11. 膻中

【定位】 前正中线,平第 4 肋间隙。

【主治】 咳嗽,气喘,胸痛,心悸,乳少,呕吐,噎膈。

【归经】 任脉。

12. 子宫穴

【定位】 中极穴旁开 3 寸。

【主治】 阴挺,疝气,腹痛。

【归经】 经外奇穴。

1.4.1.4　Acupoints on the Back

1.4.1.4.1　Dazhu (BL 11)

LOCATION　1.5 cun lateral to the lower border of the spinous process of the 1st thoracic vertebra.

（四）腰背部穴位

1. 大杼

【定位】　第 1 胸椎棘突下,旁开 1.5 寸。

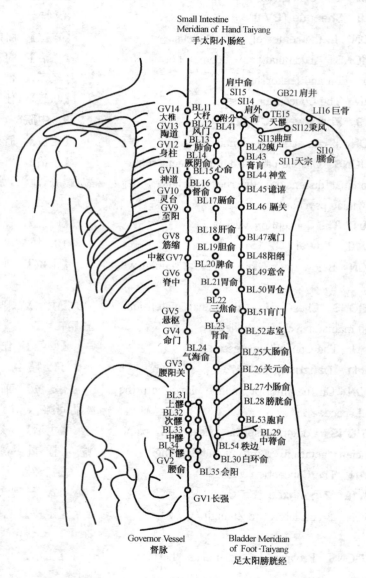

Fig. 17 - 4　Acupoints on the Shoulder, Back, Lumbus and Buttocks

图 17 - 4　肩背腰尻部穴位

INDICATIONS　Cough, fever, neck rigidity and pain in the shoulder and back.

MERIDIAN　The Bladder Meridian of Foot-*Taiyang*.

1.4.1.4.2　Fengmen (BL 12)

LOCATION　1.5 cun lateral to the lower border of the spinous process of the 2nd thoracic vertebra.

INDICATIONS　Common cold, cough, fever, headache, neck rigidity and pain in the chest and back.

MERIDIAN　The Bladder Meridian of Foot-*Taiyang*.

1.4.1.4.3　Feishu (BL 13)

LOCATION　1.5 cun lateral to the lower border of the spinous process of the 3rd thoracic vertebra.

INDICATIONS　Cough, asthma, hemoptysis, tidal fever, night sweating and nasal obstruction.

MERIDIAN　The Bladder Meridian of Foot-*Taiyang*.

1.4.1.4.4　Xinshu (BL 15)

LOCATION　1.5 cun lateral to the lower border of the spinous process of the 5th thoracic vertebra.

INDICATIONS　Cardiac pain, palpitation, haematemesis, insomnia, amnesia, night sweating, nocturnal emission and epilepsy.

MERIDIAN　The Bladder Meridian of Foot-*Taiyang*.

1.4.1.4.5　Ganshu (BL 17)

LOCATION　1.5 cun lateral to the lower border of the spinous process of the 9th thoracic vertebra.

INDICATIONS　Jaundice, pain in the hypochondriac region, hematemesis, conjunctival congestion, dizziness, night blindness, depressive and maniac psychosis, epilepsy and pain in the back along the spinal column.

MERIDIAN　The Bladder Meridian of Foot-*Taiyang*.

【主治】　咳嗽，发热，项强，肩背痛。

【归经】　足太阳膀胱经。

2. 风门

【定位】　第 2 胸椎棘突下，旁开 1.5 寸。

【主治】　伤风，咳嗽，发热头痛，项强，胸背痛。

【归经】　足太阳膀胱经。

3. 肺俞

【定位】　第 3 胸椎棘突下，旁开 1.5 寸。

【主治】　咳嗽，气喘，咯血，潮热，盗汗，鼻塞。

【归经】　足太阳膀胱经。

4. 心俞

【定位】　第 5 胸椎棘突下，旁开 1.5 寸。

【主治】　心痛，惊悸，吐血，失眠，健忘，盗汗，梦遗，癫痫。

【归经】　足太阳膀胱经。

5. 肝俞

【定位】　第 9 胸椎棘突下，旁开 1.5 寸。

【主治】　黄疸，胁痛，吐血，目赤，目眩，雀目，癫狂痫，脊背痛。

【归经】　足太阳膀胱经。

1.4.1.4.6 Danshu (BL 19)

LOCATION   1.5 cun lateral to the lower border of the spinous process of the 10th thoracic vertebra.

INDICATIONS   Jaundice, bitter taste in the mouth, pain in the hypochondriac region, pulmonary tuberculosis and tidal fever.

MERIDIAN   The Bladder Meridian of Foot-*Taiyang*.

1.4.1.4.7 Pishu (BL 20)

LOCATION   1.5 cun lateral to the lower border of the spinous process of the 11th thoracic vertebra.

INDICATIONS   Abdominal distension, jaundice, vomiting, diarrhea, dysentery, bloody stool, edema and pain in the back.

MERIDIAN   The Bladder Meridian of Foot-*Taiyang*.

1.4.1.4.8 Weishu (BL 21)

LOCATION   1.5 cun lateral to the lower border of the spinous process of the 12th thoracic vertebra.

INDICATIONS   Pain in the chest and hypochondriac region, epigastric pain, vomiting, abdominal distension and borborygmus.

MERIDIAN   The Bladder Meridian of Foot-*Taiyang*.

1.4.1.4.9 Sanjiaoshu (BL 22)

LOCATION   1.5 cun lateral to the lower border of the spinous process of the 1st lumbar vertebra.

INDICATIONS   Borborygmus, abdominal distension, vomiting, diarrhea, dysentery, edema and pain and stiffness in the back and loin.

MERIDIAN   The Bladder Meridian of Foot-*Taiyang*.

1.4.1.4.10 Shenshu (BL 23)

LOCATION   1.5 cun lateral to the lower border of

6. 胆俞

【定位】 第10 胸椎棘突下,旁开1.5寸。

【主治】 黄疸,口苦,肋痛,肺痨,潮热。

【归经】 足太阳膀胱经。

7. 脾俞

【定位】 第11 胸椎棘突下,旁开1.5寸。

【主治】 腹胀,黄疸,呕吐,泄泻,痢疾,便血,水肿,背痛。

【归经】 足太阳膀胱经。

8. 胃俞

【定位】 第12 胸椎棘突下,旁开1.5寸。

【主治】 胸胁痛,胃脘痛,呕吐,腹胀,肠鸣。

【归经】 足太阳膀胱经。

9. 三焦俞

【定位】 第1 腰椎棘突下,旁开1.5寸。

【主治】 肠鸣,腹胀,呕吐,泄泻,痢疾,水肿,腰背强痛。

【归经】 足太阳膀胱经。

10. 肾俞

【定位】 第2 腰椎棘突

the spinous process of the 2nd lumbar vertebra.

INDICATIONS Enuresis, seminal emission, impotence, irregular menstruation, leukorrhagia, edema, tinnitus, deafness and pain in the lower back.

MERIDIAN The Bladder Meridian of Foot-*Taiyang*.

1.4.1.4.11 Guanyuanshu (BL 26)

LOCATION 1.5 cun lateral to the lower border of the spinous process of the 5th lumbar vertebra.

INDICATIONS Abdominal distension, diarrhea, frequent urination or retention of urine, enuresis and pain in the lower back.

MERIDIAN The Bladder Meridian of Foot-*Taiyang*.

1.4.1.4.12 Pangguangshu (BL 28)

LOCATION 1.5 cun lateral to the lower border of the spinous process of the 2nd sacral vertebra.

INDICATIONS Retention of urine, enuresis, diarrhea, constipation, stiffness and pain in the lower back along the spinal column.

MERIDIAN The Bladder Meridian of Foot-*Taiyang*.

1.4.1.4.13 Shangliao (BL 31)

LOCATION In the 1st posterior sacral foramen.

INDICATIONS Dyschesia and dysuria, irregular menstruation, leukorrhagia, pain in the lower back, prolapse of the uterus, seminal emission and impotence.

MERIDIAN The Bladder Meridian of Foot-*Taiyang*.

1.4.1.4.14 Ciliao (BL 32)

LOCATION In the 2nd posterior sacral foramen.

INDICATIONS Hernia, irregular menstruation, dysmenorrhea, leukorrhagia, dysuria, seminal emission, pain in the lower back, numbness and flaccidity in the

下,旁开 1.5 寸。

【主治】 遗尿,遗精,阳痿,月经不调,白带,水肿,耳鸣,耳聋,腰痛。

【归经】 足太阳膀胱经。

11. 关元俞

【定位】 第 5 腰椎棘突下,旁开 1.5 寸。

【主治】 腹胀,泄泻,小便频数或不利,遗尿,腰痛。

【归经】 足太阳膀胱经。

12. 膀胱俞

【定位】 第 2 骶椎棘突下,旁开 1.5 寸。

【主治】 小便不利,遗尿,泄泻,便秘,腰脊强痛。

【归经】 足太阳膀胱经。

13. 上髎

【定位】 第1骶后孔中。

【主治】 大、小便不利,月经不调,带下,腰痛,阴挺,遗精,阳痿。

【归经】 足太阳膀胱经。

14. 次髎

【定位】 第2骶后孔中。

【主治】 疝气,月经不调,痛经,带下,小便不利,遗精,腰痛,下肢痿痹。

lower extremities.

MERIDIAN The Bladder Meridian of Foot-*Tai-yang*.

1.4.1.4.15 Zhongliao (BL 33)

LOCATION In the 3rd posterior sacral foramen.

INDICATIONS Constipation, diarrhea, dysuria, irregular menstruation, leukorrhagia and lumbago.

MERIDIAN The Bladder Meridian of Foot-*Taiy-ang*.

1.4.1.4.16 Xialiao (BL 34)

LOCATION In the 4th posterior sacral foramen.

INDICATIONS Abdominal pain, constipation, dysuria, leukorrhagia and lumbago.

MERIDIAN The Bladder Meridian of Foot-*Taiy-ang*.

1.4.1.4.17 Huangmen (BL 57)

LOCATION 3 cun lateral to the lower border of the spinous process of the 1st lumbar vertebra.

INDICATIONS Abdominal pain, constipation, abdominal mass and mammary disorders.

MERIDIAN The Bladder Meridian of Foot-*Taiyang*.

1.4.1.4.18 Changqiang (GV 1)

LOCATION 0.5 cun below the tip of the coccyx.

INDICATIONS Diarrhea, hematochezia, constipation, hemorrhoids and prolapse of the rectum.

MERIDIAN The Governor Vessel.

1.4.1.4.19 Yaoshu (GV 2)

LOCATION At the hiatus sacralis.

INDICATIONS Irregular menstruation, hemorrhoids, stiffness and pain in the lower back along the spinal column, flaccidity and arthralgia in the lower extremities and epilepsy.

MERIDIAN The Governor Vessel.

【归经】 足太阳膀胱经。

15. 中髎

【定位】 第3骶后孔中。

【主治】 便秘,泄泻,小便不利,月经不调,带下,腰痛。

【归经】 足太阳膀胱经。

16. 下髎

【定位】 第4骶后孔中。

【主治】 腹痛,便秘,小便不利,带下,腰痛。

【归经】 足太阳膀胱经。

17. 肓门

【定位】 第1腰椎棘突下,旁开3寸。

【主治】 腹痛,便秘,痞块,乳疾。

【归经】 足太阳膀胱经。

18. 长强

【定位】 尾骨尖下0.5寸。

【主治】 泄泻,便血,便秘,痔疾,脱肛。

【归经】 督脉。

19. 腰俞

【定位】 当骶管裂孔处。

【主治】 月经不调,痔疾,腰脊强痛,下肢痿痹,癫痫。

【归经】 督脉。

1.4.1.4.20   Yaoyangguan (GV 3)

LOCATION   Below the spinous process of the 4th lumbar vertebra.

INDICATIONS   Irregular menstruation, seminal emission, impotence, pain in the lumbosacral region, flaccidity and arthralgia in the lower extremities.

MERIDIAN   The Governor Vessel.

1.4.1.4.21   Mingmen (GV 4)

LOCATION   Below the spinous process of the 2nd lumbar vertebra.

INDICATIONS   Impotence, seminal emission, leukorrhagia, irregular menstruation, diarrhea and stiffness and pain in the lower back along the spinal column.

MERIDIAN   The Governor Vessel.

1.4.1.4.22   Dingchuan (EX-B 1)

LOCATION   0.5 cun lateral to Dazhui (GV 14).

INDICATIONS   Asthma and cough.

MERIDIAN   Extraordinary acupoints.

1.4.1.4.23   Jiaji (EX-B 2)

LOCATION   0.5 cun lateral to the lower border of each spinous process from the 1st thoracic vertebra to the 5th lumbar vertebra.

INDICATIONS   The Jiaji acupoints from the 1st to the 3rd thoracic vertebrae are indicated in disorders of the upper limbs; those from the 1st to the 8th thoracic vertebrae, in disorders of the chest; those from the 6th thoracic vertebra to the 5th lumbar one, in disorders of the abdomen; and those from the 1st lumbar vertebra to the 5th, in disorders of the lower limbs.

MERIDIAN   Extraordinary acupoints.

1.4.1.4.24   Yaoyan (EX-B 7)

LOCATION   In the depression 3-4 cun lateral to the

20. 腰阳关

【定位】 第4腰椎棘突下。

【主治】 月经不调,遗精,阳痿,腰骶痛,下肢痿痹。

【归经】 督脉。

21. 命门

【定位】 第2腰椎棘突下。

【主治】 阳痿,遗精,带下,月经不调,泄泻,腰脊强痛。

【归经】 督脉。

22. 定喘

【定位】 大椎穴旁开0.5寸。

【主治】 气喘,咳嗽。

【归经】 经外奇穴。

23. 夹脊

【定位】 第1胸椎至第5腰椎,各椎棘突下旁开0.5寸。

【主治】 第1胸椎至第3胸椎主治上肢疾患。
第1胸椎至第8胸椎主治胸部疾患。
第6胸椎至第5腰椎主治腹部疾患。
第1腰椎至第5腰椎主治下肢疾患。

【归经】 经外奇穴。

24. 腰眼

【定位】 第4腰椎棘突

lower border of the spinous process of the 4th lumbar vertebra.

INDICATIONS　Lumbago, irregular menstruation and leukorrhagia.

MERIDIAN　Extraordinary acupoints.

1.4.1.4.25　Shiqizhui (EX-B 8)

LOCATION　Below the spinous process of the 5th lumbar vertebra.

INDICATIONS　Pain in the lower back and extremities, paralysis of the lower extremities, metrorrhagia and metrostaxis, and irregular menstruation.

MERIDIAN　Extraordinary acupoints.

1.4.1.5　Acupoints on the Upper Extremities

1.4.1.5.1　Chize (LU 5)

LOCATION　On the transverse crease of the cubitus, near the radial border of the tendon of m. biceps brachii.

下,旁开 3～4 寸凹陷中。

【主治】　腰痛,月经不调,带下。

【归经】　经外奇穴。

25. 十七椎

【定位】　第 5 腰椎棘突下。

【主治】　腰腿痛,下肢痿痪,崩漏,月经不调。

【归经】　经外奇穴。

(五) 上肢部穴位

1. 尺泽

【定位】　肘横纹中,肱二头肌腱桡侧缘。

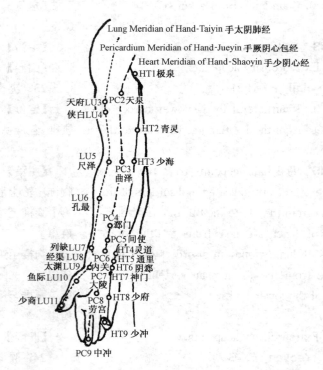

Fig. 17 - 5　Acupoints on the Medial Aspect of the Upper Limb
图 17 - 5　上肢内侧部穴位

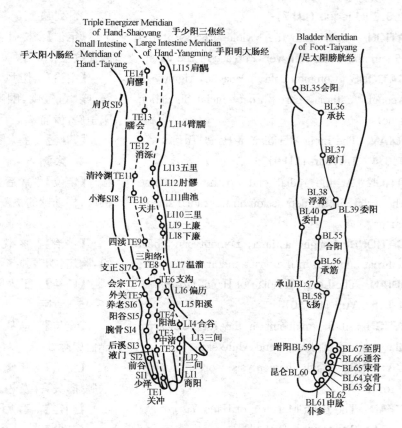

Fig. 17 - 6   Acupoints on the Lateral Aspect of the Upper Limb and the Posterior Aspect of Lower Limb

图 17 - 6   上肢外侧部和下肢后面部穴位

INDICATIONS Cough, asthma, hemoptysis, tidal fever, fullness in the chest, sore throat, infantile convulsion, vomiting, diarrhea, spasm and pain in the elbow and arm.

MERIDIAN The Lung Meridian of Hand-*Taiyin*.

1.4.1.5.2　Kongzui (LU 6)

LOCATION On the line joining Taiyuan (LU 9) and Chize (LU 5), 7 cun above the transverse crease of the wrist.

INDICATIONS Cough, asthma, hemoptysis, sore throat, spasm and pain in the elbow and arm, and hemorrhoids.

MERIDIAN The Lung Meridian of Hand-*Taiyin*.

【主治】 咳嗽,气喘,咳血,潮热,胸部胀满,咽喉肿痛,小儿惊风,吐泻,肘臂挛痛。

【归经】 手太阴肺经。

2. 孔最

【定位】 尺泽穴与太渊穴连线上,腕横纹上7寸处。

【主治】 咳嗽,气喘,咳血,咽喉肿痛,肘臂挛痛,痔疾。

【归经】 手太阴肺经。

1.4.1.5.3　Lieque（LU 7）

LOCATION　Superior to the styloid process of the radius, 1.5 cun above the transverse crease of the wrist.

INDICATIONS　Common cold, headache, rigidity of the neck, cough, asthma, sore throat, facial distortion and toothache.

MERIDIAN　The Lung Meridian of Hand-*Taiyin*.

1.4.1.5.4　Taiyuan（LU 9）

LOCATION　At the radial end of the transverse crease of the wrist, in the depression on the radial side of the radial artery.

INDICATIONS　Cough, asthma, hemoptysis, chest pain, sore throat and pain in the wrist and arm.

MERIDIAN　The Lung Meridian of Hand-*Taiyin*.

1.4.1.5.5　Yuji（LU 10）

LOCATION　At the midpoint of the 1st metacarpal bone, on the junction of the red and white skin.

INDICATIONS　Cough, hemoptysis, sore throat, aphonia and fever.

MERIDIAN　The Lung Meridian of Hand-*Taiyin*.

1.4.1.5.6　Shaoshang（LU 11）

LOCATION　On the radial side of the thumb, about 0.1 cun posterior to the corner of the nail.

INDICATIONS　Sore throat, cough, epistaxis, fever, coma, depressive and maniac psychosis.

MERIDIAN　The Lung Meridian of Hand-*Taiyin*.

1.4.1.5.7　Hegu（LI 4）

LOCATION　On the dorsum of the hand, between the 1st and 2nd metacarpal bones, level with the midpoint of the 2nd metacarpal bone on the radial side.

INDICATIONS　Headache, conjunctival congestion with swelling and pain, epistaxis, toothache, lockjaw, facial paralysis, deafness, sore throat, febrile diseases, anhidrosis or polyhidrosis, abdominal pain, constipation,

3. 列缺

【定位】　桡骨茎突上方，腕横纹上1.5寸。

【主治】　伤风，头痛，项强，咳嗽，气喘，咽喉肿痛，口眼歪斜，齿痛。

【归经】　手太阴肺经。

4. 太渊

【定位】　掌后腕横纹桡侧端，桡动脉的桡侧凹陷中。

【主治】　咳嗽，气喘，咳血，胸痛，咽喉肿痛，腕臂痛。

【归经】　手太阴肺经。

5. 鱼际

【定位】　第1掌骨中点，赤白肉际处。

【主治】　咳嗽，咳血，咽喉肿痛，失音，发热。

【归经】　手太阴肺经。

6. 少商

【定位】　拇指桡侧，指甲角旁约0.1寸。

【主治】　咽喉肿痛，咳嗽，鼻衄，发热，昏迷，癫狂。

【归经】　手太阴肺经。

7. 合谷

【定位】　手背第1、2掌骨之间，约平第2掌骨中点处。

【主治】　头痛，目赤肿痛，鼻衄，齿痛，牙关紧闭，口眼歪斜，耳聋，咽喉肿痛，热病，无汗，多汗，腹痛，便秘，经

amenorrhea and prolonged labor.

MERIDIAN The Large Intestine Meridian of Hand-*Yangming*.

1.4.1.5.8 Yangxi (LI 5)

LOCATION On the radial end of the dorsal transverse crease of the wrist, in the depression between the tendons of m. extensor pollisis longus and brevis.

INDICATIONS Headache, redness, swelling and pain of the eye, deafness, tinnitus, toothache, sore throat and pain in the wrist.

MERIDIAN The Large Intestine Meridian of Hand-*Yangming*.

1.4.1.5.9 Quchi (LI 11)

LOCATION At the midpoint of the line joining the lateral end of the transverse cubital crease and the lateral epicondyle of the humerus when the elbow is flexed to form a right angle.

INDICATIONS Sore throat, toothache, redness and pain of the eye, scrofula, urticaria, febrile disease, paralysis in the upper limb, swelling and pain in the hand and arm, abdominal pain, vomiting and diarrhea, hypertension, and maniac and depressive disorders.

MERIDIAN The Large Intestine Meridian of Hand-*Yangming*.

1.4.1.5.10 Binao (LI 14)

LOCATION On the line joining Quchi (LI 11) and Jianyu (LI 15), 7 cun above Quchi (LI 11) and at the lower end of m. deltoideus.

INDICATIONS Pain in the shoulder and arm, muscular contracture of the neck, scrofula and eye diseases.

MERIDIAN The Large Intestine Meridian of Hand-*Yangming*.

1.4.1.5.11 Jiquan (HT 1)

LOCATION In the centre of the axillary fossa, at

闭,滞产。

【归经】 手阳明大肠经。

8. 阳溪

【定位】 腕背横纹桡侧端,拇短伸肌腱与拇长伸肌腱之间的凹陷中。

【主治】 头痛,目赤肿痛,耳聋,耳鸣,齿痛,咽喉肿痛,手腕痛。

【归经】 手阳明大肠经。

9. 曲池

【定位】 屈肘,成直角,当肘横纹外端与肱骨外上髁连线的中点。

【主治】 咽喉肿痛,齿痛,目赤痛,瘰疬,瘾疹,热病,上肢不遂,手臂肿痛,腹痛吐泻,高血压,癫狂。

【归经】 手阳明大肠经。

10. 臂臑

【定位】 在曲池穴与肩髃穴连线上,曲池穴上七寸处,当三角肌下端。

【主治】 肩臂痛,颈项拘挛,瘰疬,目疾。

【归经】 手阳明大肠经。

11. 极泉

【定位】 腋窝正中,腋动

the pulsating site of the axillary artery.

INDICATIONS Pain in the cardiac region, dry throat with polydipsia, pain in the costal region, scrofula and pain in the shoulder and back.

MERIDIAN The Heart Meridian of Hand-*Shao-yin*.

1.4.1.5.12   Tongli (HT 5)

LOCATION 1 cun above the transverse crease of the wrist, on the radial side of the tendon of m. flexor carpi ulnaris.

INDICATIONS Palpitation, sudden loss of voice, aphasia due to stiffness of the tongue and pain in the wrist and forearm.

MERIDIAN The Heart Meridian of Hand-*Shaoyin*.

1.4.1.5.13   Shenmen (HT 7)

LOCATION At the ulnar end of the transverse crease of the wrist, in the depression on the radial side of the tendon of m. flexor carpi ulnaris.

INDICATIONS Angina pectoris, pavor, vexation, severe palpitation, amnesia, insomnia, depressive and maniac psychosis, and epilepsy, and pain in the chest and hypochondriac region.

MERIDIAN The Heart Meridian of Hand-*Shaoyin*.

1.4.1.5.14   Houxi (SI 3)

LOCATION On the ulnar side of the palm, proximal to the 5th metacarpophalangeal joint, at the end of the transverse crease and the junction of the red and white skin when a fist is made.

INDICATIONS Pain and rigidity in the head and nape, conjunctival congestion, deafness, sore throat, pain in the back and loin, depressive and maniac psychosis, epilepsy, and malaria.

MERIDIAN The Small Intestine Meridian of Hand-*Taiyang*.

脉搏动处。

【主治】 心痛，咽干烦渴，胁肋疼痛，瘰疬，肩背疼痛。

【归经】 手少阴心经。

12. 通里

【定位】 腕横纹上 1 寸，尺侧腕屈肌腱的桡侧。

【主治】 心悸，暴喑，舌强不语，腕臂痛。

【归经】 手少阴心经。

13. 神门

【定位】 腕横纹尺侧端，尺侧腕屈肌腱的桡侧凹陷中。

【主治】 心痛，惊悸，心烦，怔忡，健忘，失眠，癫狂痫，胸胁痛。

【归经】 手少阴心经。

14. 后溪

【定位】 握拳，第 5 掌指关节后尺侧，横纹头赤白肉际。

【主治】 头项强痛，目赤，耳聋，咽喉肿痛，腰背痛，癫狂痫，疟疾。

【归经】 手太阳小肠经。

1.4.1.5.15   Yanggu (SI 5)

LOCATION   At the ulnar end of the transverse crease on the dorsal aspect of the wrist, in the depression anterior to the styloid process of the ulna.

INDICATIONS   Headache, dizziness, tinnitus, deafness, febrile diseases, depressive and maniac psychosis, epilepsy and pain in the wrist.

MERIDIAN   The Small Intestine Meridian of Hand-*Taiyang*.

1.4.1.5.16   Yanglao (SI 6)

LOCATION   When the palm is facing the chest, the point is in the depression on the radial side of the styloid process of the ulna.

INDICATIONS   Blurred vision and aching pain in the shoulder, back, elbow and arm.

MERIDIAN   The Small Intestine Meridian of Hand-*Taiyang*.

1.4.1.5.17   Quze (PC 3)

LOCATION   In the transverse crease of the elbow, at the ulnar side of the tendon of m. biceps brachii.

INDICATIONS   Angina pectoris, palpitation, stomachache, vomiting, diarrhea, febrile diseases, contracture and pain in the elbow and arm.

MERIDIAN   The Pericardium Meridian of Hand-*Jueyin*.

1.4.1.5.18   Ximen (PC 4)

LOCATION   5 cun above the transverse crease of the wrist, between the tendons of m. palmaris longus and m. flexor carpi radialis.

INDICATIONS   Cardiac pain, palpitation, stomachache, hematemesis, haemoptysis, rooted furuncle and epilepsy.

MERIDIAN   The Pericardium Meridian of Hand-*Jueyin*.

---

15. 阳谷

【定位】 腕背横纹尺侧端,尺骨茎突前凹陷中。

【主治】 头痛,目眩,耳鸣,耳聋,热病,癫狂痫,腕痛。

【归经】 手太阳小肠经。

16. 养老

【定位】 以掌心向胸,当尺骨茎突桡侧缘凹陷中。

【主治】 目视不明,肩背肘臂酸痛。

【归经】 手太阳小肠经。

17. 曲泽

【定位】 肘横纹中,肱二头肌腱尺侧。

【主治】 心痛,心悸,胃痛,呕吐,泄泻,热病,肘臂挛痛。

【归经】 手厥阴心包经。

18. 郄门

【定位】 腕横纹上 5 寸,掌长肌腱与桡侧腕屈肌腱之间。

【主治】 心痛,心悸,胃痛,呕血,咳血,疔疮,癫痫。

【归经】 手厥阴心包经。

1.4.1.5.19　Jianshi（PC 5）

LOCATION　3 cun above the transverse crease of the wrist, between the tendons of m. palmaris longus and m. flexor carpi radialis.

INDICATIONS　Cardiac pain, palpitation, stomachache, vomiting, febrile diseases, malaria, depressive and maniac psychosis, and epilepsy.

MERIDIAN　The Pericardium Meridian of Hand-*Jueyin*.

1.4.1.5.20　Neiguan（PC 6）

LOCATION　2 cun above the transverse crease of the wrist, between the tendons of m. palmaris longus and m. flexor carpiradialis.

INDICATIONS　Angina pectoris, palpitation, stuffiness in the chest, stomachache, vomiting, epilepsy, febrile diseases, arthralgia and pain in the upper extremities, hemiplegia, insomnia, vertigo and migraine.

MERIDIAN　The Pericardium Meridian of Hand-*Jueyin*.

1.4.1.5.21　Daling（PC 7）

LOCATION　At the midpoint of the transverse crease of the wrist, between the tendons of m. palmaris longus and m. flexor carpi radialis.

INDICATIONS　Angina pectoris, palpitation, stomachache, vomiting, depressive and maniac psychosis, pyocutaneous disease and pain in the chest and hypochondriac region.

MERIDIAN　The Pericardium Meridian of Hand-*Jueyin*.

1.4.1.5.22　Laogong（PC 8）

LOCATION　Between the 2nd and 3rd metacarpal bones, just under the tip of the middle finger when a fist is clenched.

INDICATIONS　Angina pectoris, vomiting, depressive

19. 间使

【定位】　腕横纹上 3 寸，掌长肌腱与桡侧腕屈肌腱之间。

【主治】　心痛，心悸，胃痛，呕吐，热病，疟疾，癫狂痫。

【归经】　手厥阴心包经。

20. 内关

【定位】　腕横纹上 2 寸，掌长肌腱与桡侧腕屈肌腱之间。

【主治】　心痛，心悸，胸闷，胃痛，呕吐，癫痫，热病，上肢痹痛，偏瘫，失眠，眩晕，偏头痛。

【归经】　手厥阴心包经。

21. 大陵

【定位】　腕横纹中央，掌长肌腱与桡侧腕屈肌腱之间。

【主治】　心痛，心悸，胃痛，呕吐，癫狂，疮疡，胸胁痛。

【归经】　手厥阴心包经。

22. 劳宫

【定位】　第 2、3 掌骨之间，握拳，中指尖下是穴。

【主治】　心痛，呕吐，癫

and maniac psychosis, epilepsy, aphthae and foul breath.

MERIDIAN The Pericardium Meridian of Hand-*Jueyin*.

1.4.1.5.23 Zhongchong (PC 9)

LOCATION In the center of the tip of the middle finger.

INDICATIONS Angina pectoris, coma, stiffness of the tongue with swelling and pain, febrile diseases, infantile night crying, sunstroke and syncope.

MERIDIAN The Pericardium Meridian of Hand-*Jueyin*.

1.4.1.5.24 Zhongzhu (TE 3)

LOCATION In the depression between the posterior borders of the small ends of the 4th and 5th metacarpal bones when a fist is clenched.

INDICATIONS Headache, conjunctival congestion, tinnitus, deafness, sore throat, febrile diseases and difficulty in flexing and extending fingers.

MERIDIAN The Triple Energizer Meridian of Hand-*Shaoyang*.

1.4.1.5.25 Yangchi (TE 4)

LOCATION On the transverse crease of the dorsum of the wrist, in the depression on the ulnar side of the tendon of m. extensor digitorum communis.

INDICATIONS Conjunctival congestion with swelling and pain, deafness, sore throat, malaria, pain in the wrist, and diabetes.

MERIDIAN The Triple Energizer Meridian of Hand-*Shaoyang*.

1.4.1.5.26 Waiguan (TE 5)

LOCATION 2 cun above the transverse crease of the dorsum of the wrist, between the radius and ulna.

INDICATIONS Tinnitus, deafness, sudden aphonia, scrofula, pain in the hypochondriac region, numbness and pain in the upper extremities.

狂痫,口疮,口臭。

【归经】 手厥阴心包经。

23. 中冲

【定位】 中指尖端的中央。

【主治】 心痛,昏迷,舌强肿痛,热病,小儿夜啼,中暑,昏厥。

【归经】 手厥阴心包经。

24. 中渚

【定位】 握拳,第 4、5 掌骨小头后缘之间凹陷中。

【主治】 头痛,目赤,耳鸣,耳聋,咽喉肿痛,热病,手指不能屈伸。

【归经】 手少阳三焦经。

25. 阳池

【定位】 腕背纹中,指总伸肌腱尺侧缘凹陷中。

【主治】 目赤肿痛,耳聋,咽喉肿痛,疟疾,腕痛,消渴。

【归经】 手少阳三焦经。

26. 外关

【定位】 腕背横纹上 2寸,桡骨与尺骨之间。

【主治】 耳鸣,耳聋,暴喑,瘰疬,胁肋痛,上肢痹痛。

MERIDIAN The Triple Energizer Meridian of Hand-*Shaoyang*.

1.4.1.5.27　Zhigou (TE 6)

LOCATION 3 cun above the transverse crease of the dorsum of the wrist, between the radius and ulna.

INDICATIONS Tinnitus, deafness, sudden aphonia, scrofula, pain in the hypochondriac region, constipation and febrile diseases.

MERIDIAN The Triple Energizer Meridian of Hand-*Shaoyang*.

1.4.1.5.28　Laozhenxue (EX-UE 26)

LOCATION On the dorsum of the hand, between the 1st and 2nd metacarpal bones and about 0.5 cun posterior to the metacarpophalangeal joint.

INDICATIONS Stiffness in the neck, pain in the hand and arm, and stomachache.

MERIDIAN Extraordinary acupoints.

1.4.1.5.29　Yaotongxue (EX-UE 7)

LOCATION On both sides of the tendon of m. extensor digitorum communis of the dorsum of the hand and 1 cun below the transverse crease of the wrist. Two acupoints on each hand.

INDICATION Acute lumbar sprain.

MERIDIAN Extraordinary acupoints.

1.4.1.6　Acupoints on the Lower Extremities

1.4.1.6.1　Biguan (ST 31)

LOCATION On the line joining the anterior superior iliac spine and lateral border of the basis patella, level with the gluteal groove.

INDICATIONS Lumbago, cold sensation in the knee, Wei-syndrome, Bi-syndrome, and abdominal pain.

MERIDIAN The Stomach Meridian of Foot-*Yangming*.

【归经】　手少阳三焦经。

27. 支沟

【定位】　腕背横纹上 3 寸,桡骨与尺骨之间。

【主治】　耳鸣,耳聋,暴喑,瘰疬,胁肋痛,便秘,热病。

【归经】　手少阳三焦经。

28. 落枕穴

【定位】　手背,第 2、3 掌骨间,指掌关节后约 0.5 寸。

【主治】　落枕,手臂痛,胃痛。

【归经】　经外奇穴。

29. 腰痛穴

【定位】　手背,指总伸肌腱的两侧,腕横纹下 1 寸处,一手 2 穴。

【主治】　急性腰扭伤。

【归经】　经外奇穴。

(六) 下肢部穴位

1. 髀关

【定位】　髂前上棘与髌骨外缘连线上,平臀下横纹处。

【主治】　腰痛膝冷,痿痹,腹痛。

【归经】　足阳明胃经。

1.4.1.6.2 Futu (ST 32)

LOCATION On the line joining the anterior superior iliac spine and the lateral border of the patella, 6 cun above the laterosuperior border of the patella.

INDICATIONS Lumbago, cold sensation in the knee, Wei-syndrome, Bi-syndrome, and abdominal pain.

MERIDIAN The Stomach Meridian of Foot-*Yangming*.

1.4.1.6.3 Liangqiu (ST 34)

LOCATION On the line joining the anterior superior iliac spine and lateral border of the patella, 2 cun above the laterosuperior border of the patella.

2. 伏兔

【定位】 在髂前上棘与髌骨外缘连线上,髌骨外上缘上6寸。

【主治】 腰痛膝冷,痿痹,腹痛。

【归经】 足阳明胃经。

3. 梁丘

【定位】 在髂前上棘与髌骨外缘连线上,髌骨外上缘上2寸。

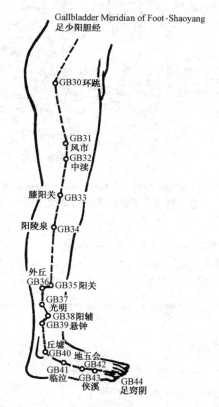

Fig. 17－7 Acupoints on the Lateral Aspect of the Lower Limb

图 17－7 下肢外侧部穴位

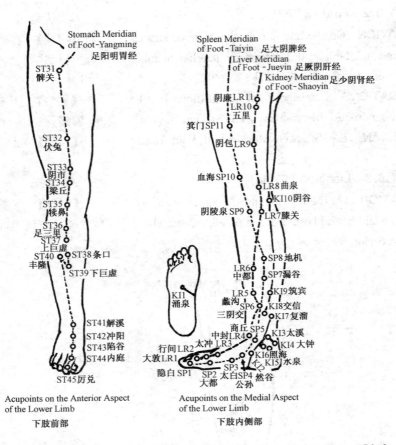

Fig. 17 - 8   Acupoints on the Anterior and Medical Aspect of the Lower Limb

图 17 - 8   下肢前面及内侧面穴位

INDICATIONS   Pain and swelling in the knee, motor impairment of the lower extremities, gastric pain, mastitis and hematuria.

MERIDIAN   The Stomach Meridian of Foot-*Yangming*.

1.4.1.6.4   Dubi（ST 35）

LOCATION   At the lateral border of the patella and in the depression lateral to the patellar ligament.

INDICATIONS   Pain in the knee, paralysis of the lower limb with difficulty in flexion and extension, and

【主治】 膝肿痛,下肢不遂,胃痛,乳痈,血尿。

【归经】 足阳明胃经。

4. 犊鼻

【定位】 髌骨外缘,髌韧带外侧凹陷中。

【主治】 膝痛,下肢麻痹,屈伸不利,脚气。

beriberi.

MERIDIAN   The Stomach Meridian of Foot-*Yang-ming*.

1.4.1.6.5   Zusanli (ST 36)

LOCATION   3 cun below Dubi (ST 35), one finger-breadth away from the anterior crest of the tibia.

INDICATIONS   Gastric pain, vomiting, dysphagia, abdominal distension, diarrhea, dysentery, constipation, mastitis, acute appendicitis, numbness and pain in the lower extremities, edema, depressive and maniac psychosis, beriberi and emaciation due to asthenic consumption.

MERIDIAN   The Stomach Meridian of Foot-*Yang-ming*.

1.4.1.6.6   Shangjuxu (ST 37)

LOCATION   3 cun below Zusanli (ST 36).

INDICATIONS   Borborygmus, abdominal pain, diarrhea, constipation, acute appendicitis, Wei-syndrome and Bi-syndrome in the lower extremities, and beriberi.

MERIDIAN   The Stomach Meridian of Foot-*Yang-ming*.

1.4.1.6.7   Xiajuxu (ST 39)

LOCATION   3 cun below Shangjuxu (ST 37).

INDICATIONS   Pain in the lower abdomen, diarrhea, dysentery, mastitis, Wei-syndrome and Bi-syndrome of the lower extremities, and lower back pain involving the testicle.

MERIDIAN   The Stomach Meridian of Foot-*Yang-ming*.

1.4.1.6.8   Fenglong (ST 40)

LOCATION   8 cun superior to the external malleolus, 1 cun lateral to Tiaokou (ST 38).

INDICATIONS   Headache, vertigo, cough with

【归经】 足阳明胃经。

5. 足三里

【定位】 犊鼻穴下 3 寸，胫骨前嵴外 1 横指处。

【主治】 胃痛，呕吐，噎膈，腹胀，泄泻，痢疾，便秘，乳痈，肠痈，下肢痹痛，水肿，癫狂，脚气，虚劳羸弱。

【归经】 足阳明胃经。

6. 上巨虚

【定位】 足三里穴下 3 寸。

【主治】 肠鸣，腹痛，泄泻，便秘，肠痈，下肢痿痹，脚气。

【归经】 足阳明胃经。

7. 下巨虚

【定位】 上巨虚穴下 3 寸。

【主治】 小腹痛，泄泻，痢疾，乳痈，下肢痿痹，腰脊痛引睾丸。

【归经】 足阳明胃经。

8. 丰隆

【定位】 外踝高点上 8 寸，条口穴外 1 寸。

【主治】 头痛，眩晕，痰

excessive sputum, vomiting, constipation, edema, depressive and maniac psychosis, epilepsy, Wei-syndrome and Bi-syndrome in the lower extremities.

MERIDIAN The Stomach Meridian of Foot-*Yangming*.

1.4.1.6.9　Jiexi (ST 41)

LOCATION On the dorsum of the foot, at the midpoint of the transverse crease of the ankle joint, in the depression between the tendons of m. extensor hallucis longus and digitorum longus.

INDICATIONS Headache, vertigo, depressive and maniac psychosis, abdominal distension, constipation, Wei-syndrome and Bi-syndrome in the lower extremities.

MERIDIAN The Stomach Meridian of Foot-*Yangming*.

1.4.1.6.10　Neiting (ST 44)

LOCATION On the dorsum of the foot, at the end of the web striation between the 2nd and 3rd toes.

INDICATIONS Toothache, sore throat, distorted mouth, gastric pain, abdominal distension, constipation and diarrhea.

MERIDIAN The Stomach Meridian of Foot-*Yangming*.

1.4.1.6.11　Gongsun (SP 4)

LOCATION At the border anterior and inferior to the base of the 1st metatarsal bone, at the junction of the red and white skin.

INDICATIONS Stomachache, vomiting, abdominal pain, diarrhea and dysentery.

MERIDIAN The Spleen Meridian of Foot-*Taiyin*.

1.4.1.6.12　Shangqiu (SP 5)

LOCATION In the depression anterior and inferior to the medial malleolus.

INDICATIONS Abdominal distension, diarrhea,

多咳嗽,呕吐,便秘,水肿,癫狂痫,下肢痿痹。

【归经】　足阳明胃经。

9. 解溪

【定位】　足背踝关节横纹的中央,踇长伸肌腱与指长伸肌腱之间。

【主治】　头痛,眩晕,癫狂,腹胀,便秘,下肢痿痹。

【归经】　足阳明胃经。

10. 内庭

【定位】　足背第 2、3 趾间缝纹端。

【主治】　齿痛,咽喉肿痛,口歪,胃痛,腹胀,便秘,腹泻。

【归经】　足阳明胃经。

11. 公孙

【定位】　第1跖骨基底部的前下缘,赤白肉际。

【主治】　胃痛,呕吐,腹痛,泄泻,痢疾。

【归经】　足太阴脾经。

12. 商丘

【定位】　内踝前下方凹陷中。

【主治】　腹胀,泄泻,便

constipation, jaundice and pain in the ankle.

MERIDIAN The Spleen Meridian of Foot-*Taiyin*.

1.4.1.6.13 Sanyinjiao (SP 6)

LOCATION 3 cun directly above the tip of the medial malleolus, on the posterior border of the medial aspect of the tibia.

INDICATIONS Borborygmus, abdominal distension, diarrhea, irregular menstruation, leukorrhagia, prolapse of the uterus, sterility, prolonged labor, seminal emission, impotence, enuresis, hernia, insomnia, Wei-syndrome and Bi-syndrome in the lower extremities and beriberi.

MERIDIAN The Spleen Meridian of Foot-*Taiyin*.

1.4.1.6.14 Diji (SP 8)

LOCATION 3 cun below Yinlingquan (SP 9).

INDICATIONS Abdominal pain, dysuria, diarrhea, edema, irregular menstruation, dysmenorrhea and seminal emission.

MERIDIAN The Spleen Meridian of Foot-*Taiyin*.

1.4.1.6.15 Yinlingquan (SP 9)

LOCATION In the depression of the lower border of the medial condyle of the tibia.

INDICATIONS Abdominal distension, diarrhea, edema, jaundice, dysuria or incontinence of urination and pain in the knee.

MERIDIAN The Spleen Meridian of Foot-*Taiyin*.

1.4.1.6.16 Xuehai (SP 10)

LOCATION 2 cun above the medial and superior border of the patella.

INDICATIONS Irregular menstruation, metrorrhagia and metrostaxis, amenorrhea, urticaria, eczema and erysipelas.

MERIDIAN The Spleen Meridian of Foot-*Taiyin*.

秘,黄疸,足踝痛。

【归经】 足太阴脾经。

13. 三阴交

【定位】 内踝高点上 3 寸,胫骨内侧面后缘。

【主治】 肠鸣腹胀,泄泻,月经不调,带下,阴挺,不孕,滞产,遗精,阳痿,遗尿,疝气,失眠,下肢痿痹,脚气。

【归经】 足太阴脾经。

14. 地机

【定位】 阴陵泉穴下 3寸。

【主治】 腹痛,小便不利,泄泻,水肿,月经不调,痛经,遗精。

【归经】 足太阴脾经。

15. 阴陵泉

【定位】 胫骨内侧髁下缘凹陷中。

【主治】 腹胀,泄泻,水肿,黄疸,小便不利或失禁,膝痛。

【归经】 足太阴脾经。

16. 血海

【定位】 髌骨内上缘上 2寸。

【主治】 月经不调,崩漏,经闭,瘾疹,湿疹,丹毒。

【归经】 足太阴脾经。

1.4.1.6.17 Chengfu (BL 36)

LOCATION At the midpoint of the transverse gluteal fold.

INDICATIONS Pain in the lower back, sacral, gluteal and femoral regions and hemorrhoids.

MERIDIAN The Bladder Meridian of Foot-*Taiyang*.

1.4.1.6.18 Yinmen (BL 37)

LOCATION 6 cun below Chengfu (BL 36), on the line joining Chengfu (BL 36) and Weizhong (BL 40).

INDICATIONS Lumbago, Wei-syndrome and Bi-syndrome in the lower extremities.

MERIDIAN The Bladder Meridian of Foot-*Taiyang*.

1.4.1.6.19 Weiyang (BL 39)

LOCATION At the lateral end of the popliteal transverse crease, on the medial border of the tendon of m. biceps femoris.

INDICATIONS Abdominal fullness, dysuria, pain and stiffness in the lower back along the spinal column, spasm and pain in the leg and foot.

MERIDIAN The Bladder Meridian of Foot-*Taiyang*.

1.4.1.6.20 Weizhong (BL 40)

LOCATION At the midpoint of the popliteal transverse crease.

INDICATIONS Lumbago, Wei-syndrome and Bi-syndrome in the lower extremities, abdominal pain, vomiting and diarrhea, dysuria, enuresis and erysipelas.

MERIDIAN The Bladder Meridian of Foot-*Taiyang*.

1.4.1.6.21 Chengshan (BL 57)

LOCATION At the top of the fossa of the belly between the two gastrocnemius muscles.

17. 承扶

【定位】 臀横纹中央。

【主治】 腰骶臀部疼痛，痔疾。

【归经】 足太阳膀胱经。

18. 殷门

【定位】 承扶穴与委中穴连线上，承扶穴下 6 寸。

【主治】 腰痛，下肢痿痹。

【归经】 足太阳膀胱经。

19. 委阳

【定位】 腘横纹外端，股二头肌腱内缘。

【主治】 腹满，小便不利，腰脊强痛，腿足挛痛。

【归经】 足太阳膀胱经。

20. 委中

【定位】 腘横纹中央。

【主治】 腰痛，下肢痿痹，腹痛，吐泻，小便不利，遗尿，丹毒。

【归经】 足太阳膀胱经。

21. 承山

【定位】 腓肠肌两肌腹之间凹陷的顶端。

INDICATIONS Hemorrhoids, beriberi, constipation, contracture and pain in the lower back and leg.

MERIDIAN The Bladder Meridian of Foot-*Taiyang*.

1.4.1.6.22 Kunlun (BL 60)

LOCATION In the depression between the tip of the external malleolus and tendo calcaneus.

INDICATIONS Headache, neck rigidity, dizziness, epistaxis, epilepsy, dystocia, pain in the lumbosacral region, pain and swelling in the heel.

MERIDIAN The Bladder Meridian of Foot-*Taiyang*.

1.4.1.6.23 Zhiyin (BL 67)

LOCATION On the lateral side of the small toe, about 0.1 cun lateral to the corner of the nail.

INDICATIONS Headache, pain in the eye, nasal obstruction, epistaxis, malposition of fetus and dystocia.

MERIDIAN The Bladder Meridian of Foot-*Taiyang*.

1.4.1.6.24 Yongquan (KI 1)

LOCATION At the anterior 1/3 of the sole (the length of the toe is not included), in the depression appearing on the sole when the foot is in plantar flexion.

INDICATIONS Headache, dizziness, insomnia, giddiness, sore throat, aphonia, constipation, dysuria, infantile convulsion, depressive and maniac psychosis and syncope.

MERIDIAN The Kidney Meridian of Foot-*Shaoyin*.

1.4.1.6.25 Taixi (KI 3)

LOCATION In the depression between the tip of the medial malleolus and the tendo calcaneous.

INDICATIONS Irregular menstruation, seminal emission, impotence, frequent micturition, constipation,

【主治】 痔疾,脚气,便秘,腰腿拘急疼痛。

【归经】 足太阳膀胱经。

22. 昆仑

【定位】 外踝高点与跟腱之间凹陷中。

【主治】 头痛,项强,目眩,鼻衄,癫痫,难产,腰骶疼痛,脚跟肿痛。

【归经】 足太阳膀胱经。

23. 至阴

【定位】 足小趾外侧趾甲角旁约0.1寸。

【主治】 头痛,目痛,鼻塞,鼻衄,胎位不正,难产。

【归经】 足太阳膀胱经。

24. 涌泉

【定位】 于足底(去趾)前1/3处,足趾跖屈时呈凹陷。

【主治】 头痛,头昏,失眠,目眩,咽喉肿痛,失音,便秘,小便不利,小儿惊风,癫狂,昏厥。

【归经】 足少阴肾经。

25. 太溪

【定位】 内踝高点与跟腱之间凹陷中。

【主治】 月经不调,遗精,阳痿,小便频数,便秘,消

diabetes, hemoptysis, asthma, sore throat, toothache, insomnia, lumbago, deafness and tinnitus.

MERIDIAN The Kidney Meridian of Foot-*Shaoyin*.

1.4.1.6.26　Zhaohai (KI 6)

LOCATION In the depression at the lower border of the medial malleolus.

INDICATIONS Irregular menstruation, leukorrhagia, prolapse of the uterus, frequent micturition, retention of urine, dry sore throat, epilepsy and insomnia.

MERIDIAN The Kidney Meridian of Foot-*Shaoyin*.

1.4.1.6.27　Fengshi (GB 31)

LOCATION On the midline of the lateral aspect of the thigh, 7 cun above the transverse popliteal crease.

INDICATIONS Wei-syndrome and Bi-syndrome in the lower extremities, general pruritus and beriberi.

MERIDIAN The Gallbladder Meridian of Foot-*Shaoyang*.

1.4.1.6.28　Xiyangguan (GB 33)

LOCATION 3 cun above Yanglingquan (GB 34), in the depression superior to the external epicondyle of the femur.

INDICATIONS Swelling, pain and contracture in the knee joint and numbness in the shank.

MERIDIAN The Gallbladder Meridian of Foot-*Shaoyang*.

1.4.1.6.29　Yanglingquan (GB 34)

LOCATION In the depression anterior and inferior to the small head of the fibula.

INDICATIONS Hypochondriac pain, bitter taste in the mouth, vomiting, Wei-syndrome and Bi-syndrome in the lower extremities, beriberi, jaundice and infantile convulsion.

MERIDIAN The Gallbladder Meridian of Foot-

渴,咳血,气喘,咽喉肿痛,齿痛,失眠,腰痛,耳聋,耳鸣。

【归经】　足少阴肾经。

26. 照海

【定位】　内踝下缘凹陷中。

【主治】　月经不调,带下,阴挺,小便频数,癃闭,咽喉干痛,癫痫,失眠。

【归经】　足少阴肾经。

27. 风市

【定位】　大腿外侧正中,腘横纹水平线上7寸。

【主治】　下肢痿痹,遍身瘙痒,脚气。

【归经】　足少阳胆经。

28. 膝阳关

【定位】　阳陵泉穴上3寸,股骨外上髁上方的凹陷中。

【主治】　膝关节肿痛挛急,小腿麻木。

【归经】　足少阳胆经。

29. 阳陵泉

【定位】　腓骨小头前下方凹陷中。

【主治】　胁痛,口苦,呕吐,下肢痿痹,脚气,黄疸,小儿惊风。

【归经】　足少阳胆经。

Shaoyang.

1.4.1.6.30   Xuanzhong (Juegu, GB 39)

LOCATION   3 cun above the tip of the external malleolus, at the posterior border of the fibula.

INDICATIONS   Stiffness in the nape, distending pain in the chest and hypochondrium, Wei-symdrome and Bi-symdrome in the lower extremities, soreness and swelling in the throat, beriberi and hemorrhoids.

MERIDIAN   The Gallbladder Meridian of Foot-*Shaoyang*.

1.4.1.6.31   Qiuxu (GB 40)

LOCATION   Anterior and inferior to the external malleolus, in the depression on the lateral side of the tendon of m. extensor digitorum longus.

INDICATIONS   Distending pain in the chest and hypochondrium, Wei-syndrome and Bi-syndrome in the lower extremities and malaria.

MERIDIAN   The Gallbladder Meridian of Foot-*Shaoyang*.

1.4.1.6.32   Dadun (LR 1)

LOCATION   On the lateral aspect of the dorsum of the great toe, about 0.1 cun lateral to the corner of the nail.

INDICATIONS   Hernia, enuresis, amenorrhea, metrorrhagia and metrostaxis, prolapse of the uterus and epilepsy.

MERIDIAN   The Liver Meridian of Foot-*Jueyin*.

1.4.1.6.33   Xingjian (LR 2)

LOCATION   On the dorsum of the foot, at the end of the web striation between the 1st and 2nd toes.

INDICATIONS   Headache, dizziness, conjunctival congestion with swelling and pain, glaucoma, pain in the hypochondriac region, hernia, dysuria, metrorrhagia and metrostaxis, irregular menstruation, dysmenorrhea, leu-

30. 悬钟(绝骨)

【定位】 外踝高点上 3 寸,腓骨后缘。

【主治】 项强,胸胁胀痛,下肢痿痹,咽喉肿痛,脚气,痔疾。

【归经】 足少阳胆经。

31. 丘墟

【定位】 外踝前下方,趾长伸肌腱外侧凹陷中。

【主治】 胸胁胀痛,下肢痿痹,疟疾。

【归经】 足少阳胆经。

32. 大敦

【定位】 姆趾外侧趾甲角旁约0.1寸。

【主治】 疝气,遗尿,经闭,崩漏,阴挺,癫痫。

【归经】 足厥阴肝经。

33. 行间

【定位】 足背,第 1、2 趾间缝纹端。

【主治】 头痛,目眩,目赤肿痛,青盲,胁痛,疝气,小便不利,崩漏,月经不调,痛经,带下,中风。

korrhagia and apoplexy.

MERIDIAN The Liver Meridian of Foot-*Jueyin*.

1.4.1.6.34　Taichong (LR 3)

LOCATION On the dorsum of the foot, in the depression at the articulation of the 1st and 2nd metatarsals.

INDICATIONS Headache, vertigo, conjunctival congestion with swelling and pain, pain in the hypochondriac region, enuresis, hernia, metrorrhagia and metrostaxis, irregular menstruation, epilepsy, vomiting, infantile convulsion, Wei-syndrome and Bi-syndrome in the lower limbs.

MERIDIAN The Liver Meridian of Foot-*Jueyin*.

1.4.1.6.35　Baichongwo (EX-LE 3)

LOCATION 1 cun above Xuehai (SP 10)

INDICATIONS Itching and pain due to wind and dampness, and sore in the vulva.

MERIDIAN Extraordinary acupoints.

1.4.1.6.36　Dannangxue (EX-LE 6)

LOCATION 1 to 2 cun below Yanglingquan (GB 34)

INDICATIONS Acute or chronic cholecystitis, cholelithiasis, biliary ascariasis, Wei-syndrome and Bi-syndrome in the lower extremities.

MERIDIAN Extraordinary acupoints.

1.4.1.6.37　Lanweixue (EX-LE 7)

LOCATION About 2 cun below Zusanli (ST 36).

INDICATIONS Acute or chronic appendicitis, indigestion, paralysis in the lower extremities.

MERIDIAN Extraordinary acupoints.

All the above acupoints are shown in Fig. 17.

1.4.2　Acupoints for Infantile Tuina

In infantile Tuina treatment, besides reference to or

【归经】　足厥阴肝经。

34. 太冲

【定位】　足背,第1、2跖骨结合部之间凹陷中。

【主治】　头痛,眩晕,目赤肿痛,胁痛,遗尿,疝气,崩漏,月经不调,癫痫,呕逆,小儿惊风,下肢痿痹。

【归经】　足厥阴肝经。

35. 百虫窝

【定位】　血海穴上1寸。

【主治】　风湿痒痛,下部生疮。

【归经】　经外奇穴。

36. 胆囊穴

【定位】　阳陵泉穴下1~2寸处。

【主治】　急、慢性胆囊炎,胆石症,胆道蛔虫症,下肢痿痹。

【归经】　经外奇穴。

37. 阑尾穴

【定位】　足三里穴下约2寸处。

【主治】　急、慢性阑尾炎,消化不良,下肢瘫痪。

【归经】　经外奇穴。

（以上穴位均见图17）

二、小儿穴位

小儿推拿穴位,除在治疗

employment of some adult meridian acupoints and extra-ordinary acupoints there are some specific acupoints for infantile tuina, which are gradually developed and summed up according to the physiological and pathological charac-teristics of infants. Although they are not on the routes of the regular meridians, these acupoints are mostly distrib-uted under elbow and knee joints of the limbs, where the meridian qi is comparatively active and abundant, espe-cially on the palm and dorsum of the hands. As an old say-ing goes: "All the meridians and collaterals in children converge in the hands." The specific acupoints are very sensitive to stimuli from tuina manipulations and other outside factors, liable to accept and transmit the thera-peutic stimuli to related viscera, so can produce preven-tive and curative effect on diseases. The forms of acu-points used for infantile tuina have developed from point form to linear form and regional form. Infantile tuina acu-points are mostly named after zang and fu organs such as points Xinjing, Dachang and Pangguang and parts of the human body such as Wuzhijie, Fu and Ji. They are also given names after the theory of five elements such as spleen-earth and liver-wood, function of acupoints such as Duanzheng and Jingning. Rivers and mountains such as Shangen, Hongchi, buildings such as Tianting, Sanguan, animals' names such as Laolong, Guiwei, and some philo-sophical words such as Yinyang, Bagua, are used as names of infantile tuina acupoints, too. Because acupoints are continuously being discovered and new names are given to some operated portions with compound manipulations, up to now there have been as many as two hundred acu-points, which greatly enrich clinical practice of infantile tuina. Here is an introduction to the most commonly used specific acupoints for infantile tuina.

中,可参考运用成人的经穴和奇穴外,尚有根据小儿生理、病理特点逐渐形成和归纳出的一些特定穴位,这些穴位虽多不在经脉的循行线上,但亦多分布在经气相对活跃的四肢肘膝关节以下,尤其是古人所说的"小儿百脉汇于两掌"的手掌与手背部位。这些特定穴位对于手法等外界刺激的感觉比较敏感,故易于接收并传递这些治疗信息至体内有关脏腑,从而发挥治病和防病的作用。小儿推拿特定穴位的形态,从经穴的点状进而发展形成线状和面状,多根据脏腑名称(如心经、大肠、膀胱等),人体部位(如五指节、腹、脊等),五行学说(如脾土、肝木等),作用功能(如端正、精宁等),山川河流(如山根、洪池等),还有建筑物体(如天庭、三关等),动物名称(如老龙、龟尾等),哲学名词(如阴阳、八卦等)来命名的,这些穴位的不断发现和因复式手法操作的部位而定名的,迄今为止已达 200 个之多,现将最常用的部分小儿推拿特定穴位介绍如下。

1.4.2.1 Acupoints on the Upper Limbs

1.4.2.1.1 Pijing

LOCATION The ungual whorl surface of the thumb.

MANIPULATION Pushing rotationally or pushing along the radial border of the thumb towards the wrist with the infantile thumb bent is reinforcing, called reinforcing Pijing. Pushing straight from the tip to the base of the thumb is clearing, called clearing Pijing. Reinforcing and clearing Pijing are generally known as pushing Pijing.

TIMES 100 to 500.

INDICATIONS Diarrhea, constipation, dysentery, inappetence, and jaundice, etc.

（一）上肢部穴位

1. 脾经

【定位】 拇指末节螺纹面。

【操作】 旋推或将患儿拇指屈曲,循拇指桡侧边缘向掌根方向直推为补,称补脾经;由指端向指根方向直推为清,称清脾经。补脾经、清脾经,统称推脾经。

【次数】 100～500 次。

【主治】 腹泻,便秘,痢疾,食欲不振,黄疸等。

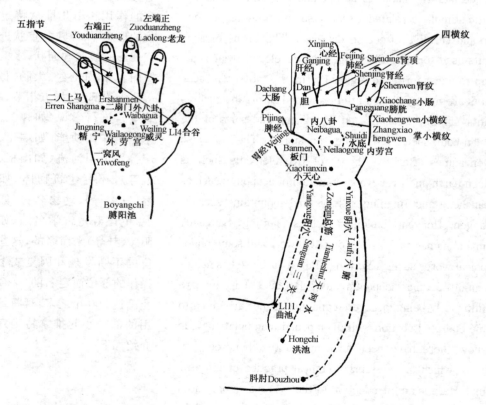

Fig. 18 - 1 Specific Acupoints for Infantile Tuina (on the Upper Limb)

图 18 - 1 小儿推拿特定穴位(上肢)

CLINICAL APPLICATION

(1) Reinforcing Pijing has the function of invigorating the spleen and stomach, replenishing qi and blood, and is used to treat inappetence, emaciation of muscles, and indigestion, etc. caused by splenogastric asthenia and deficiency of qi and blood.

(2) Clearing Pijing has the action of eliminating damp heat and resolving phlegm to stop vomiting, which is used to treat yellowish skin, nausea and vomiting, diarrhea and dysentery caused by fumigation of pathogenic damp heat. Reinforcing Pijing is commonly used for infants, whose spleen and stomach are delicate and unable to stand forceful purging or clearing therapy. Clearing Pijing can only be used for children with stronger constitution or sthenia pathogenic factors.

(3) Infants are generally weak with deficiency of healthy qi. When they are suffering from skin eruption and febrile disease, pushing and reinforcing Pijing may let out skin eruption of measles, but the manipulations should be quick and forceful.

1.4.2.1.2 Ganjing

LOCATION The ungual whorl surface of the index finger.

MANIPULATION Pushing rotationally is reinforcing, called reinforcing Ganjing. Pushing straight towards the base of the finger is clearing, called clearing Ganjing. Reinforcing and clearing Ganjing are all known as pushing Ganjing.

TIMES 100 to 500.

INDICATIONS Restlessness, infantile convulsion, conjunctival congestion, feverish sensation over five centres, bitter taste in the mouth, and dry throat, etc.

CLINICAL APPLICATION

(1) Clearing Ganjing plays the roles of calming the

【临床应用】

（1）补脾经能健脾胃，补气血。用于脾胃虚弱，气血不足而引起的食欲不振、肌肉消瘦、消化不良等症。

（2）清脾经能清热利湿，化痰止呕。用于湿热薰蒸所致的皮肤发黄、恶心呕吐、腹泻痢疾等症。小儿脾胃薄弱，不宜攻伐太甚，在一般情况下，脾经穴多用补法，体壮邪实者方能用清法。

（3）小儿体虚，正气不足，患斑疹热病时，推补本穴，可使隐疹透出，但手法宜快，用力宜重。

2. 肝经

【定位】 食指末节螺纹面。

【操作】 旋推为补，称补肝经；向指根方向直推为清，称清肝经。补肝经和清肝经统称推肝经。

【次数】 100～500 次。

【主治】 烦躁不安，惊风，目赤，五心烦热，口苦，咽干等。

【临床应用】

（1）清肝经能平肝泻火，

liver and purging pathogenic fire, relieving convulsion and spasm, alleviating liver stagnation and removing restlessness. It is often used for infantile convulsion, spasm, restlessness and feverish sensation over five centres, etc.

(2) Ganjing should be cleared rather than reinforced. When the liver is asthenia and needs reinforcing, clearing must be added after reinforcing. Or reinforcing Shenjing is employed instead, which is known as nourishing the kidney to reinforce the liver.

1.4.2.1.3　Xinjing

LOCATION　The ungual whorl surface of the middle finger.

MANIPULATION　Pushing rotationally is reinforcing, called reinforcing Xinjing. Pushing straight towards the base of the finger is clearing, called clearing Xinjing. Reinforcing and clearing Xinjing are generally known as pushing Xinjing.

TIMES　100 to 500.

INDICATIONS　Hyperpyretic coma, feverish sensation over five centres, orolingual ulceration, hot and difficult urination, asthenia of cardiac blood, and terrified restlessness, etc.

CLINICAL APPLICATION

(1) Clearing Xinjing functions as clearing away heat and purging pathogenic fire in the heart, and is often used for unconsciousness due to high fever, reddened face, oral ulceration, scanty and hot urine due to hyperactivity of heart fire. The manipulation is usually applied together with clearing Tianheshui and Xiaochang.

(2) Xinjing is suitable for clearing rather than reinforcing methods, in case heart fire should be induced. If reinforcing manipulation is needed for symptoms such as restlessness, sleep with eyes open due to insufficiency of qi and blood, clearing must be given after reinforcing. Or

熄风镇惊,解郁除烦。常用于惊风、抽搐、烦躁不安、五心烦热等症。

(2) 肝经宜清不宜补,若肝虚应补时则需补后加清,或以补肾经代之,称为滋肾养肝法。

3. 心经

【定位】　中指末节螺纹面。

【操作】　旋推为补,称补心经;向指根方向直推为清,称清心经。补心经和清心经统称推心经。

【次数】　100～500 次。

【主治】　高热神昏,五心烦热,口舌生疮,小便赤涩,心血不足,惊惕不安等。

【临床应用】

(1) 清心经能清热退心火。常用于心火旺盛而引起的高热神昏、面赤口疮、小便短赤等。多与清天河水、清小肠等合用。

(2) 本穴宜用清法,不宜用补法,乃恐动心火之故。若气血不足而见心烦不安、睡卧露睛等症,需用补法时,可补后加清,或以补脾经代之。

reinforcing Pijing is employed instead.

1.4.2.1.4　Feijing

LOCATION　The ungual whorl surface of the ring finger.

MANIPULATION　Pushing rotationally is reinforcing, called reinforcing Feijing; pushing straight towards the base of the finger is called clearing Feijing. Reinforcing and clearing Feijing are generally known as pushing Feijing.

TIMES　100 to 500.

INDICATIONS　Common cold, fever, cough, stuffiness in the chest, dyspnea, sweating due to asthenia, and prolapse of the rectum, etc.

CLINICAL APPLICATION

(1) Reinforcing Feijing has the function of nourishing pulmonary qi, and is used to treat asthenia cold syndrome of the lung meridian manifested as asthenic impairment of pulmonary qi, cough, dyspnea, deficient perspiration and aversion to cold.

(2) Clearing Feijing plays the roles of dispersing the lung to clear away heat from it, dispersing wind to relieve the exterior and resolving phlegm to stop cough, and is used for exterior fever and sthenia-heat syndrome with symptoms of cough, dyspnea and wheezy phlegm.

1.4.2.1.5　Shenjing

LOCATION　The ungual whorl surface of the little finger.

MANIPULATION　Pushing straight from the base of the finger towards its tip is reinforcing, called reinforcing Shenjing. Pushing straight towards the base of the finger is called clearing Shenjing. Reinforcing and clearing Shenjing are generally known as pushing Shenjing.

TIMES　100 to 500.

INDICATIONS　Congenital defect, weakness due to

4. 肺经

【定位】　无名指末节螺纹面。

【操作】　旋推为补,称补肺经;向指根方向直推为清,称清肺经。补肺经和清肺经统称推肺经。

【次数】　100～500 次。

【主治】　感冒,发热,咳嗽,胸闷,气喘,虚汗,脱肛等。

【临床应用】

(1) 补肺经能补益肺气。用于肺气虚损,咳嗽气喘,虚汗怕冷等肺经虚寒证。

(2) 清肺经能宣肺清热,疏风解表,化痰止咳。用于感冒发热及咳嗽、气喘、痰鸣等属肺经实热证者。

5. 肾经

【定位】　小指末节螺纹面。

【操作】　由指根向指尖方向直推为补,称补肾经;向指根方向直推为清,称清肾经。补肾经和清肾经统称推肾经。

【次数】　100～500 次。

【主治】　先天不足,久病

lingering illness, diarrhea due to kidney-deficiency, enuresis, deficient asthma, heat in the bladder, and dribbling urination with stabbing pain, etc.

CLINICAL APPLICATION

（1）Reinforcing Shenjing functions to replenish the kidney and brain, warm and nourish the primordial qi. It is used to treat congenital defect, weakness due to lingering illness, chronic diarrhea resulting from renal asthenia, polyuria, enuresis, sweating due to asthenia, and dyspnea, etc.

（2）Clearing Shenjing has the function of clearing away damp heat in the lower energizer, and is used to treat hot and difficult urination, etc. due to accumulated heat in the bladder. Clinically, Shenjing is often treated with reinforcing method. Clearing Shenjing, if needed, is often replaced by clearing Xiaochang.

1.4.2.1.6　Dachang

LOCATION　On the radial edge of the index finger, the line from the tip of the finger to Hukou.

MANIPULATION　Pushing straight from the tip of the finger to Hukou is called reinforcing Dachang. Pushing in the opposite direction is called clearing Dachang. Reinforcing and clearing Dachang are generally known as pushing Dachang.

TIMES　100 to 300.

INDICATIONS　Diarrhea, prolapse of the rectum, dysentery and constipation.

CLINICAL APPLICATION

（1）Reinforcing Dachang has the action of astringing the intestine to arrest prolaspe and warming the middle energizer to stop diarrhea, and is used for diarrhea, prolapse of the rectum and other symptoms due to asthenia cold.

（2）Clearing Dachang functions to cool the intestine, eliminate damp heat and promote defecation, and is used

体虚,肾虚腹泻,遗尿,虚喘,膀胱蕴热,小便淋沥刺痛等。

【临床应用】

（1）补肾经能补肾益脑,温养下元。用于先天不足、久病体虚、肾虚久泻、多尿、遗尿、虚汗喘息等。

（2）清肾经能清利下焦湿热。用于膀胱蕴热所致的小便赤涩等症。临床上肾经穴一般多用补法,需用清法时,也多以清小肠代之。

6. 大肠

【定位】　食指桡侧缘,自食指尖至虎口成一直线。

【操作】　从食指尖直推向虎口为补,称补大肠;反之为清,称清大肠。补大肠和清大肠统称推大肠。

【次数】　100～300 次。

【主治】　腹泻,脱肛,痢疾,便秘。

【临床应用】

（1）补大肠能涩肠固脱,温中止泻。用于虚寒腹泻、脱肛等病症。

（2）清大肠能清利肠腑,除湿热,导积滞。多用于湿

for fever, abdominal pain, dysentery, and constipation, etc. due to damp heat and retention of food in the intestine.

(3) The acupoint Dachang is also known as Zhisanguan and can be used for diagnosis (for details see the Diagnosis Chapter).

1.4.2.1.7 Xiaochang

LOCATION On the ulnar edge of the little finger, the line from the tip of the finger to its base.

MANIPULATION Pushing straight from the tip of the finger to its base is called reinforcing Xiaochang, while pushing in the opposite direction is called clearing Xiaochang. Reinforcing and clearing Xiaochang are generally known as pushing Xiaochang.

TIMES 100 to 300.

INDICATIONS Hot and difficult urination, watery diarrhea, enuresis, and anuria, etc.

CLINICAL APPLICATION Clearing Xiaochang has the function of clearing away damp heat in the lower energizer and separating purity from turbidity, and is used to treat scanty, hot and difficult urination, anuresis and watery diarrhea. Combined with clearing Tianheshui, this manipulation is also used to strengthen the action of clearing away pathogenic heat and inducing diuresis when pathogenic heat exists in the heart meridian and has transferred to the small intestine. Reinforcing Xiaochang is selected if the problem is of polyuria and enuresis caused by asthenia cold in the lower energizer.

1.4.2.1.8 Shending

LOCATION On the tip of the little finger.

MANIPULATION Pressing and kneading the point with the tip of the thumb or index finger is called kneading Shending.

TIMES 100 to 500.

热、积食滞留肠道,身热腹痛,痢下赤白,大便秘结等症。

(3) 本穴又称指三关,尚可用于诊断,详见诊断章。

7. 小肠

【定位】 小指尺侧边缘,自指尖到指根成一直线。

【操作】 从指尖直推向指根为补,称补小肠;反之则为清,称清小肠。补小肠和清小肠统称推小肠。

【次数】 100～300 次。

【主治】 小便赤涩,水泻,遗尿,尿闭等。

【临床应用】 清小肠能清利下焦湿热,分清别浊,多用于小便短赤不利、尿闭、水泻等症。若心经有热,移热于小肠,以本法配合清天河水,能加强清热利尿的作用。若属下焦虚寒所致的多尿、遗尿则宜用补小肠。

8. 肾顶

【定位】 小指顶端。

【操作】 以中指或拇指端按揉,称揉肾顶。

【次数】 100～500 次。

INDICATIONS Spontaneous perspiration, night sweating, and infantile metopism, etc.

CLINICAL APPLICATION Kneading Shending has the action of astringing primordial qi and consolidating the exterior to stop perspiration. It has certain therapeutic effect on spontaneous perspiration, night sweating or polyhidrosis.

1.4.2.1.9 Shenwen

LOCATION On the palmar surface of the hand, at the area of the cross striation of the 2nd interphalangeal joint of the little finger.

MANIPULATION Pressing and kneading the point with the tip of the thumb or index finger is called kneading Shenwen.

TIMES 100 to 500.

INDICATIONS Conjunctival congestion, thrush, and toxic heat sinking into the interior, etc.

CLINICAL APPLICATION Kneading Shenwen functions to expel wind, improve acuity of vision and dissipate mass. The manipulation is mainly used for conjunctival congestion with swelling and pain, high fever, sensation of cold air while breathing, cold hands and feet caused by interiorly-sunken and stagnated toxic heat.

1.4.2.1.10 Sihengwen

LOCATION On the palmar surface of the hand, at the area of the cross striations of the 1st interphalangeal joints of the index, middle, ring and little fingers.

MANIPULATION Nipping and kneading the points with the nail of the thumb is called nipping Sihengwen; while pushing from the cross striation of the index finger to that of the little finger with the infants' four fingers put closely alongside is called pushing Sihengwen.

TIMES Nip each acupoint 5 times and push 100 to 300 times.

【主治】 自汗,盗汗,解颅等。

【临床应用】 揉肾顶能收敛元气,固表止汗,对自汗、盗汗或大汗淋漓不止等症均有一定的疗效。

9. 肾纹

【定位】 手掌面,小指第2指间关节横纹处。

【操作】 中指或拇指端按揉,称揉肾纹。

【次数】 100~500 次。

【主治】 目赤,鹅口疮,热毒内陷等。

【临床应用】 揉肾纹能祛风明目、散瘀结。主要用于目赤肿痛或热毒内陷,瘀结不散所致的高热、呼吸气凉、手足逆冷等症。

10. 四横纹

【定位】 掌面食、中、无名、小指第 1 指间关节横纹处。

【操作】 拇指甲掐揉,称掐四横纹;四指并拢从食指横纹处推向小指横纹处,称推四横纹。

【次数】 掐各 5 次,推100~300 次。

INDICATIONS Infantile malnutrition, abdominal distension and pain, disharmony of qi and blood, indigestion, convulsion, dyspnea and fissure on the lip.

CLINICAL APPLICATION Nipping the acupoint has the effect of abating fever, relieving vexation and dissipating mass. And pushing the point can regulate the middle energizer to promote circulation of qi, regulate qi and blood and relieve abdominal flatulence, and is often used clinically to treat infantile malnutrition, abdominal distension, disharmony between qi and blood, indigestion. Pushing the acupoint is often combined with reinforcing Pijing and kneading Zhongwan (CV 12) in clinic. Pricking the point with a filiform needle or a three-edged needle to cause bleeding can also produce a good result in treating infantile malnutrition.

1.4.2.1.11 Xiaohengwen

LOCATION On the palmar surface of the hand, at the area of the cross striations of the metacarpophalangeal articulation of the index, middle, ring and little fingers.

MANIPULATION Nipping the point with the nail of the thumb is called nipping Xiaohengwen, and pushing it with the lateral aspect of the thumb is known as pushing Xiaohengwen.

TIMES Nip each point 5 times and push 100 to 300 times.

INDICATIONS Restlessness, oral ulceration, fissures on the lip, and abdominal distension, etc.

CLINICAL APPLICATION Pushing and nipping the acupoint has the action of reducing fever, relieving distension and removing stasis, and is mainly used for ulceration of the lip, and abdominal distension, etc. due to splenogastric heat stagnation. In clinic, pushing Xiaohengwen is effective in treating pulmonary dry rale.

【主治】 疳积，腹胀腹痛，气血不和，消化不良，惊风，气喘，口唇破裂等。

【临床应用】 本穴掐之能退热除烦，散瘀结；推之能调中行气，和气血，消胀满。临床上多用于疳积、腹胀、气血不和、消化不良等。常与补脾经、揉中脘等合用。用毫针或三棱针点刺本穴出血以治疗疳积，效果也好。

11. 小横纹

【定位】 掌面食、中、无名、小指掌指关节横纹处。

【操作】 以拇指甲掐，称掐小横纹；拇指侧推，称推小横纹。

【次数】 掐各 5 次，推100～300 次。

【主治】 烦躁，口疮，唇裂，腹胀等。

【临床应用】 推掐本穴能退热、消胀、散结。主要用于脾胃热结所致的口唇破烂及腹胀等症。临床上用推小横纹治疗肺部干性啰音，有一定疗效。

1.4.2.1.12　Zhangxiaohengwen

LOCATION　At the end of the ulnar palm striation, below the base of the little finger on the palmar aspect.

MANIPULATION　Pressing and kneading the point with the tip of the thumb or middle finger is called kneading Zhangxiaohengwen.

TIMES　100 to 500.

INDICATIONS　Cough and asthma due to phlegm-heat, orolingual ulcer, whooping cough, and salivation, etc.

CLINICAL APPLICATION　Kneading the acupoint plays the roles of clearing away heat and dissipating mass, soothing chest oppression, dispersing lung and resolving phlegm to stop cough. The point is mainly used to treat dyspnea, cough and orolingual ulcer, but it is also an important acupoint for whooping cough and pneumonia. In clinic, kneading Zhangxiaohengwen has some therapeutic effects on pulmonary moist rale.

1.4.2.1.13　Weijing

LOCATION　On the palmar surface of the thumb knuckle next to the palm.

MANIPULATION　Pushing rotationally is called reinforcing Weijing. Pushing straight towards the base of the thumb is called clearing Weijing. Reinforcing and clearing Weijing are all known as pushing Weijing.

TIMES　100 to 500.

INDICATIONS　Vomiting, nausea, belching, polydipsia, bulimia, inappetence, haematemesis, and epistaxis, etc.

CLINICAL APPLICATION

(1) Clearing Weijing has the action of clearing away damp heat in the middle energizer, regulating the stomach to direct adverse qi downward, purging fire in the stomach, relieving restlessness and thirst and treating

12．掌小横纹

【定位】　掌面小指根下，尺侧掌纹头。

【操作】　中指或拇指端按揉，称揉掌小横纹。

【次数】　100～500 次。

【主治】　痰热喘咳，口舌生疮，顿咳，流涎等。

【临床应用】　揉掌小横纹能清热散结，宽胸宣肺，化痰止咳。主要用于喘咳、口舌生疮等，为治疗百日咳、肺炎的要穴。临床上用揉掌小横纹治疗肺部湿性啰音，有一定的疗效。

13．胃经

【定位】　拇指掌面近掌端第 1 节。

【操作】　旋推为补，称补胃经；向指根方向直推为清，称清胃经。补胃经和清胃经统称推胃经。

【次数】　100～500 次。

【主治】　呕恶嗳气，烦渴善饥，食欲不振，吐血，衄血等。

【临床应用】

（1）清胃经能清中焦湿热，和胃降逆，泻胃火，除烦止渴。亦可用于胃火上亢引起的衄血等症。临床上多与清

epistaxis caused by flaring up of stomach fire as well. Clinically, clearing Weijing is often used to treat nausea and vomiting due to splenogastric damp heat or disharmony of gastric qi in combination with clearing Pijing, pushing Tianzhugu and pushing from Hengwen to Banmen. The method is also combined with clearing Dachang, reducing Liufu, kneading Tianshu (ST 25) and pushing down Qijiegu to treat gastrointestinal sthenia heat marked by gastric and abdominal distension, fever, polydipsia, constipation and anorexia.

(2) Reinforcing Weijing has the function of invigorating the spleen and stomach to promote transportation and transformation. In clinic, it is often used together with reinforcing Pijing, kneading Zhongwan (CV 12), rotationally rubbing Fu and pressing and kneading Zusanli (ST 36) to treat splenogastric asthenia marked by indigestion, anorexia and abdominal distension.

1.4.2.1.14 Banmen

LOCATION   On the flat surface of the major thenar eminence of the palm.

MANIPULATION   Kneading with the end of a finger is called kneading Banmen or arc-pushing Banmen. Pushing from the base of the thumb to the transverse crease of the wrist with pushing manipulation is called pushing from Banmen to Hengwen. Otherwise, it is called pushing from Hengwen to Banmen.

TIMES   100 to 300.

INDICATIONS   Indigestion, abdominal distension, inappetence, vomiting, diarrhea, asthma, belching and infantile malnutrition as well.

CLINICAL APPLICATION

(1) Kneading Banmen plays the role of invigorating the spleen and stomach to promote digestion and eliminate food retention, and free qi activities. It is used for trea-

脾经、推天柱骨、横纹推向板门等合用,治疗脾胃湿热,或胃气不和所引起的呕恶等症;若胃肠实热、脘腹胀满、发热烦渴、便秘纳呆,多与清大肠、退六腑、揉天枢、推下七节骨等合用。

(2) 补胃经能健脾胃,助运化,临床上常与补脾经、揉中脘、摩腹、按揉足三里等合用,治疗脾胃虚弱、消化不良、纳呆腹胀等。

14. 板门

【定位】 手掌大鱼际平面。

【操作】 指端揉,称揉板门或运板门;用推法自指根推向腕横纹,称板门推向横纹,反之称横纹推向板门。

【次数】 100～300 次。

【主治】 食积,腹胀,食欲不振,呕吐,腹泻,气喘,嗳气等。还可用于治疗疳积。

【临床应用】

(1) 揉板门能健脾和胃、消食化滞,运达上下之气。多用于乳食停积,食欲不振或嗳

ting indigestion, inappetence, belching, abdominal distension, diarrhea and vomiting.

(2) Pushing from Banmen to Hengwen can stop diarrhea, while pushing from Hengwen to Banmen is able to
stop vomiting.

1.4.2.1.15 Neilaogong

LOCATION　In the centre of the palm, at the midpoint between the bent middle and ring fingers.

MANIPULATION　Kneading with the tip of the middle finger is called kneading Neilaogong. Nipping and arc-
pushing from the base of the little finger through Zhangxiaohengwen and Xiaotianxin to Neilaogong is called arc-
pushing Neilaogong or Shuidi Laomingyue (Fishing up the
Bright Moon from the Bottom of Water).

TIMES　Knead 100 to 300 times; arc-push 10 to 30
times.

INDICATIONS　Fever, polydipsia, aphthae, gum ulcer, interior heat with deficient dysphoria, etc.

CLINICAL APPLICATION

(1) Kneading Neilaogong has the action of clearing a-
way heat and relieving dysphoria, and is used for orolingual ulcer, fever and polydipsia resulting from heat in the
heart meridian.

(2) Arc-pushing Neilaogong is the compound manipulation of arc-pushing Zhangxiaohengwen, kneading Xiaotianxin and arc-pushing Neilaogong. It is effective in
clearing away asthenia heat, therefore is mostly suitable
for treating asthenia heat in the heart meridian and kidney
meridian.

1.4.2.1.16 Neibagua

LOCATION　On the palmar surface. Taking the centre of the palm as the centre of a circle and 2/3 the distance from the centre of the circle to the cross striation on
the middle finger base as the radius, draw a circle. The

气、腹胀、腹泻、呕吐等症。

（2）板门推向横纹能止
泻,横纹推向板门能止呕吐。

15．内劳宫

【定位】　掌心中,屈指时
在中指、无名指之间的中点。

【操作】　中指端揉,称揉
内劳宫;自小指根掐运起,经
掌小横纹、小天心至内劳宫,
称运内劳宫(水底捞明月)。

【次数】　揉 100～300
次,运 10～30 次。

【主治】　发热,烦渴,口
疮,齿龈糜烂,虚烦内热等。

【临床应用】

（1）揉内劳能清热除烦,
用于心经有热而致的口舌生
疮、发热、烦渴等症。

（2）运内劳为运掌小横
纹、揉小天心、运内劳宫的复
合手法,能清虚热,对心、肾两
经虚热最为适宜。

16．内八卦

【定位】　手掌面,以掌心
为圆心,从圆心至中指根横纹
约 2/3 处为半径所作的圆周。

circle is acupoint Neibagua.

MANIPULATION Nipping and pushing clockwise with arc-pushing manipulation is called arc-pushing Neibagua or Bagua.

TIMES   100 to 300.

INDICATIONS Cough with phlegmatic asthma, chest stuffiness, poor appetite, abdominal distension, and vomiting, etc.

CLINICAL APPLICATION Arc-pushing Neibagua functions to relieve chest stuffiness, regulate qi and resolve phlegm, remove food retention and promote digestion. It is mainly used to treat cough and dyspnea due to stagnated phlegm, dyspepsia, chest stuffiness, abdominal distension, vomiting and poor appetite. Arc-pushing Neibagua is commonly used together with pushing Pijing and Feijing, kneading Banmen and Zhongwan(CV 12).

1.4.2.1.17 Xiaotianxin

LOCATION In the depression of the junction between the major and minor thenar eminences.

MANIPULATION Kneading with the tip of the middle finger is called kneading Xiaotianxin. Nipping with the nail of the thumb is called nipping Xiaotianxin. Striking with the tip of the middle finger or its flexed interphalangeal joint is called pounding Xiaotianxin.

TIMES   Knead 100 to 300 times; nip and pound 5 to 20 times respectively.

INDICATIONS Infantile convulsion with spasm, restlessness, night crying, hot and difficult urination, strabismus, conjunctival congestion with pain, measles with incomplete eruption.

CLINICAL APPLICATION

(1) Kneading Xiaotianxin has the effect of clearing away heat, relieving convulsion, promoting urination and improving vision. It is mainly used for conjunctival

【操作】 用运法,顺时针方向掐运,称运内八卦或运八卦。

【次数】 100～300 次。

【主治】 咳嗽痰喘,胸闷纳呆,腹胀,呕吐等。

【临床应用】 运内八卦能宽胸利膈,理气化痰,行滞消食。主要用于痰结喘嗽、乳食内伤、胸闷、腹胀、呕吐、纳呆等,多与推脾经、推肺经、揉板门、揉中脘等合用。

17. 小天心

【定位】 大小鱼际交接处凹陷中。

【操作】 中指端揉,称揉小天心;拇指甲陷,称掐小天心;以中指尖或屈曲的指间关节捣,称捣小天心。

【次数】 揉 100～300 次;掐、捣 5～20 次。

【主治】 惊风,抽搐,烦躁不安,夜啼,小便赤涩,斜视,目赤痛,疹痘欲出不透。

【临床应用】

(1) 揉小天心能清热、镇惊、利尿、明目,主要用于心经有热而致的目赤肿痛、口舌生

congestion with swelling and pain, orolingual ulcer and terrified restlessness caused by heat in the heart meridian, or scanty brown urine, etc. caused by heat moved from the heart meridian into the small intestine meridian. Additionally, the manipulation is also effective against scleroderma neonatorum, jaundice, enuresis, edema, furuncle, measles with incomplete eruption.

（2）Nipping and pounding Xiaotianxin can relieve convulsion and tranquilize the mind, which is chiefly used for infantile convulsion with spasm, night crying, terrified restlessness, etc. If convulsion with superduction and strabismus occurs, pounding Laolong, nipping Renzhong (CV 26) and clearing Ganjing are combined with this manipulation. Nipping and pounding downward is for superduction. Nipping and pounding to the left side is for right strabismus, otherwise, operating to the right for left strabismus.

1.4.2.1.18 Zongjin

LOCATION At the midpoint of the palmar transverse crease of the wrist.

MANIPULATION Pressing and kneading the acupoint is called kneading Zongjin. Nipping it with the nail of the thumb is called nipping Zongjin.

TIMES Knead 100 to 300 times and nip 3 to 5 times.

INDICATIONS Infantile convulsion with spasm, night crying, orolingual ulcer, tidal fever, and toothache, etc.

CLINICAL APPLICATION Kneading Zongjin has the effect of clearing away pathogenic heat in the heart meridian, removing obstruction, relieving spasm and regulating qi activity in the body. Clinically it is often combined with clearing Tianheshui and Xinjing to treat sthenia-heat syndrome manifested as orolingual ulcer, tidal fever, night crying. The manipulation should be quick and a

疮、惊惕不安或心经有热，移热于小肠而致的小便短赤等症。此外对新生儿硬皮症、黄疸、遗尿、水肿、疮疖、痘疹欲出不透亦有效。

（2）掐、捣小天心能镇惊安神。主要用于惊风抽搐、夜啼、惊惕不安等症。若见惊风眼翻、斜视，可与捣老龙、掐人中、清肝经等合用。眼上翻者则向下掐、捣；若右斜视者则向左掐、捣；左斜视者则向右掐、捣。

18. 总筋

【定位】 掌后腕横纹中点。

【操作】 按揉本穴称揉总筋；用拇指甲掐称掐总筋。

【次数】 揉 100～300 次；掐 3～5 次。

【主治】 惊风，抽掣，夜啼，口舌生疮，潮热，牙痛等。

【临床应用】 揉总筋能清心经热，散结止痉，通调周身气机。临床上多与清天河水、清心经配合，治疗口舌生疮、潮热、夜啼等属实热证者。操作时手法宜快，并稍有力。治疗惊风抽掣多用掐法。

little forceful. Nipping manipulation is used for infantile convulsion with spasm.

1.4.2.1.19 Dahengwen

LOCATION On the posterior palmar transverse crease of the wrist, Its end close to the thumb is known as Yangchi and that close to the small finger Yinchi.

MANIPULATION Pushing separately from the centre of the posterior palmar transverse crease of the wrist (where Zongjin is located) towards both sides with the two thumbs is called parting-pushing Dahengwen, also known as separating Yinyang (Yinchi and Yangchi). Pushing jointly from Yinchi and Yangchi towards Zongjin is called joining Yinyang (Yinchi and Yangchi).

TIMES 30 to 50.

INDICATIONS Alternate fever and chill, diarrhea, abdominal distension, dysentery, vomiting, food retention, restlessness and retention of excessive phlegm fluid.

CLINICAL APPLICATION

(1) Separating Yinyang functions to balance yin and yang, regulate qi and blood and promote digestion, and is commonly used for alternate fever and chill, restlessness due to imbalance between yin and yang and disharmony between qi and blood, as well as milk and food retention, abdominal distension, diarrhea and vomiting.

(2) Joining Yinyang has the action of resolving phlegm and eliminating obstruction, and is often used to treat cough and dyspnea due to stagnated phlegm, and stuffiness in the chest, etc. In combination with kneading Shenwen and clearing Tianheshui, the manipulation is able to enhance the effect of resolving phlegm and removing obstruction.

1.4.2.1.20 Shixuan (EX-UE 11, also called Shiwang)

LOCATION On the red-white border of the tips of

19. 大横纹

【定位】 仰掌,掌后横纹。近拇指端称阳池,近小指端称阴池。

【操作】 两拇指自掌后横纹中(总筋)向两旁分推,称分推大横纹,又称分阴阳;自两旁(阴池、阳池)向总筋合推,称合阴阳。

【次数】 30～50 次。

【主治】 寒热往来,腹泻,腹胀,痢疾,呕吐,食积,烦躁不安,痰涎壅盛等。

【临床应用】

(1)分阴阳功能平衡阴阳,调和气血,行滞消食。多用于阴阳不调,气血不和而致的寒热往来、烦躁不安,以及乳食停滞、腹胀、腹泻、呕吐等。

(2)合阴阳能化痰散结,多用于痰结喘嗽、胸闷等症。配合揉肾纹,清天河水能加强化痰散结的作用。

20. 十宣(十王)

【定位】 十指尖指甲内

the ten fingers, in the inner part of the nail.

MANIPULATION　Nipping the points is called nipping Shixuan.

TIMES　Nip each point 5 times or until consciousness is regained.

INDICATIONS　Convulsion, high fever and syncope.

CLINICAL APPLICATION　Nipping Shixuan is mainly used for emergency treatment and has the effect of clearing away pathogenic heat, restoring consciousness and inducing resuscitation. It is commonly used together with nipping Laolong, Renzhong (GV 26) and Xiaotianxin.

1.4.2.1.21　Laolong

LOCATION　0.1 cun posterior to the nail of the middle finger.

MANIPULATION　Nipping the acupoint with nipping manipulation is called nipping Laolong.

TIMES　Nip 5 times or until consciousness is regained.

INDICATION　Acute convulsion.

CLINICAL APPLICATION　Nipping Laolong is mainly used for first aid and has the action of restoring consciousness and inducing resuscitation. For the infant patient who has acute convulsion with sudden syncope or high fever with spasm, if the treatment can cause the infant to feel pain or make it utter any words, the problem is easy to treat. Otherwise, difficult.

1.4.2.1.22　Duanzheng

LOCATION　At the red-white junctions of both aspects of the nail base of the middle finger. The one on the radial aspect is called Zuoduanzheng, while the other on the ulnar aspect is Youduanzheng.

MANIPULATION　Nipping the acupoint with the nail

赤白肉际处。

【操作】　用掐法，称掐十宣。

【次数】　各掐5次，或醒后即止。

【主治】　惊风、高热、昏厥。

【临床应用】　掐十宣主要用于急救，有清热、醒神、开窍的作用，多与掐老龙、掐人中、掐小天心等合用。

21．老龙

【定位】　中指甲后1分处。

【操作】　用掐法，称掐老龙。

【次数】　掐5次，或醒后即止。

【主治】　急惊风。

【临床应用】　掐老龙主要用于急救，有醒神开窍的作用。若小儿急惊暴厥，或高热抽搐，掐之知痛有声者，较易治，不知痛而无声者，一般难治。

22．端正

【定位】　中指甲根两侧赤白肉处，桡侧称左端正，尺侧称右端正。

【操作】　用拇指甲掐或

of the thumb is called nipping Duanzheng. Kneading it with the whorl surface of the thumb is called kneading Duanzheng.

TIMES Nip 5 times and knead 50 times.

INDICATIONS Epistaxis, convulsion, vomiting, diarrhea and dysentery.

CLINICAL APPLICATION

(1) Kneading Youduanzheng functions to descend the adverse qi to stop vomiting and is mainly used for nausea, vomiting and other symptoms caused by adverse rising of gastric qi. Kneading Zuoduanzheng has the function of raising the middle energizer qi and is mainly used for watery diarrhea and dysentery, etc.

(2) Nipping Duanzheng is commonly used to treat infantile convulsion, which is often combined with nipping Laolong and clearing Ganjing. The point is also effective against epistaxis. The way of treating the problem is to tie up the infant's middle finger with a thin string from the cross striation of the 3rd knuckle to the end of the finger (not too tight), and then keep the infant lying in bed.

1.4.2.1.23 Wuzhijie

LOCATION On the dorsum of the hand, the 1st interphalangeal joints of the five fingers.

MANIPULATION Nipping the acupoint with the nail of the thumb is called nipping Wuzhijie. Kneading and twisting it with the thumb and index finger is called kneading Wuzhijie.

TIMES Nip each acupoint 3 to 5 times, knead and twist 30 to 50 times.

INDICATIONS Convulsion, salivation, terrified restlessness, and cough with expectoration due to wind, etc.

CLINICAL APPLICATION Nipping and kneading Wuzhijie function to relieve convulsion and calm the mind, expel wind phlegm, smooth joint movement and dredge

拇指螺纹面揉称掐、揉端正。

【次数】 掐5次,揉50次。

【主治】 鼻衄,惊风,呕吐,泄泻,痢疾。

【临床应用】

(1) 揉右端正能降逆止呕,主要用于胃气上逆而引起的恶心呕吐等症;揉左端正功能升提,主要用于水泻、痢疾等症。

(2) 掐端正多用于治疗小儿惊风,常与掐老龙、清肝经等配合。同时本穴对鼻衄有效,方法:用细绳由中指第3节横纹起扎至指端(不可太紧),扎后让患儿静卧即可。

23. 五指节

【定位】 掌背五指第1指间关节。

【操作】 拇指甲掐,称掐五指节;用拇、食指揉搓称揉五指节。

【次数】 各掐3~5次;揉搓30~50次。

【主治】 惊风,吐涎,惊惕不安,咳嗽风痰等。

【临床应用】 掐、揉五指节能安神镇惊,祛风痰,通关窍。掐五指节主要用于惊惕

orifices. Nipping Wuzhijie is mainly used for terrified restlessness and convulsion, and commonly combined with clearing Ganjing and nipping Laolong. While kneading Wuzhijie is chiefly used for stuffiness in the chest, phlegmatic dyspnea and cough, and it is often combined in use with arc-pushing Neibagua, pushing and kneading Danzhong (CV 17).

1.4.2.1.24 Ershanmen

LOCATION On the dorsum of the hand, in the depression on both sides of the base of the middle phalanx.

MANIPULATION Nipping the acupoint with the nail of the thumb is called nipping Ershanmen. Pressing and kneading it with the lateral hump of the thumb is called kneading Ershanmen.

TIMES Nip 5 times and knead 100 to 500 times.

INDICATIONS Convulsion with spasm and fever without sweating.

CLINICAL APPLICATION Nipping or kneading Ershanmen functions to relieve the exterior with diaphoresis, reduce fever and relieve asthma. It is an effective manipulation for diaphoresis. Kneading the acupoint is often used to treat invasion by exogenous wind cold, but the operation should be quick and slightly forceful. Used in combination with kneading Shending, reinforcing Pijing and Shenjing, the manipulation is applicable to patients who are of general debility and suffer from exogenous wind cold.

1.4.2.1.25 Shangma

LOCATION On the dorsum of the hand, in the depression posterior to the metacarpophalangeal articulations of the ring and little fingers.

MANIPULATION Kneading the acupoint with the tip of the thumb is called kneading Shangma and nipping it

不安、惊风等症，多与清肝经、掐老龙等合用；揉五指节主要用于胸闷、痰喘、咳嗽等症，多与运内八卦、推揉膻中等合用。

24. 二扇门

【定位】　掌背中指根本节两侧凹陷处。

【操作】　拇指甲掐，称掐二扇门；拇指偏峰按揉，称揉二扇门。

【次数】　掐5 次，揉100～500 次。

【主治】　惊风抽搐，身热无汗。

【临床应用】　掐、揉二扇门能发汗透表，退热平喘，是发汗效法。揉时要稍用力，速度宜快，多用于风寒外感。本法与揉肾顶、补脾经、补肾经等配合应用，适宜于平素体虚外感者。

25. 上马

【定位】　手背无名及小指掌指关节后陷中。

【操作】　拇指端揉和拇指甲掐称揉上马或掐上马。

with the nail of the thumb is called nipping Shangma.

TIMES　Nip 3 to 5 times and knead 100 to 500 times.

INDICATIONS　Asthenia heat with cough and asthma, hot and dribbling urination, abdominal pain, toothache, and grinding teeth at night, etc.

CLINICAL APPLICATION　Kneading Shangma is frequently used in clinic, which has the function of nourishing kidney yin, promoting circulation of qi to remove obstruction, inducing diuresis for treating stranguria. It is a principal method for replenishing vital essence to tonify kidney, which is mainly used for symptoms of tidal fever, restlessness, toothache, hot and dribbling urination resulting from asthenic yin and resultant predominant yang. Combined with kneading Xiaohengwen and operated many times, this manipulation is effective against infantile patients with weak constitution, who suffer from pulmonary infection with dry rale, which is lingering and does not disappear. While for moist rale kneading the point should be combined with kneading Zhangxiaohengwen.

1.4.2.1.26　Wailaogong

LOCATION　In the centre of the dorsum of the hand, opposite to Neilaogong.

MANIPULATION　Kneading the acupoint is called kneading Wailaogong and nipping it called nipping Wailaogong.

TIMES　Nip 5 times and knead 100 to 500 times.

INDICATIONS　Common cold of wind cold type, distension and pain in the abdomen, borborygmus, diarrhea, dysentery, prolapse of the rectum, enuresis and hernia.

CLINICAL APPLICATION　The acupoint is warm in nature and an acupoint for warming yang and expelling

【次数】　掐3～5次，揉100～500次。

【主治】　虚热喘咳，小便赤涩淋沥，腹痛，牙痛，睡时磨牙等。

【临床应用】　临床上用揉法为多，揉上马能滋阴补肾，顺气散结，利水通淋，为补肾滋阴的要法。主要用于阴虚阳亢所致的潮热烦躁、牙痛、小便赤涩淋沥等症。本法对体质虚弱，肺部感染有干性啰音，久不消失者配揉小横纹；湿性啰音配揉掌小横纹，多揉有一定疗效。

26. 外劳宫

【定位】　掌背中，与内劳宫相对处。

【操作】　用揉法，称揉外劳，用掐法称掐外劳。

【次数】　掐5次，揉100～300次。

【主治】　风寒感冒，腹痛腹胀，肠鸣腹泻，痢疾，脱肛，遗尿，疝气。

【临床应用】　本穴性温，为温阳散寒、升阳举陷佳穴，

cold, invigorating splenic yang to raise visceroptosis. And it is also effective for relieving the exterior with diaphoresis. Kneading Wailaogong is often seen in clinic and mainly used for all kinds of cold syndrome such as invasion of exogenous wind cold, nasal obstruction with discharge, visceral cold retention, indigestion, borborygmus, diarrhea, abdominal pain due to cold dysentery and hernia. The manipulation can also invigorate yang to raise visceroptosis, so clinically it is often used to treat prolapse of the rectum, enuresis and other symptoms in combination with reinforcing Pijing and Shenjing, pushing Sanguan and kneading Dantian.

1.4.2.1.27　Weiling

LOCATION　On the dorsum of the hand, in the depression between the 2nd and 3rd metacarpal bones.

MANIPULATION　Nipping the acupoint is called nipping Weiling.

TIMES　Nip 5 times or until consciousness is regained.

INDICATION　Convulsion.

CLINICAL APPLICATION　Nipping Weiling has the effect of inducing resuscitation and restoring consciousness. It is mainly used for emergency treatment of acute convulsion, sudden syncope and coma.

1.4.2.1.28　Jingning

LOCATION　On the dorsum of the hand, in the suture between the 4th and 5th metacarpal bones.

MANIPULATION　Nipping the acupoint is called nipping Jingning.

TIMES　5 to 10.

INDICATIONS　Phlegmatic asthma with croup, retching, infantile malnutrition, and intra-ocular ulcer polyp, etc.

CLINICAL APPLICATION　Nipping Jingning func-

兼能发汗解表。临床上用揉法为多，揉外劳宫主要用于一切寒证，不论外感风寒，鼻塞流涕以及脏腑积寒，完谷不化，肠鸣腹泻，寒痢腹痛，疝气等皆宜，且能升阳举陷，故临床上也多配合补脾经、补肾经、推三关、揉丹田等治疗脱肛、遗尿等症。

27．威灵

【定位】　手背第 2、3 掌骨歧缝间。

【操作】　用掐法，称掐威灵。

【次数】　掐 5 次，或醒后即止。

【主治】　惊风。

【临床应用】　掐威灵有开窍醒神的作用。主要用于急惊暴厥、昏迷不醒时的急救。

28．精宁

【定位】　手背第 4、5 掌骨歧缝间。

【操作】　用掐法，称掐精宁。

【次数】　5～10 次。

【主治】　痰喘气吼，干呕，疳积，眼内胬肉等。

【临床应用】　掐精宁能

tions to promote flow of qi, remove stagnation, resolve phlegm, which is commonly used for dyspepsia, phlegmatic retention, croup and phlegmatic asthma, retching and infantile malnutrition. But the method should be used with great care for weak infants. If needed, it should be combined with reinforcing Pijing, pushing Sanguan and pinching Ji to avoid overpurgation impairing primordial qi. In the treatment of acute convulsion and syncope, the method is often combined with nipping Weiling to enhance the effect of inducing resuscitation and restoring consciousness.

1.4.2.1.29 Waibagua

LOCATION On the dorsum of the hand, around Wailaogong and opposite to Neibagua.

MANIPULATION Nipping and arc-pushing the acupoint clockwise with the thumb is called arc-pushing Waibagua.

TIMES 100 to 300.

INDICATIONS Chest distress, abdominal distension, and constipation, etc.

CLINICAL APPLICATION Arc-pushing Waibagua has the action of regulating qi to alleviate chest distress, dissipating stasis to eliminate mass. In clinic, it is applied together with rubbing Fu, pushing-kneading Danzhong (CV 17) to treat stuffiness in the chest, abdominal distension and constipation.

1.4.2.1.30 Yiwofeng

LOCATION On the dorsum of the hand, in the depression of the middle of the transverse crease of the wrist.

MANIPULATION Kneading the acupoint with the tip of a finger is called kneading Yiwofeng.

TIMES 100 to 300.

INDICATIONS Abdominal pain, borborygmus,

行气, 破结, 化痰。多用于痰食积聚、气吼痰喘、干呕、疳积等症。本法于体虚者宜慎用, 如必须应用时则多与补脾经、推三关、捏脊等同用, 以免克伐太甚, 元气受损。用于急惊昏厥时, 本法多与掐威灵配合, 能加强开窍醒神的作用。

29. 外八卦

【定位】 掌背外劳宫周围, 与内八卦相对处。

【操作】 拇指作顺时针方向掐运, 称运外八卦。

【次数】 100～300 次。

【主治】 胸闷, 腹胀, 便结等。

【临床应用】 运外八卦能宽胸理气, 通滞散结。临床上多与摩腹、推揉膻中等合用, 治疗胸闷、腹胀、便结等症。

30. 一窝风

【定位】 手背腕横纹正中凹陷处。

【操作】 指端揉, 称揉一窝风。

【次数】 100～300 次。

【主治】 腹痛, 肠鸣, 关

arthralgia and common cold.

CLINICAL APPLICATION Kneading Yiwofeng has the function of warming the middle energizer to promote qi circulation, relieving arthralgia and smoothing joint movement, which is indicated in abdominal pain caused by cold or food retention, and commonly used together with grasping Dujiao, pushing Sanguan and kneading Zhongwan (CV 12). The manipulation can also dispel wind cold, disperse qi stagnation of the interior and exterior, so it is effective against arthralgia due to cold in meridians or common cold due to exogenous pathogenic wind and cold.

1.4.2.1.31 Boyangchi

LOCATION On the dorsum of the forearm, 3 cun posterior to Yiwofeng.

MANIPULATION Nipping the acupoint with the nail of the thumb is called nipping Boyangchi, and kneading it with the tip of a finger is called kneading Boyangchi.

TIMES Nip 3 to 5 times and knead 100 to 300 times.

INDICATIONS Constipation, hot urination and headache.

CLINICAL APPLICATION Nipping and kneading Boyangchi play the role of relieving headache, promoting defecation and urination. Kneading more times is especially effective against constipation, but the method must not be applied to incontinent defecation. When it is used to treat common cold, headache and scanty hot urination, kneading Boyangchi is often combined with other methods of relieving the exterior and inducing diuresis.

1.4.2.1.32 Sanguan

LOCATION On the radial aspect of the forearm, the line between Yangchi and Quchi (LI 11).

MANIPULATION Pushing the acupoint from the wrist towards the elbow with the radial side of the thumb

节痹痛,伤风感冒。

【临床应用】 揉一窝风能温中行气,止痹痛,利关节。常用于受寒、食积等原因而引起的腹痛等症,多与拿肚角、推三关、揉中脘等合用。本法亦能发散风寒,宣通表里,对寒滞经络引起的痹痛或感冒风寒等也有效。

31. 膊阳池

【定位】 在手背一窝风后3寸处。

【操作】 拇指甲掐或指端揉,称掐膊阳池或揉膊阳池。

【次数】 掐3～5次,揉100～300次。

【主治】 便秘,溲赤,头痛。

【临床应用】 掐、揉膊阳池能止头痛,通大便,利小便,特别是对大便秘结,多揉之有显效,对大便滑泻者禁用;用于感冒头痛,或小便赤涩短少,多与其他解表、利尿法同用。

32. 三关

【定位】 前臂桡侧,阳池至曲池成一直线。

【操作】 用拇指桡侧面或食、中指面自腕推向肘,称

or the faces of the index and middle fingers is called pushing Sanguan. Pushing it from the lateral end of the thumb to the elbow with the infant's thumb flexed is called pushing Sanguan greatly (Datuisanguan).

TIMES 100 to 300.

INDICATIONS Deficiency of qi and blood, deuteropathic weakness, yang asthenia with cold limbs, abdominal pain, diarrhea, eruptive macule and sudamina crystallina, measles with incomplete eruption, common cold due to wind-cold and all other asthenia cold syndromes.

CLINICAL APPLICATION

(1) Pushing Sanguan is warm and hot in nature, and has the function of invigorating qi and promoting its circulation, warming yang and dispelling cold, relieving the exterior with diaphoresis. The technique is indicated in all asthenia cold syndromes, but should be careful with all syndromes which are not asthenia cold diseases. While treating cold limbs, pale complexion, inappetence, infantile malnutrition, vomiting and diarrhea caused by asthenic qi and blood, decline of fire in mingmen, asthenia-cold of the kidney and asthenic yang qi clinically, the manipulation is commonly used together with reinforcing Pijing and Shenjing, kneading Dantian, pinching Ji and rubbing Fu.

(2) The method is often combined in use with clearing Feijing, pushing Cuanzhu (BL 2), nipping-kneading Ershanmen to treat common cold with wind-cold syndrome, aversion to cold without perspiration and measles with incomplete eruption. It is also effective for invasion of the interior by rash toxin, jaundice, and puerperal jaundice, etc.

1.4.2.1.33 Liufu

LOCATION On the ulnar aspect of the forearm, the line between Yinchi and the elbow.

MANIPULATION Pushing from the elbow to the

推三关；屈患儿拇指，自拇指外侧端推向肘称为大推三关。

【次数】 100～300 次。

【主治】 气血虚弱，病后体弱，阳虚肢冷，腹痛，腹泻，斑疹白痦，疹出不透以及感冒风寒等一切虚寒病证。

【临床应用】

(1) 推三关性温热，能补气行气，温阳散寒，发汗解表，主治一切虚寒病证，对非虚寒病证宜慎用。临床上治疗气血虚弱，命门火衰，下元虚冷，阳气不足引起的四肢厥冷、面色无华、食欲不振、疳积、吐泻等症。多与补脾经、补肾经、揉丹田、捏脊、摩腹等合用。

(2) 对感冒风寒，怕冷无汗或疹出不透等症，多与清肺经、推攒竹、掐揉二扇门等合用。此外对疹毒内陷、黄疸、阴疸等亦有疗效。

33. 六腑

【定位】 前臂尺侧，阴池至肘成一直线。

【操作】 用拇指面、中指

wrist with the faces of the thumb or middle finger is called reducing Liufu or pushing Liufu.

TIMES   100 to 300.

INDICATIONS   All kinds of sthenia-heat syndromes including high fever, polydipsia, convulsion, sore throat, and constipation, etc.

CLINICAL APPLICATION

(1) Reducing Liufu is cold in nature and functions to clear away pathogenic heat, cool blood and detoxicate. It can be applied to all sthenia-heat syndromes such as invasion of yingfen (nutrient-system) and xuefen (blood system) by SFC pathogens, visceral heat stasis and food retention, high fever and polydipsia. Reducing Liufu combined with reinforcing Pijing has the effect of stopping sweat. But for infants with loose stools or diarrhea due to splenic asthenia, this method should be used with great care.

(2) Reducing Liufu is strongly cold in nature, while pushing Sanguan is greatly hot. They can be used singly or in combination. If an infant patient is of debility with asthenia qi and aversion to cold, pushing Sanguan is given alone; if high fever, polydipsia and macular eruption occur to a child, reducing Liufu is singly operated. When used together, manipulating the two acupoints can balance yin and yang, avoid injuring healthy qi with strong cold or heat. If the problem is cold-heat complicated syndrome and heat is the dominant, the manipulation is done in the way of reducing Liufu 3 times plus pushing Sanguan once, otherwise pushing Sanguan 3 times and reducing Liufu once for cases with cold as the dominant.

1.4.2.1.34 Tianheshui

LOCATION   In the middle of the forearm, the line between Zongjin and Quze (PC 3).

MANIPULATION   Pushing the acupoint from the

面自肘推向腕,称退六腑或推六腑。

【次数】   100～300 次。

【主治】   一切实热病证。高热,烦渴,惊风,咽痛,大便秘结干燥等。

【临床应用】

(1) 退六腑性寒凉,能清热、凉血、解毒。对温病邪入营血,脏腑郁热积滞,壮热烦渴等实热证均可应用。本穴与补脾经合用,有止汗之效。若患儿平素大便溏薄或脾虚腹泻者,慎用本法。

(2) 本法与推三关为大凉大热之法,可单用,亦可合用。若患儿气虚体弱,畏寒怕冷,可单用推三关,如高热烦渴、发斑等可单用退六腑。而两穴合用能平衡阴阳,防止大凉大热,伤其正气。如寒热夹杂,以热为主,则可以退六腑三数,推三关一数之比推之;若以寒为重,则可以推三关三数,退六腑一数之比推之。

34. 天河水

【定位】   前臂正中,总筋至曲泽成一直线。

【操作】   用食、中二指面

wrist to the elbow with the faces of the index and middle fingers is called clearing Tianheshui. The manipulation of striking up and down with the index and middle fingers dipped into water from Zongjin to Quze (PC 3) just like plucking a string and giving cold puffs to the acupoint while striking is called Dama Guotianhe (Beating the Horse to Cross the Heaven River).

TIMES　100 to 300.

INDICATIONS　Exogenous fever, tidal fever, endopyrexia, restlessness, thirst, wagging tongue, sublingual swelling, convulsion and all other pyretic symptoms.

CLINICAL APPLICATION

(1) Clearing Tianheshui is slightly cool and moderate in nature, which has the action of clearing away heat, relieving the exterior, removing fire and relieving restlessness. When it is used to treat heat syndromes, it clears away heat without injuring yin, so it is often used to treat feverish sensation over five centres, dry throat, ulcer on the lip and tongue, night crying. The method is also used together with opening Tianmen, pushing Kangong and arc-pushing Taiyang (EX-HN5) to treat common cold with fever.

(2) Dama Guotianhe has stronger effect in clearing away pathogenic heat than clearing Tianheshui, so it is commonly used for sthenia fever and high fever.

1.4.2.2　Acupoints on the Head and Face

1.4.2.2.1　Tianmen (Cuanzhu)

LOCATION　The line from the midpoint between the two eyebrows up to the anterior hairline.

MANIPULATION　Pushing the acupoint straight upward with both thumbs alternately is called pushing Cuanzhu.

TIMES　30 to 50.

INDICATIONS　Fever, headache, cold, listlessness, and terrified restlessness, etc.

自腕推向肘,称清天河水;用食、中二指沾水自总筋处,一起一落弹打如弹琴状,边打边吹凉气随之,直至曲泽,称打马过天河。

【次数】　100～300 次。

【主治】　外感发热,潮热,内热,烦躁不安,口渴,弄舌,重舌,惊风等一切热证。

【临床应用】

(1) 清天河水性微凉,较平和,能清热解表,泻火除烦,用于治疗热性病证,清热而不伤阴分。多用于五心烦热、口燥咽干、唇舌生疮、夜啼等症;对于感冒发热,常与开天门、推坎宫、运太阳等合用。

(2) 打马过天河清热之力大于清天河水,多用于实热、高热等症。

(二) 头面部穴位

1. 天门(攒竹)

【定位】　两眉中间至前发际成一直线。

【操作】　两拇指自下而上交替直推,称开天门或推攒竹。

【次数】　30～50 次。

【主治】　发热,头痛,感冒,精神委靡,惊惕不安等。

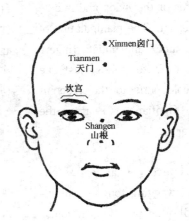

Fig. 18 - 2　Specific Acupoints for Infantile Tuina（on the Face）
图 18 - 2　小儿推拿特定穴位（面部）

CLINICAL APPLICATION　Pushing Cuanzhu functions to dispel wind and relieve the exterior, restore consciousness and induce resuscitation, tranquilize and ease the mind, which is often used together with pushing Kangong and kneading Taiyang（EX-HN 5）to treat exogenous fever and headache, etc. Terrified restlessness and dysphoria are treated with the method in combination with clearing Ganjing and pressing-kneading Baihui（GV 20）.

1.4.2.2.2　Kangong

LOCATION　The transverse line from the inner end to the outer end of the eyebrow.

MANIPULATION　Pushing the acupoints separately from the inner end of the eyebrow to the outer end with both thumbs is called pushing Kangong.

TIMES　30 to 50.

INDICATIONS　Exogenous fever, convulsion, headache and conjunctival congestion with pain.

CLINICAL APPLICATION　Pushing Kangong has an action of dispelling wind and relieving the exterior, restoring

【临床应用】　推攒竹能疏风解表，开窍醒脑，镇静安神。常用于外感发热、头痛等症，多与推坎宫、揉太阳等合用；若惊惕不安，烦躁不宁多与清肝经、按揉百会等合用。

2. 坎宫

【定位】　自眉头起沿眉向眉梢成一横线。

【操作】　两拇指自眉心向眉梢作分推，称推坎宫。

【次数】　30~50 次。

【主治】　外感发热，惊风，头痛，目赤痛。

【临床应用】　推坎宫能疏风解表，醒脑明目，止头痛。

consciousness and improving vision, relieving headache, which is often used together with pushing Cuanzhu, kneading Taiyang（EX-HN5）to treat exogenous fever and headache. When used for conjunctival congestion with pain, it is often combined in use with clearing Ganjing, nipping-kneading Xiaotianxin and clearing Tianheshui. Or after pushing, pricking the acupoint to let out blood or nipping and pressing method is added to reinforce the therapeutic effect.

1.4.2.2.3　Shangen

LOCATION　Between the inner canthi of both eyes.

MANIPULATION　Nipping the acupoint with the nail of the thumb is called nipping Shangen.

TIMES　3 to 5.

INDICATIONS　Convulsion and twitch.

CLINICAL APPLICATION　Nipping Shangan has the effect of inducing resuscitation, activating the eye and tranquilizing the mind, which is often used together with nipping Renzhong（GV 26）and Laolong to treat convulsion, coma and twitch. In addition to treating diseases, the acupoint can also be used in diagnosis. For example, occurrence of visible bluish vein on the acupoint indicates splenogastric asthenia cold or convulsion.

1.4.2.2.4　Yaguan

LOCATION　1 cun inferior to the ear, in the depression of the lower jaw bone.

MANIPULATION　Pressing the acupoint with the thumb is called pressing Yaguan, and kneading it with the index finger is called kneading Yaguan.

TIMES　5 to 10.

INDICATIONS　Trismus and facial distortion.

CLINICAL APPLICATION　Pressing Yaguan is mainly used for trismus, while kneading Yaguan

常用于外感发热、头痛,多与推攒竹、揉太阳等合用;若用于治疗目赤痛,多和清肝经、掐揉小天心、清河水等合用。亦可推后点刺放血或用掐按法,以增强疗效。

3. 山根

【定位】　两目内眦之间。

【操作】　拇指甲掐,称掐山根。

【次数】　3~5 次。

【主治】　惊风,抽搐。

【临床应用】　掐山根有开关窍,醒目定神的作用,对惊风、昏迷、抽搐等症多与掐人中、掐老龙等合用。本穴除用于治疗疾病外,还用于诊断,如见山根处青筋显露为脾胃虚寒或惊风。

4. 牙关

【定位】　耳下 1 寸、下颌骨陷中。

【操作】　拇指按或中指揉,各按牙关或揉牙关。

【次数】　5~10 次。

【主治】　牙关紧闭,口眼歪斜。

【临床应用】　按牙关主要用于牙关紧闭;若口眼歪

commonly for facial distortion.

1.4.2.2.5 Xinmen

LOCATION   2 cun above the midpoint of the anterior hairline, in the depression of the bone anterior to Baihui (GV 20).

MANIPULATION   Hold the infant's head with both hands, push alternately with the two thumbs from the anterior hairline towards the acupoint (only push to the border of the point if the fontanel hasn't been closed). This manipulation is called pushing Xinmen. Kneading gently with the tip of the thumb is called kneading Xinmen.

TIMES   Push or knead 50 to 100 times respectively.

INDICATIONS   Headache, convulsion, dizziness and restlessness, nasal obstruction, and epistaxis, etc.

CLINICAL APPLICATION   Pushing or kneading the acupoint functions to relieve convulsion, tranquilize the mind and induce resuscitation, which is often used for headache, convulsion and nasal obstruction. The front fontanel is normally closed 12 to 18 months after birth. Manipulations on this acupoint should be gently performed. Forceful pressing must be avoided in clinic.

1.4.2.2.6 Erhougaogu

LOCATION   In the depression inferior to the postauditory process and superior to the retroauricular hairline.

MANIPULATION   Kneading the acupoint with the tip of the thumbs or middle fingers is called kneading Erhougaogu.

TIMES   30 to 50.

INDICATIONS   Headache, convulsion and restlessness.

CLINICAL APPLICATION   Kneading Erhougaogu has the action of dispelling wind and relieving the exterior, so it can treat common cold with headache. It is often

斜,则多用揉牙关。

5. 囟门

【定位】 前发际正中直上 2 寸,百会前骨陷中。

【操作】 两手扶儿头,两拇指自前发际向该穴轮换推之(囟门未合时,仅推至边缘),称推囟门。拇指端轻揉本穴称揉囟门。

【次数】 推或揉均 50～100 次。

【主治】 头痛,惊风,神昏烦躁,鼻塞,衄血等。

【临床应用】 推、揉囟门能镇惊安神通窍。多用于头痛、惊风、鼻塞等症。正常前囟在生后 12～18 个月之间才闭合,故临床操作时手法需注意,不可用力按压。

6. 耳后高骨

【定位】 耳后入发际高骨下凹陷中。

【操作】 两拇指或中指端揉,称揉耳后高骨。

【次数】 30～50 次。

【主治】 头痛,惊风,烦躁不安。

【临床应用】 揉耳后高骨主要能疏风解表,治感冒头痛,多与推攒竹、推坎宫、揉太

used in combination with pushing Cuanzhu and Kangong and kneading Taiyang (EX-HN5). The acupoint also has the effect of easing the mind and removing restlessness, so it can treat dizziness and restlessness, too.

1.4.2.2.7 Tianzhugu

LOCATION The line from the midpoint of the posterior hairline to Dazhui (GV 14).

MANIPULATION Pushing the acupoint straight downward with the thumb or the index and middle fingers is called pushing Tianzhugu. Scraping it downward with a spoon dipped in water is called scraping Tianzhugu.

TIMES Push 100 to 500 times or scrape until mild ecchymoma appears.

INDICATIONS Nausea and vomiting, stiff nape, fever, convulsion, and sore throat, etc.

CLINICAL APPLICATION Pushing or scraping Tianzhugu plays the role of descending the adverse qi and stopping vomiting, expelling wind and removing cold, which is mainly used to treat vomiting, nausea, exogenous fever and stiff nape. To treat vomiting or nausea the manipulation is often coordinated with pushing from Hengwen to Banmen and kneading Zhongwan (CV 12). The manipulation itself is effective too, but more times of pushing are needed. To treat exogenous fever and stiffness and pain in the nape it is commonly combined with grasping Fengchi (GB 20) and nipping-kneading Ershanmen. Scraping Tianzhugu is done with the edge of a small Chinese wine cup dipped in ginger juice or cool water, scraping it downward until mild ecchymoma appears in local areas.

1.4.2.3 Acupoints on the Chest and Abdomen

1.4.2.3.1 Rugen

LOCATION 0.2 cun below the breast.

MANIPULATION Kneading the acupoint with the tip of the middle finger is called kneading Rugen.

阳等合用；亦能安神除烦，治疗神昏烦躁等症。

7. 天柱骨

【定位】 颈后发际正中至大椎穴成一直线。

【操作】 用拇指或食中指自上向下直推，称推天柱。或用汤匙边蘸水自上向下刮。

【次数】 推 100～500 次，刮至皮下轻度瘀血即可。

【主治】 呕恶，项强，发热，惊风，咽痛等症。

【临床应用】 推、刮天柱骨能降逆止呕，祛风散寒，主要治疗呕吐、恶心和外感发热、项强等症。治疗呕恶多与横纹推向板门、揉中脘等合用，单用本法亦有效，但推拿次数须多才行；治疗外感发热、颈项强痛等症多与拿风池、掐揉二扇门等同用；用刮法多以酒盅边蘸姜汁或凉水自上向下刮，至局部皮下有轻度瘀血即可。

（三）胸腹部穴位

1. 乳根

【定位】 乳下 2 分。

【操作】 中指端揉，称揉乳根。

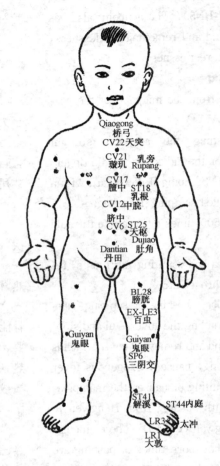

Fig. 18 - 3　Specific Acupoints for Infantile Tuina (on the Anterior Aspect of the Body)
图 18 - 3　小儿推拿特定穴位(全身正面)

TIMES　20 to 50.

INDICATIONS　Cough, asthma and stuffiness in the chest.

CLINICAL APPLICATION　See acupoint Rupang.

1.4.2.3.2　Rupang

LOCATION　0.2 cun lateral to the breast.

MANIPULATION　Kneading the acupoint with the tip of the middle finger is called kneading Rupang.

【次数】　20～50 次。

【主治】　喘咳,胸闷。

【临床应用】　见乳旁穴。

2. 乳旁

【定位】　乳外旁开 2 分。

【操作】　中指端揉,称揉乳旁。

TIMES 20 to 50.

INDICATIONS Stuffiness in the chest, cough, wheezing and vomiting.

CLINICAL APPLICATION Both kneading Rupang and kneading Rugen have the function of relieving chest distress to regulate qi, stopping cough and resolving phlegm. In clinic, the two acupoints are often used in combination and performed with the index and middle fingers together.

1.4.2.3.3 Xielei

LOCATION From the two hypochondria under the armpits to Tianshu (ST 25).

MANIPULATION Palm-twisting and rubbing the acupoints with both palms from the hypochondria under the armpits to Tianshu (ST 25) is called palm-twisting and rubbing Xielei, also known as Anxian Zoucuomo (palm-twisting and rubbing while touching strings).

TIMES 50 to 100.

INDICATIONS Stuffiness in the chest, pain in the hypochondriac region, phlegmatic dyspnea, infantile malnutrition, and hepatosplenomegaly, etc.

CLINICAL APPLICATION Palm-twisting and rubbing Xielei is opening and descending in nature, which has the action of guiding qi downward, resolving phlegm, relieving chest stuffiness and removing accumulation and mass in the abdomen. It is effective for chest stuffiness and abdominal distension resulted from indigestion, phlegm accumulation and adverse qi. For hepatosplenomegaly, long time of palm-twisting and rubbing is needed. But for patients with sinking of splenic qi and failure of kidney to promote inspiration the method should be used precautiously.

1.4.2.3.4 Fu (abdomen)

LOCATION On the abdomen.

【次数】 20~50 次。

【主治】 胸闷,咳嗽,痰鸣,呕吐。

【临床应用】 揉乳旁与揉乳根均有宽胸理气,止咳化痰的作用,临床上多两穴配用,以食、中两指同时操作。

3. 胁肋

【定位】 从腋下两胁至天枢处。

【操作】 以两手掌从两胁腋下搓摩至天枢处,称搓摩胁肋,又称按弦走搓摩。

【次数】 50~100 次。

【主治】 胸闷,胁痛,痰喘气急,疳积,肝脾肿大等。

【临床应用】 搓摩胁肋,性开而降,能顺气化痰,除胸闷,开积聚,对小儿由于食积、痰壅、气逆所致的胸闷、腹胀等有效。若肝脾肿大,则须久久搓摩,非一日之功。对中气下陷,肾不纳气者宜慎用。

4. 腹

【定位】 腹部。

MANIPULATION Pushing the acupoint along the border of the xiphoid angles or from Zhongwan (CV 12) to the umbilicus, then toward both sides of the abdomen is called parting-pushing Fuyinyang. Rubbing with the palm or the four fingers is called rubbing Fu.

TIMES Push separately 100 to 200 times and rub for 5 minutes.

INDICATIONS Abdominal pain and distension, indigestion, nausea and vomiting.

CLINICAL APPLICATION Rubbing Fu and parting-pushing Fuyinyang have the function of invigorating the spleen and stomach and regulating qi to promote digestion. They are very effective for disorders in infantile digestive function such as diarrhea, vomiting, nausea, constipation, abdominal distension and anorexia. In combination with nipping Ji and pressing-kneading Zusanli (ST 36), the manipulations may be used as a method of infantile health care.

1.4.2.3.5 Qi (umbilicus)

LOCATION On the umbilicus.

MANIPULATION Kneading the acupoint with the tip of the middle finger or the palmar base is called kneading Qi (the umbilicus). Rubbing it with the fingers or palm is called rubbing Qi. Holding the umbilicus with the thumb, index and middle fingers, shaking and kneading it is also called kneading Qi.

TIMES Knead 100 to 600 times and rub for 5 minutes.

INDICATIONS Abdominal pain and distension, indigestion, constipation, borborygmus, vomiting and diarrhea.

CLINICAL APPLICATION Rubbing Qi and kneading Qi have the action of warming yang to dispel cold, invigorating qi and blood, strengthening the spleen and

【操作】 沿肋弓角边缘或自中脘至脐,向两旁分推,称分推腹阴阳;掌或四指摩称摩腹。

【次数】 分推 100～200 次,摩 5 分钟。

【主治】 腹痛,腹胀,消化不良,呕吐恶心。

【临床应用】 摩腹、分推腹阴阳能健脾和胃,理气消食。对于小儿腹泻、呕吐、恶心、便秘、腹胀、厌食等消化功能紊乱效果较好,常与捏脊、按揉足三里合用,作为小儿保健手法。

5. 脐

【定位】 肚脐。

【操作】 用中指端或掌根揉,称揉脐;指摩或掌摩称摩脐;用拇指和食、中两指抓住肚脐抖揉,亦称揉脐。

【次数】 揉 100～600 次,摩 5 分钟。

【主治】 腹胀,腹痛,食积,便秘,肠鸣,吐泻。

【临床应用】 揉脐、摩脐能温阳散寒,补益气血,健脾和胃,消食导滞。多用于腹

stomach and promoting digestion to eliminate stagnation. They are often used to treat diarrhea, constipation, abdominal pain and infantile malnutrition. In clinic, kneading Qi, rubbing Fu, pushing up Qijiegu and kneading Guiwei are commonly used in combination, and they are chiefly known as kneading Guiwei, pushing Qijie, rubbing Fu and kneading Qi (Guiwei Qijie, Mofu Rouqi), which are very effective in treating diarrhea.

1.4.2.3.6　Dantian

LOCATION　On the lower abdomen, 2 or 3 cun under the umbilicus.

MANIPULATION　Kneading or rubbing it, which is respectively called kneading Dantian or rubbing Dantian.

TIMES　Knead 50 to 100 times and rub for 5 minutes.

INDICATIONS　Diarrhea, abdominal pain, enuresis, prolapse of the rectum, hernia and uroschesis.

CLINICAL APPLICATION　Kneading and rubbing Dantian function to reinforce the kidney to strengthen the body resistance, warm and reinforce kidney yang, and separate purity from turbidity. The manipulations are often used to treat abdominal pain, hernia, enuresis and prolapse of rectum due to infantile congenital insufficiency and cold accumulation in the lower abdomen, which are frequently combined with reinforcing Shenjing, pushing Sanguan and kneading Waiguan (TE 5). Kneading Dantian has certain therapeutic effect on uroschesis when it is used in combination with pushing Jimen and clearing Xiaochang in clinic.

1.4.2.3.7　Dujiao

LOCATION　On the large tendons, 2 cun under the umbilicus and 2 cun lateral to Shimen (CV 5).

MANIPULATION　Grasping the acupoint with the thumb, index and middle fingers is called grasping Dujiao.

泻、便秘、腹痛、疳积等症。临床上揉脐、摩腹、推上七节骨、揉龟尾常配合应用,简称"龟尾七节,摩腹揉脐",治疗腹泻效果较好。

6. 丹田

【定位】　小腹部（脐下2～3寸之间）。

【操作】　或揉或摩,称揉丹田或摩丹田。

【次数】　揉50～100次,摩5分钟。

【主治】　腹泻,腹痛,遗尿,脱肛,疝气,尿潴留。

【临床应用】　揉、摩丹田能培肾固本,温补下元,分清别浊。多用于小儿先天不足,寒凝少腹所致的腹痛、疝气、遗尿、脱肛等症,常与补肾经、推三关、揉外关等合用。揉丹田对尿潴留有一定效果,临床上常与推箕门、清小肠等合用。

7. 肚角

【定位】　脐下2寸（石门）旁开2寸之大筋。

【操作】　用拇、食、中三指作拿法,称拿肚角,或用中

Pressing it with the tip of the middle finger is called pressing Dujiao.

TIMES 3 to 5.

INDICATIONS Abdominal pain and diarrhea.

CLINICAL APPLICATION Pressing and grasping Dujiao are effective manipulations of relieving abdominal pain, which can be used for pain caused by all kinds of factors and is especially good for cold pain and abdominal pain due to improper diet. The manipulation can produce strong stimulations, so it is enough to grasp 3 or 5 times in short duration. In order to avoid infant patient's crying and not to hinder the performance, the manipulation may be done after all other manipulations have finished.

1.4.2.4 Acupoints on the Back

1.4.2.4.1 Jianjing (GB 21)

LOCATION At the midpoint from Dazhui (GV 14) to the acromion, on the tendon and muscle of the shoulder.

MANIPULATION Lifting and grasping the tendon of the shoulder symmetrically with the thumb and the index and middle fingers forcefully is called grasping Jianjing. Pressing the acupoint with a finger tip is called pressing Jianjing.

TIMES 5.

INDICATIONS Common cold, convulsion and difficulty in raising the upper limbs.

CLINICAL APPLICATION Pressing and grasping Jianjing play the role of facilitating the flow of qi and blood and relieving the exterior with diaphoresis, which is commonly used as a finishing manipulation at ending treatment in clinic. It can also be used to treat common cold and obstructive pain of the upper limbs.

1.4.2.4.2 Dazhui (GV 14)

LOCATION Refer to the adult acupoints.

指端按,称按肚角。

【次数】 3～5次。

【主治】 腹痛,腹泻。

【临床应用】 按、拿肚角是止腹痛的要法,对各种原因引起的腹痛均可应用,特别是对寒痛、伤食痛效果更好。本法刺激较强,一般拿3～5次即可,不可拿得时间太长。为防止患儿哭闹而影响手法的进行,可在诸手法推毕,再拿此穴。

(四) 背部

1. 肩井

【定位】 在大椎与肩峰连线之中点,肩部筋肉处。

【操作】 用拇指与食、中二指对称用力提拿肩筋,称拿肩井;用指端按其穴称按肩井。

【次数】 5次。

【主治】 感冒,惊厥,上肢抬举不利。

【临床应用】 按、拿肩井能宣通气血,发汗解表。临床上多用于治疗结束后的总收法(结束手法),也可用于治疗感冒、上肢痹痛等。

2. 大椎

【定位】 见成人穴位。

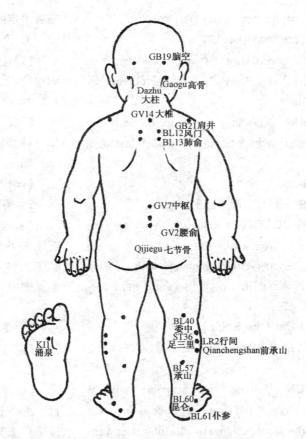

Fig. 18 - 4 Specific Acupoints for Infantile Tuina (on the Posterior Aspect of the Body)

图 18 - 4 小儿推拿特定穴位(全身背面)

MANIPULATION Kneading the acupoint with the tip of the middle finger is called kneading Dazhui.

TIMES 20 to 30.

INDICATIONS Fever, stiff nape and cough.

CLINICAL APPLICATION Kneading Dazhui (GV 14) has an action of clearing away heat and relieving the exterior, which is mainly used for cold, fever and stiff nape. Besides, lifting-pinching manipulation has certain effect on whooping-cough by lifting and pinching the acupoint with flexed index and middle fingers dipped in water

【操作】 中指端揉,称揉大椎。

【次数】 20～30 次。

【主治】 发热,项强,咳嗽。

【临床应用】 揉大椎有清热解表的作用,主要用于感冒、发热、项强等。此外用提捏法,以屈曲的食、中两指蘸清水在穴位上提捏,至局部皮下出现轻度瘀血为止,对百日

until mild ecchymoma appears in the local area.

1.4.2.4.3　Fengmen (BL 12)

LOCATION　1.5 cun lateral to the space between the processes of the 2nd and 3rd thoracic vertebrae, below the 2nd vertebra.

MANIPULATION　Kneading the acupoint with the tip of the index and middle fingers is called kneading Fengmen (BL 12).

TIMES　20 to 30.

INDICATIONS　Cold, cough and dyspnea.

CLINICAL APPLICATION　Kneading Fengmen (BL 12) is mainly used to treat exogenous wind cold, cough and dyspnea. In clinic, it is often combined with clearing Feijing, kneading Feishu (BL 13) and pushing and kneading Danzhong (CV 17).

1.4.2.4.4　Jizhu (the Spine)

LOCATION　The line between Dazhui (GV 14) and Changqiang (GV 1).

MANIPULATION　Pushing the acupoint straight downward with the faces of the index and middle fingers is called pushing Ji (the spinal column). Pinching it upward is called pinching Ji, which is commonly done 3 to 5 times. Pinching Ji 3 times then lifting the skin of the spine once is called Niesantiyifa, a method of pinching three times and lifting once. Press and rub softly several times on the back to relax the muscles on this area before doing pinching Ji manipulation.

TIMES　Push 100 to 300 times, and pinch 3 to 5 times.

INDICATIONS　Fever, convulsion, night crying, infantile malnutrition, diarrhea, vomiting, abdominal pain, and constipation, etc.

CLINICAL APPLICATION

（1）The acupoint Jizhu belongs to the governor

咳有一定的疗效。

3. 风门

【定位】　第2椎下（第2胸椎与第3胸椎棘突间）旁开1.5寸。

【操作】　食、中两指端揉，称揉风门。

【次数】　20～30次。

【主治】　感冒,咳嗽,气喘。

【临床应用】　揉风门主要用于外感风寒、咳嗽气喘。临床上多与清肺经、揉肺俞、推揉膻中等配合应用。

4. 脊柱

【定位】　大椎至长强成一直线。

【操作】　用食、中二指面自上而下作直推,称推脊;用捏法自下而上称为捏脊。捏脊一般捏3～5遍,每捏三下再将背脊皮提一下,称为捏三提一法。在捏脊前先在背部轻轻按摩几遍,使肌肉放松。

【次数】　推100～300次,捏3～5次。

【主治】　发热,惊风,夜啼,疳积,腹泻,呕吐,腹痛,便秘等。

【临床应用】

（1）脊柱穴属督脉经,督

vessel, which goes through the spinal column, pertains to the brain, connects the kidney, and has the function of governing yang qi and controlling renal yang. Pinching Jizhu upward has the effect of regulating yin and yang, smoothing qi and blood, regulating zang and fu organs, dredging the meridians, cultivating primordial qi and strengthening the body, which is one of the commonly used manipulations for child health care. Clinically it is often used in coordination with reinforcing Pijing, reinforcing Shenjing, pushing Sanguan, rubbing Fu, pressing and kneading Zusanli (ST 36) to treat some chronic diseases due to congenital insufficiency and postnatal deficiency with certain effect. When used alone, the method is known as the therapy of pinching the spine, which is used not only for infantile malnutrition and diarrhea, but also for insomnia, gastrointestinal diseases and irregular menstruation in adult. While performed, the manipulation may involve the bladder meridian of foot-taiyang. So selection of lifting heavily this point or pressing and kneading corresponding Back-Shu acupoints may be used to enhance curative results according to different cases clinically.

(2) Pushing Jizhu from top to bottom has the effect of clearing away pathogenic heat, which often combines in use with clearing Tianheshui, reducing Liufu and pushing Yongquan (KI 1).

1.4.2.4.5 Qijiegu

LOCATION   The line from the 4th lumbar vertebra to the end of the coccyx, or Changqiang (GV 1).

MANIPULATION   Pushing the acupoint straight upward with the radial side of the thumb or the faces of the index and middle fingers is called pushing-up Qijiegu, and pushing downward is called pushing-down Qijiegu.

TIMES   100 to 300.

INDICATIONS   Diarrhea, constipation and prolapse

脉贯脊属脑络肾,督率阳气,统摄真元。用捏脊法自下而上能调阴阳,理气血,和脏腑,通经络,培元气,具有强健身体的功能,是小儿保健常用主要手法之一。临床上多与补脾经、补肾经、推三关、摩腹、按揉足三里等配合应用,治疗先、后天不足的一些慢性病证,均有一定的效果。本法单用名捏脊疗法,不仅常用于小儿疳积、腹泻等,还可应用于成人失眠、肠胃病、月经不调等。本法操作时亦旁及足太阳膀胱经脉,临床应用时可根据不同的病情,重提或按揉相应的背部俞穴,能加强疗效。

(2) 推脊柱穴从上至下,能清热,多与清河水、退六腑、推涌泉等合用。

5. 七节骨

【定位】 第4腰椎至尾骨端(长强)成一直线。

【操作】 用拇指桡侧面或食、中二指面自下向上或自上向下作直推,分别称为推上七节和推下七节。

【次数】 100~300次。

【主治】 泄泻,便秘,脱

of the rectum.

CLINICAL APPLICATION

(1) Pushing-up Qijiegu has the function of warming yang to relieve diarrhea, which is commonly used for asthenia-cold diarrhea and chronic dysentery, etc. It is often used clinically with pressing and kneading Baihui (GV 20) and kneading Dantian to treat enuresis and prolapse of the rectum caused by sinking of spleen qi. This method is not suitable for disorders of sthenia-heat syndrome because it may induce abdominal distension or other problems in infant patients.

(2) Pushing-down Qijiegu has an action of purging heat to promote defecation and is often used for constipation and dysentery, etc. due to heat accumulation in the intestine. If diarrhea belongs to asthenia-cold syndrome, pushing-down Qijiegu must not be used in case chronic diarrhea could be induced.

1.4.2.4.6　Guiwei

LOCATION　At the end of the coccyx.

MANIPULATION　Kneading the acupoint with the tip of the thumb or the middle finger is called kneading Guiwei.

TIMES　100 to 300.

INDICATIONS　Diarrhea, constipation, prolapse of the rectum and enuresis.

CLINICAL APPLICATION　Guiwei is just the acupoint Changqiang (GV 1) of the governor vessel. Kneading it has the effect of regulating qi of the governor vessel and the function of the large intestine. The acupoint is moderate in nature and can stop diarrhea or promote defecation, which is often used together with kneading Ji and pushing Qijiegu in the treatment of diarrhea and constipation.

1.4.2.5　Acupoints on the Lower Limbs.

1.4.2.5.1　Jimen

LOCATION　On the medial aspect of the thigh, the

肛。

【临床应用】

(1) 推上七节骨能温阳止泻,多用于虚寒腹泻、久痢等症。临床上常与按揉百会、揉丹田等合用治疗气虚下陷所致的脱肛、遗尿等症。若属实热证,则不宜用本法,用后多令儿腹胀或出现其他变症。

(2) 推下七节骨能泻热通便,多用于肠热便秘、痢疾等症。若腹泻属虚寒者,不可用本法,以防滑泄。

6. 龟尾

【定位】　尾骨端。

【操作】　拇指端或中指端揉,称揉龟尾。

【次数】　100~300次。

【主治】　泄泻,便秘,脱肛,遗尿。

【临床应用】　龟尾穴即督脉经之长强穴,揉之有通调督脉之经气,调理大肠的作用。该穴性平和,能止泻,也能通便;多与揉脐、推七节骨配合应用,以治腹泻、便秘等症。

(五) 下肢部穴位

1. 箕门

【定位】　大腿内侧,膝盖

line from the superior border of the knee to the groin.

MANIPULATION　Pushing the acupoint straight from the medial superior border of the knee to the groin with the index and middle fingers is called pushing Jimen.

TIMES　100 to 300.

INDICATIONS　Hot and difficult urination, anuria, and watery diarrhea, etc.

CLINICAL APPLICATION　Pushing Jimen is moderate in nature and has good effect of diuresis. In the treatment of uroschesis it is often used with kneading Dantian and pressing and kneading Sanyinjiao (SP 6). For hot and difficult urination, it is commonly combined in use with clearing Xiaochang.

1.4.2.5.2　Baichong

LOCATION　On the thick muscles of the medial aspect above the knee.

MANIPULATION　Pressing or grasping the acupoint is called pressing Baichong or grasping Baichong.

TIMES　5 to 10.

INDICATIONS　Spasm in the limbs, flaccidity and lameness in the lower extremities.

CLINICAL APPLICATION　Pressing and grasping Baichong has the function of activating the meridians and relieving spasm. In the treatment of paralysis and arthralgia of the lower limbs the method is often used together with grasping Weizhong (BL 40), pressing and kneading Zusanli (ST 36). To treat convulsion and spasm forceful manipulation should be given.

1.4.2.5.3　Qianchengshan

LOCATION　Lateral to the tibia of the foreleg, opposite to Houchengshan.

MANIPULATION　Nipping or kneading the acupoint is called nipping Qianchengshan or kneading Qianchengshan.

上缘至腹股沟成一直线。

【操作】　用食、中二指自膝盖内上缘至腹股沟部作直推法,称推箕门。

【次数】　100～300 次。

【主治】　小便赤涩不利,尿闭,水泻等。

【临床应用】　推箕门性平和,有较好的利尿作用。用于尿潴留多与揉丹田、按揉三阴交等合用,用于小便赤涩不利多与清小肠等合用。

2. 百虫

【定位】　膝上内侧肌肉丰厚处。

【操作】　或按或拿,称按百虫或拿百虫。

【次数】　5～10 次。

【主治】　四肢抽搐,下肢痿躄。

【临床应用】　按、拿百虫能通经络,止抽搐,多用于下肢瘫痪及痹痛等症,常与拿委中、按揉足三里等合用。若用于惊风、抽搐,手法刺激宜重。

3. 前承山

【定位】　前腿胫骨旁,与后承山相对处。

【操作】　掐或揉本穴,称掐前承山或揉前承山。

TIMES Nip 5 times and knead 30 times.

INDICATIONS Convulsion and spasm in the lower limb.

CLINICAL APPLICATION Nipping and kneading the acupoint is mainly used to treat spasm. The method is often used together with grasping Weizhong（BL 40）, pressing Baichong and nipping Jiexi（ST 41）in the treatment of opisthotonus and spasm in the lower limb, etc.

1.4.2.5.4 Pucan（BL 61）

LOCATION In the depression below the lateral malleolus of the heel.

MANIPULATION Grasping the acupoint is called grasping Pucan and nipping it called nipping Pucan.

TIMES 5 to 10.

INDICATIONS Syncope and convulsion.

CLINICAL APPLICATION In the treatment of infantile asthma, vomiting and diarrhea, pushing upward and nipping downward the acupoint are used. There was ancient record about biting the acupoint to treat infantile shock, which has the function of reviving yang for resuscitation. This method is also called Laohu Tunshi（Tiger swallowing its prey）.

1.4.2.5.5 Houchengshan

LOCATION In the depression below the m. gastrocnemius.

MANIPULATION Grasping the acupoint is called grasping Chengshan.

TIMES 5.

INDICATIONS Pain and cramp of the leg and flaccidity of the lower extremity.

CLINICAL APPLICATION Grasping Houchengshan stops twitch and activates the meridians and collaterals. In combination with grasping Weizhong（BL 40）it can be

【次数】 掐 5 次，揉 30 次。

【主治】 惊风，下肢抽搐。

【临床应用】 掐揉本穴主治抽搐。常与拿委中、按百虫、掐解溪等合用治疗角弓反张、下肢抽搐等症。

4. 仆参

【定位】 足跟外踝下凹陷中。

【操作】 用拿法，称拿仆参；或用掐法称掐仆参。

【次数】 5～10 次。

【主治】 昏厥，惊风。

【临床应用】 治小儿哮喘，上吐下泻。用上推下掐法。古有记载小儿休克，以口咬此穴，可急救回阳，这种方法又叫老虎吞食。

5. 后承山

【定位】 腓肠肌腹下陷中。

【操作】 用拿法，称拿承山。

【次数】 5 次。

【主治】 腿痛转筋，下肢痿软。

【临床应用】 拿后承山，能止抽搐，通经络，常与拿委中等配合治疗惊风抽搐、下肢

used to treat convulsion and twitch, flaccidity of the lower limbs, pain and cramp of the lower limb.

All the above acupoints can be seen in Fig. 18.

1.5 Commonly Used Diagnostic Approaches in Tuina

Tuina therapy has a wide scope of indications. It involves diseases in traumatology, surgery, internal medicine, gynecology and pediatrics. In clinical practice, its examination and treatment should be conducted under the guidance of the basic theory of TCM and in combination with modern medical knowledge. That is to say, tuina treatment should be based on an overall understanding of a patient's general condition and local symptoms, a comprehensive analysis and a correct diagnosis by means of inspection, auscultation and olfaction, inquiring and palpation diagnoses in TCM as well as modern medical physical and laboratory examinations.

The common knowledge of inspection, auscultation and olfaction, inquiring and palpation diagnoses can be gained by reference to diagnostics of TCM. The diagnosis and examination of the spinal column and the limbs included in inspection and palpation diagnoses of TCM are important means of tuina diagnosis.

1.5.1 Physical Examinations of the Spinal Region

1.5.1.1 The normal functions of the spinal column

A normal spine has the function of ventriflexion, retroflexion, lateroflexion to the right and left and rotation. The cervical vertebrae can normally ventriflex 35°, retroflex 35°, lateroflex 45°and rotate 30°. The normal lumbar

---

痿软、腿痛转筋等。

（以上穴位均见图18）

第五节　推拿常用诊断方法

推拿疗法的适应范围广，涉及伤、外、内、妇、儿各科疾病，临床上在检查和治疗过程中强调以中医基础理论为指导，结合现代医学知识，即通过中医的望、闻、问、切四诊及现代医学的物理、实验室检查等手段，全面了解患者的全身情况和局部症状，对疾病进行综合分析，得出正确诊断，再加以治疗。

望、闻、问、切的一般内容，可参阅中医诊断学。在推拿诊治的望诊和切诊中，其对脊柱和四肢部疾病的诊查更具有特殊的临床价值。

一、脊柱部检查

（一）正常功能

正常脊柱有前屈、后伸、左右侧屈及旋转功能。其中，颈椎活动的范围是前屈35°，后伸35°，侧屈45°，旋转30°；

vertebrae ventriflex 90°, retroflex 30°, lateroflex 20°and rotate 30°.

1.5.1.2 Inspection diagnosis

Inspection diagnosis of the spinal area should be first concentrated in whether there is any change in the spinal physiological curve and whether there is any deformity of the spinal column. The normal spine has four physiological curves, i. e. the cervical anterior curvature, thoracic posterior curvature, lumbar anterior curvature and sacrococcygeal posterior curvature. In examinations, inspection should also be made on the abnormal conditions of a patient's posture such as spinal lateral curvature (scoliosis) or inclination, humpback, aggravation or lessening of the lumbar anterior curvature, pelvic obliquity.

Deformity of the spinal anterior curvatures (lordosis) mostly results from poor posture or infantile poliomyelitis. Deformity of the spinal posterior curvatures manifested in angular form like a hump is often seen in infantile rickets and tuberculosis of the spine. Deformity of the spinal posterior curvatures shaped as an arc with a stiff posture is often seen in rheumatoid spondylitis. Kyphosis in old patients commonly occurs in the thoracic section. Scoliosis often results from improper posture, different lengths of the lower limbs, deformity of the shoulder, rupture of the fibrous rings of the thoracic intervertebral disk, infantile poliomyelitis and chronic pathologic changes of the thoracic cavity or thorax. Scoliosis caused by improper posture may disappear on lying flat and bending the waist.

Attention should also be paid to the color of the skin, fine hair, swelling of local soft tissues. For example, coffee-color spots of different shape on the lower back indicate the existence of neurofibroma or proliferative fibrosis.

腰椎正常的活动范围是前屈90°，后伸 30°，侧屈 20°，旋转30°。

(二) 望诊

脊柱部的望诊，首先要注意脊柱的生理曲线是否改变，脊柱有无畸形。正常脊柱有四个生理弯曲，即颈椎前凸、胸椎后凸、腰椎前凸和骶尾椎后凸。诊查中要观察姿势有无异常，如脊柱侧弯或倾斜、驼背、腰前凸增大或减小，骨盆歪斜等。

脊柱前凸畸形多由于姿势不良或小儿麻痹症。脊柱后凸畸形，表现为成角如驼峰状，多见于小儿佝偻病和脊柱结核，后凸畸形为圆弧形、姿势强直，多见于类风湿脊柱炎；老年人后凸畸形多在胸椎一段。脊柱侧突畸形大多由姿势不良、下肢不等长、肩部畸形、胸椎间盘纤维环破裂症、小儿麻痹症及慢性胸腔或胸廓病变所引起。姿势不良引起的侧突畸形，可在平卧及弯腰时消失。

脊柱望诊时还要注意皮肤颜色、汗毛和局部软组织肿胀情况。如背腰部不同形状的咖啡色斑点，反映了神经纤

Too long fine hair in the lumbosacral area and dark skin suggest congenital sacral rupture. Swelling of the mesal soft tissue in the waist indicates bulge of the dura mater of spinal cord, and swelling in lumbar trigone of one side often means multiple abscess.

1.5.1.3 Palpation diagnosis

When palpation diagnosis is conducted, the patient takes a standing position or a lying position. Pressure pain points in spinal examinations are divided into superficial, deep and indirect tenderness. Superficial tenderness shows pathologic changes in the superficial layer such as that in the supraspinal and interspinal ligaments, while deep and indirect tenderness indicates that pathologic changes take place in the deep areas such as in the vertebral body, small joints, intervertebral discs. In most cases of strain of soft tissues in the back, myospasm and tenderness can be found in the affected area. For instance, strain of the interspinal ligaments can cause interspinous tenderness. Strain of the supraspinal ligaments has supraspinal tenderness. Strain of the lumbar fascia commonly causes tenderness and thick sense or myospasm or streak node beside the transverse process of the third lumbar vertebra. Strain of the lumbodorsal muscles has the reflection of tenderness and spasm of local muscles. In the case of rupture of the fibrous rings of the cervical and lumbar intervertebral disk, there can be found deep tenderness and radiating pain in the interspinal area and both sides of the diseased intervertebral discs. If there is only aching pain, or vague pressure pain point, or no tenderness at all, or a comfortable sense when the waist is being stricken with a fist, that is the sign of symptomatic lumbago of retroversion of uterus, nephroptosia, neurosism, etc. Pressure pain points on the back and lumbar regions

维瘤或纤维异样增殖综合征的存在；腰骶部汗毛过长，皮肤色深，多有先天性骶椎裂；腰部中线软组织肿胀，多为硬脊膜膨出；一侧腰三角区肿胀，多为流注脓肿。

（三）触诊

脊柱部触诊取站位或卧位。检查脊柱压痛点要分别浅、深压痛和间接压痛。浅压痛表示浅部病变，如棘上、棘间韧带等组织。深压痛和间接压痛表示深部的病变，如椎体、小关节和椎间盘等组织。腰背部的软组织劳损，大多数在病变部位找到肌痉挛和压痛，如棘间韧带劳损在棘突之间有压痛，棘上韧带劳损在棘上有压痛；腰筋膜劳损多在第三腰椎横突旁有压痛和肥厚感，或是肌痉挛，或有条索状结节。腰背肌劳损常伴有局部肌肉压痛或痉挛。颈、腰椎间盘纤维环破裂症，在病变椎间盘的棘突间及两旁有深压痛和放射痛。如果腰部只有酸痛，压痛点不明确，或者根本没有压痛点，用拳叩击腰部反觉舒适，往往是子宫后倾、肾下垂、神经衰弱等引起的症状性腰痛。背腰部的压痛点，亦应注意区别是否为内脏疾病在背腰部的反射性疼痛点。如心脏疾患有时可在左侧心

should also be identified whether they are the reflected pain points of the visceral diseases in this area. For example, heart diseases may sometimes have tenderness around the left acupoint Xinshu (BL 15), while the pressure pain point of diseases of the liver and gallbladder may appear at the right acupoints Ganshu (BL 18) and Danshu (BL 19). In clinic, therefore, careful and overall observation and examination are quite necessary.

1.5.1.4 Specific examinations

1.5.1.4.1 Percussion test on the vertex

The patient sits straight, and the doctor knocks the patient's vertex with one hand in fist separated by the palm of the other hand. If that causes pain in the neck, serial pain and numb sensation in the upper limb or pain in the lower back and lower limb of the affected side, the test proves to be positive, which indicates that the cervical or lumbar nerve roots are being compressed.

1.5.1.4.2 Test of squeezing and pressing the intervertebral foramen

The patient sits vertically, and the doctor presses the patient's vertex with both hands overlapped together and makes the cervical vertebrae squeezed and pressed from different directions. If that causes pain in the neck or nape or radiating pain, it indicates that the test is positive and the cervical nerve roots are being compressed.

1.5.1.4.3 Test of traction of the brachial plexus

The patient bends his or her neck forward. The doctor sustains the patient's head with one hand, holds the wrist of the affected side with the other and pulls in opposite direction. Pain and numbness in the diseased limb prove that the test is positive, which suggests that brachial plexus is being compressed and pathologic change in the cervical vertebrae exists.

俞穴处有压痛,胆、肝疾患可表现在右侧胆、肝俞穴位置处压痛,因此临床上必须要详细、全面地诊察。

(四)特殊检查

1. 叩顶试验

患者正坐,医者用拳隔手掌叩击患者头顶,如引起颈痛并有上肢串痛和麻木感,或引起患侧腰腿痛,均属阳性,提示颈或腰神经根受压。

2. 椎间孔挤压试验

患者正坐,医者用双手重叠按压患者头顶,并控制颈椎在不同角度下进行挤压,如引起颈项疼痛和放射痛者为阳性,提示颈神经根受压。

3. 臂丛神经牵拉试验

患者颈部前屈,医者以一手抵住患者头部,一手握患肢腕部,反方向牵拉,患肢有疼痛或麻木感为阳性,提示臂丛神经受压和颈椎病变。

1.5.1.4.4   Test of bending the neck

The patient is in a supine position and bends the neck actively or passively for 1 - 2 minutes. If pain is caused in the lumbar and lower limb regions, the result of the test is positive, which indicates that the lumbar nerve roots are being compressed.

1.5.1.4.5   Test of sticking out the abdomen

The patient lies on his back, sticks out the abdomen to cause the lower back and pelvis to leave the bed and gives a cough. Pain in the lumbus and leg shows a positive reaction, which indicates that the lumbar nerve roots are being compressed.

1.5.1.4.6   Test of lifting a straightened leg

The patient lies on his back with his legs and knee joints stretching straight, and then does raising leg movement one leg after the other. Measure the indolent angle of raising legs i. e. the angle between the bed and the lifted leg. The angle less than 60° shows the positive reaction, which indicates that the lumbar nerve roots are being compressed and lumbar vertebral pathologic changes exist.

1.5.1.4.7   Test of dorsiflexion of the great toe

The patient is in a supine position with his lower limbs stretching. The doctor presses the patient's great toes with his two thumbs, meanwhile asks the patient to flex them backward with force to cause counteraction in reverse directions. If the patient's strength of dorsiflexion decreases or disappears at the moment, it indicates that the test is positive and the 4th and 5th lumbar intervertebral nerve roots are being compressed and some pathologic changes have occurred in the lumbar vertebrae.

1.5.1.4.8   Test of the great toe's plantar flexion

The patient lies on his back and straightens the lower limbs. The doctor supports the palmar aspect of the

4. 屈颈试验

患者仰卧,主动或被动屈颈1～2分钟,引起腰腿痛为阳性,提示腰部神经根受压。

5. 挺腹试验

患者仰卧,将腹部挺起,腰部及骨盆离开床面同时咳嗽一声,如引起腰腿痛为阳性,提示腰部神经根受压。

6. 直腿抬高试验

患者仰卧,两腿伸直,在保持膝关节伸直的情况下,分别作直腿抬高动作。测量抬高时无痛的角度范围(抬高肢体与床面的夹角)。当夹角在60°以下,直腿抬高阳性时,提示腰神经根受压,腰椎病变。

7. 踇趾背伸试验

患者仰卧,下肢伸直,医者以两拇指下压患者两踇趾甲,同时嘱患者用力背伸踇趾,作相对对抗,如此时患者踇趾背伸力量减弱或消失,提示此试验阳性,为腰$_{4\sim5}$椎间神经根受压病变。

8. 踇趾蹠屈试验

患者仰卧,下肢伸直,医者以两拇指顶住患者两踇趾

patient's great toes with his hands and asks the patient to flex the great toes forcefully to cause counteraction in reverse directions. If the patient's strength of plantar flexion decreases or disappears at the moment, it indicates that the test is positive and the intervertebral nerve roots between the 5th lumbar and 1st sacral vertebrae are being compressed and some pathologic changes have occurred.

1.5.2　Physical Examinations of the Upper Extremities

1.5.2.1　The normal function of the upper limbs

Physical examinations of the upper limbs include the tests of the shoulder, elbow wrist joints. When the scapula is kept unmoved, the normal activity range of the shoulder joint is as follows: abduction, 90°; adduction, 45°; ventriflexion, 90°; retroflexion, 45°; internal rotation 70°-90°; external rotation, 30° and raising, 180°(abduction or procuration including rotating activity of the scapula). The activity range of the elbow joint includes flexion, 130°-150°; pronation, 80°-90°; supination, 80°-90°. While the dorsiflexion of the wrist joint is 30°-60°, volar flexion, 50°-60°, abduction, 15°-20°and adduction, 30°-40°.

1.5.2.2　Inspection diagnosis

Contrast examinations should be done in inspection diagnosis. Observations are first made on whether both shoulders are of the same height and whether both upper limbs are of the same thickness and length. Physical observations are also made on color of the skin and on whether there is deformity, swelling, phyma, and atrophy, etc. Erection of the scapula indicates congenital erect scapula. If the inner edge of the scapula stands backward, especially apparent when the hands are placed

掌侧,同时嘱患者用力跖屈蹈趾,作相对对抗,如此时患者蹈趾蹠屈力量减弱或消失,提示此试验阳性,为腰$_5$骶$_1$椎间神经根受压病变。

二、上肢部检查

(一)正常功能

对上肢部的检查,包括肩、肘关节等重点诊察部位。正常情况下,肩关节活动自如,当肩胛骨不动时,其活动范围外展90°,内收45°,前屈90°,后伸45°,内旋70°～90°,外旋30°,上举180°(外展或前屈加肩胛骨旋转活动)。肘关节屈曲130°～150°,旋前80°～90°,旋后80°～90°。腕关节背伸30°～60°,掌屈50°～60°,外展15°～20°,内收30°～40°。

(二)望诊

上肢部望诊必须两侧对比检查,首先要观察两肩部是否等高,两上肢是否等粗等长。外观其皮肤颜色情况,有无畸形、肿胀、肿块、肌肉萎缩等。若肩胛骨高耸,多为先天性肩胛骨高耸症,若肩胛骨内缘向后突起,尤在用手抵墙时更为明显,则为前锯肌瘫痪,

on a wall, it suggests paralysis of the serratus anterior muscle, also known as pterygoid muscle. In cases with acute injury, apparent swelling on the back part of the shoulder suggests dislocation of the shoulder joint or fracture of the scapula. Disappearance of deltoid tuberosity and formation of a square shoulder mostly indicates luxation of the shoulder. Compare the two shoulders and see whether the outer end of the clavicle has been stuck out and the affected shoulder has displaced downward, forward or inward. The former shows dislocation of the acromioclavicular joints or fracture of the outer end of the clavicle, and the latter is the sign of dislocation of the sternoclavicular joint or fracture of the clavicle. The elbow joint has a portable angle of 5° to 7° in a normal straightened position, and the angle in women is generally larger than that in men. Increase of the angle means cubitus valgus of the elbow, while decrease of the portable angle or inclination of the forearm to the ulnar side indicates cubitus varus of the elbow. The medial condyle and lateral condyle of the humerus and the olecranon of the ulna form an isosceles triangle, called elbow triangle in 90° flexion of the elbow. When the elbow joint dislocates, the normal relationship of the elbow triangle will be broken. When supracondylar fracture occurs, the affected arm often keeps a semiflexion position. When supracondylar extension fracture of the humerus or dislocation of the rear part of the elbow joint occur, the olecranon clearly sticks backward. In infant patients with semiluxation of capitulum radii, deformity of forward rotation of the forearm is often seen. Silver-fork shaped or bayonet-shape deformity is often seen in distal fracture of the radius. Radial nerve injury may cause ptosis of the wrist joint. Median nerve injury makes the thumb unable to do actions of opposing vola and abduction, the thumb and index finger unable to flex and do hyperextension. Atrophy of the major thenar results in monkey

又称翼状肌。对于急性损伤患者,如果在肩后部有明显肿胀,则提示可能有肩关节脱位或肩胛骨骨折。三角肌膨隆消失成"方肩",多提示肩关节脱位。对比两肩,看锁骨外端是否高突,患肩是否向下、前、内移位,前者说明肩锁关节脱位或锁骨外端骨折,后者则为胸锁关节脱位或锁骨骨折。正常肘关节伸直位时,有5°～7°的携带角,一般女性比男性度数稍大,携带角增大为肘外翻,减小或前臂尺偏则为肘内翻。肱骨内髁、外髁和尺骨鹰嘴在屈肘90°时呈一等腰三角形,称为肘三角,肘关节脱位时,肘三角即失去正常关系。髁上骨折时,患肢常处于半屈肘位,肱骨髁上伸直型骨折或肘关节后方脱位时,鹰嘴后突明显,小儿桡骨头半脱位者,以前臂旋前畸形多见。桡骨远端骨折可见到银叉状畸形或枪刺状畸形,桡神经损伤出现腕下垂;正中神经损伤,拇指不能作对掌、外展动作,拇指和食指不能弯曲,亦不能过伸,大鱼际萎缩,呈猿手畸形;尺神经损伤后,拇指不能内收,其余四指不能作内收和外展运动,第四、五手指指掌关节不能屈曲,小鱼际萎缩,呈爪形手。两侧近端指间关节呈对称性棱形肿胀,多为类

paw. Ulnar nerve injury causes the thumb unable to adduction, the other fingers unable to do adduction and abduction and the 4th and 5th metacarpophalangeal articulations unable to flex and extend. Atrophy of the minor thenar leads to claw hand. Symmetric rhomboid swelling of the interphalangeal joints of the proximal end on both sides indicates rheumatoid arthritis. Clubbed finger of the whole finger suggests pulmonary heart disease or bronchiectasis, or cyanotic congenital heart disease etc. As for diseases of infants under three years old, color of the finger vein (i. e. the radial superficial venules on the palmar surface of the index finger) may be used as references to determine severity of diseace. The 1st knuckle of the index finger is called wind pass, the 2nd qi pass and the 3rd life pass in pediatrics diagnosis. Normal finger vein is light red in color and looms in wind pass. Bright red finger vein is due to invasion of exogenous pathogen. Purple finger vein indicates pyretic pathogen. Dark blue suggests convulsion. And pale color is of asthenia cold syndrome. Abnormal color of finger vein seen in wind pass is the sign of mild diseases. When it gets to qi pass, the disease has been very serious. Its penetration through life pass shows a critical condition of the disease.

1.5.2.3　Palpation diagnosis

In palpation diagnosis of the shoulder area, it is necessary to understand its normal anatomic structure, movement range and bony marks. The acromion is at the highest bony projection of outer shoulder. Inferior to the acromion, the bony projection is the greater tuberosity of humerus. Anterior to the acromion is the outer end of the clavicle. The coracoid process is at the place superior medial to the head of the humerus and one-finger breadth inferior to 1/3 the crossing spot of the outer and middle clavicle. In palpation diagnosis, careful examination

风湿性关节炎；整个手指呈杵状指，多为肺原性心脏病，支气管扩张或发绀型先天性心脏病等疾患，3 岁以下的婴幼儿疾病，望指纹（在食指掌面桡侧的浅表静脉）的颜色可作为辨别病情轻重的参考。食指第 1 节为风关，第 2 节为气关，第 3 节为命关。正常指纹，色呈浅红，隐现于风关之内。如纹色鲜红为感受外邪，色紫为热，色青为惊风，色淡多属虚寒证。纹色见于风关为病轻，至气关为病重，透过命关则病笃。

（三）触诊

肩部触诊，首先要了解肩部的正常解剖结构、活动幅度及其骨性标志。肩峰在肩外最高点骨性突出处；其下方的骨性高突处为肱骨大结节；肩峰前方为锁骨外端，锁骨外、中 1/3 交界处的下方一横指、肱骨头内上方为喙突。

肩部触诊时，用拇指详细检查，寻找压痛点，并注意关

should be made with the thumb to seek for tenderness point, to take notice of whether the joint structure is normal, whether there is abnormal condition on movement, friction sound and also to look out to exclude fracture. Examination of the tenderness point on the shoulder should be combined with that of functions of the shoulder joint to determine the locality of pathologic change. Tenderness point on the anterior inferior area to the acromion denotes pathologic change around the minor tuberosity of the humerus. That on the external aspect of the acromion indicates pathologic change around the greater tuberosity of the humerus. Noticeable tenderness on the external humeral epicondyle suggests external humeral epicondylitis (tennis elbow), while noticeable tenderness on the internal humeral epicondyle shows internal humeral epicondylitis. Pathologic change of the ulnar nerve causes local significant tenderness and thickening sensation on the ulnar side lateral to the elbow and serial numbness on the upper arm. Limitation to abduction and adduction of the forearm indicates injury of the originating end of the internal and external flexor and extensor of the forearm or injury of collateral ligaments or avulsion fracture of the internal and external epicondyles. Tenderness on the styloid process of the radius is mostly caused by tenosynovitis of the short extensor muscle and long abductor muscle of the thumb. Tenderness on the palmar surface of the metacarpophalangeal joints is often seen in tenosynovitis of the 1st, 2nd, 3rd and 4th fingers. Tenderness on the central part of the wrist transverse bracelet of the palmar aspect accompanied by radiating pain and numbness of the fingers is the symptoms of carpal tunnel syndrome. Localized mass, which is palpable on the dorsal aspect of the wrist and can slightly move along the muscle tendon in vertical direction, but can not move in parallel direction, is usually thecal cyst.

节结构是否正常,活动时有无异常状态及摩擦音等,并应注意排除骨折。对肩部压痛点,须和肩关节功能检查结合,来判断病变的部位。如压痛点在肩峰前下方,一般是肱骨小结节附近的病变;压痛点在肩峰外侧,多见于肱骨大结节附近的病变。肱骨外上髁压痛明显,提示肱骨外上髁炎(网球肘);肱骨内上髁压痛明显,提示肱骨内上髁炎;尺神经病变,在肘后尺侧局部压痛明显且有肥厚感和上肢的串麻现象;若前臂外展或内收活动受限,则表示内、外侧前臂屈、伸肌起点或侧副韧带的损伤或内、外上髁撕脱骨折。桡骨茎突处压痛多系拇短伸肌、拇长展肌腱鞘炎;掌指关节掌侧处压痛,多见于第 1、2、3、4 指腱鞘炎。掌侧腕横纹中央区压痛且伴手指放射痛和麻木感,为腕管综合征。腕部背侧触及局限性肿块,且肿块可顺肌腱的垂直方向轻微移动,但不能平行移动者,通常为腱鞘囊肿。

1.5.2.4 Specific examinations

1.5.2.4.1 Abduction test of the shoulder joint

Loss of function of the shoulder joint accompanied by severe pain indicates dislocation and fracture of the shoulder joint. Necessity of careful abduction accompanied by abrupt pain suggests clavicular fracture. Feeling no pain at the beginning of abduction and worse pain as the shoulder raises horizontally indicates adhesion of the shoulder joint. Pain felt in the course of abduction and no pain felt during raising shows subdeltoid bursitis. Pain felt during abduction and within the range of 60°–120°raising, yet no pain beyond the range indicates tendinitis of supraspinatus muscle. Pain felt in the course of abduction and raising suggests periarthritis of the shoulder.

1.5.2.4.2 Test of the long tendon of the biceps muscle

Ask the patient to do extreme internal rotation, that is, with the elbow flexed to put the forearm at the back. If that causes pain in the shoulder area, it proves tenosynovitis of long head of biceps brachii.

1.5.2.4.3 Test of tennis elbow

The patient slightly bends his forearm and clenches a half fist first and tries to flex the wrist joint as much as possible, and then does complete pronation of the forearm and finally straightens the elbow. If at that time, pain is brought forth in the lateral aspect of the humeroradial articulation, the test proves positive, which indicates pathologic changes of the external humeral epicondyle.

1.5.2.4.4 Resistive test

The patient stretches his fingers and does dorsiflexion of the wrist joint, the examiner presses the patient's palm with his hand, and the patient flexes his wrist against the resistance. If pain is felt, the test proves to be

（四）特殊检查

1. 肩关节外展试验

肩关节功能丧失并伴有剧痛时，提示肩关节脱位或骨折。外展动作小心翼翼，并有突然疼痛者，提示锁骨骨折。外展开始不痛，越近水平位时肩越痛，提示肩关节粘连。外展过程中疼痛上举时反而不痛，提示三角肌下滑囊炎。外展到上举60°～120°范围内有剧痛，超过120°时反而疼痛消失，提示可能是冈上肌肌腱炎。外展至上举过程中皆有疼痛，可能为肩关节周围炎。

2. 肱二头肌长腱试验

让患者主动作肩极度内旋活动，即在屈肘位、前臂置于背后，引起肩痛者，提示肱二头肌长头腱鞘炎。

3. 网球肘试验

前臂稍弯曲，手半握拳，腕关节尽量屈曲，然后将前臂完全旋前，再将肘伸直，此时肱桡关节的外侧发生疼痛即为阳性，提示为肱骨外上髁病变。

4. 抗阻力试验

患者伸手指和背伸腕关节，检查者以手按压患者手掌，患者抗阻力屈腕，肘内侧痛为阳性，提示肱骨内上髁

positive and pathologic change proves to have occurred in the medial epicondyle of humerus.

1.5.2.4.5   Test of clenching a fist

The patient's diseased hand clenches a fist with the thumb inside and the four fingers outside and flexes the wrist joint toward the ulnar side. Pain in the styloid process of the radius proves the test to be positive, which indicates tenosynovitis stenosans.

1.5.2.4.6   Test of flexing the wrist

If flexing the patient's wrist joint to the extreme limit brings about numbness to his fingers, the test indicates carpal tunnel syndrome.

1.5.3   Physical Examinations of the Lower Extremities

1.5.3.1   The normal functions of the lower limbs

In the physical examination of the lower extremities, the focal point should be put on the test of moving extent of the joint as well as accompanied symptoms.

The normal functions of the hip joint are: flexion $130°-140°$, retroflexion $10°-30°$, abduction $45°-60°$, external rotation $40°-50°$, and internal rotation, $30°-45°$; those of the knee joint are: flexion $120°-150°$; while the ankle joint: dorsiflexion $35°$ and plantar flexion $45°$.

1.5.3.2   Inspection diagnosis

Observations are made on whether there are hyperadduction, shortness and deformity in abduction, abnormal conditions of length and thickness and atrophy of muscles in the lower limbs. Swelling of the hip joint can lead to plumpness of the groin. Lateral superior protuberance of the hip joint mostly results from congenital dislocation or semiluxation. Lateral inferior swelling of the hip joint chiefly belongs to pathologic change of the greater

病变。

5. 握拳试验

患手握拳（拇指在里，四指在外），腕关节向尺侧屈曲，桡骨茎突处疼痛为阳性，提示桡骨茎突狭窄性腱鞘炎。

6. 屈腕试验

将患者腕关节极度屈曲，即引起手指麻痛，提示腕管综合征。

三、下肢部检查

（一）正常功能

下肢关节的活动范围及其伴随症状，是下肢检查的重点。在正常情况下，髋关节屈曲130°～140°，后伸10°～30°，外展45°～60°，外旋40°～50°，内旋30°～45°，膝关节屈曲120°～150°，踝关节背屈35°，跖屈（向足底方向屈）45°。

（二）望诊

观察下肢有无过度内收，外展短缩畸形以及长短、粗细及肌肉萎缩，髋关节肿胀可见到腹股沟饱满；髋关节外上方突起多由先天性脱位或半脱位引起；而外下方肿胀多属大转子病变或因腰骶部感染，脓液流注引起。婴幼儿双侧臀

trochanter or is caused by infusion of pus because of lumbosacral infection. Asymmetry of the bilateral buttock rugae in infants often indicates congenital dislocation of the hip. A normal knee joint has only 5° of hyperextension. Hyperextension of more than 5° belongs to retroextension deformity or back knee, while inability to stretch straight is flexion deformity. Under normal conditions, the thigh and shank have slight eversion at 5° to 8°. If eversion is more or less than 5° to 8°, it is eversion deformity or inversion deformity. Swelling of the synovial bursa superior to the patella suggests bursal synovitis. Plumpness of the two Xiyan (pitting on both sides of the knee) and swelling around the knee is because of hydrarthrosis. Swelling of the tibia and the condyle of the femur or swelling of the metaphysis suggest bone tumor. Swelling of the tibial tubercle denotes osteochondritis. Rhomboid swelling in the knee area indicates tuberculosis of the knee joint or rheumatoid arthritis. Swelling in the medial and lateral ankles and severe pain caused by dorsiflexion suggest fracture of malleolus. Disappearance of the pitting inferior to the ankle, broardened calcaneus and pain in the ending point of the Achilles tendon suggests fracture of the calcaneus. Disappearance of the normal pittings inferior to both ankles and on both sides of the Achilles tendon accompanied by wavy sensation indicates hydrarthrosis or hematoma. If swelling is limited to one side, injury of the collateral ligament is often seen. Swelling in the posterior area of the foot indicates Achilles tendinitis, bursal synovitis, and hyperosteogeny, etc.

1.5.3.2 Palpation diagnosis

The patient is in a supine position. The examiner touches and presses forcefully with both his thumbs the area 2 cm around the midpoint of the inguinal ligaments on both sides and observes the response, or strikes the greater

皱襞不对称,常提示先天性脱髋。正常膝关节仅有 5°的过伸,过伸超过 5°为后翻畸形(或膝反张)。不能伸直则为屈曲畸形。正常情况下,大腿和小腿有 5°～8°的轻度外翻,如外翻超过或者小于 5°～8°则为外翻或内翻畸形。髌上滑囊区肿胀,提示滑囊炎,两侧膝眼饱满及膝周隆起肿大为关节积液;胫骨和股骨髁部及干骺端的肿大提示骨肿瘤;胫骨结节肿大提示骨软骨炎;膝部棱形肿胀,提示膝关节结核或类风湿关节炎。内、外踝处肿胀、背屈剧痛,提示踝骨骨折。踝下凹陷消失,跟骨增宽,跟腱止点处疼痛,提示跟骨骨折;内外踝下方及跟腱两侧的正常凹陷消失,兼有波动感,提示关节内积液或者血肿;肿胀局限于一侧,多见于侧副韧带损伤;足后部肿胀多属跟腱炎、滑囊炎、骨质增生等。

(三) 触诊

患者仰卧,检查者两拇指用力触压其两腹股沟韧带中点 2 cm 处,观察其反应,或用拳叩击大转子或足跟,若引起

trochanter or the heel with a fist. If pain in the hip joint is caused, pathologic change in this area is suggested. Superficial tenderness on the lateral side of the greater tochanter indicates bursal synovitis in this part. Tenderness on the edge of the whirbone denotes malacoplakia of the hip bone. Tenderness on the tubercle of the tibia indicates osteochondritis of the tibial tubercle. Tenderness on the point of attachment of the collateral ligament shows injury of the collateral ligament. Tenderness on Achilles tendon suggests pathologic change of the tendon itself or the membrane beside the tendon. Tenderness on the medial and lateral parts of the calcaneus indicates pathologic change of the calcaneus itself. Tenderness directly below the medial and lateral ankles on both sides of the calcaneus denotes pathologic change of the subtalar joint.

1.5.3.4   Specific examinations

1.5.3.4.1   Flexion test of both knees and hips

The patient is in a supine position and flexes his both knees and hips. Occurrence of pain at less than 90° of flexion indicates pathologic change in the hip joint. Pain between 90°- 120° flexion suggests pathologic change of the sacro-iliac articulation, and pain at more than 120° shows pathologic change of the lumbar vertebrae or lumbosacral joint.

1.5.3.4.2   Hyperextension test of the hip joint

The patient is in a prone position and straightens both legs. The doctor presses the patient's sacroposterior part to fix his or her pelvis with one hand and supports up the affected shank to make his or her hip joint hyperextend. Occurrence of pain at that time indicates pathologic change of the hip joint.

1.5.3.4.3   Percussion test of the foot heel

The patient is in a supine position and stretches both legs. The doctor raises the diseased leg with one hand and

髋关节痛，提示该部病变；外侧大转子浅表压痛，提示该部滑囊炎；髌骨边缘压痛，提示髌骨软化症；胫骨结节压痛，提示胫骨结节软骨炎；侧副韧带附着点压痛，提示侧副韧带损伤；跟腱压痛，提示腱本身或腱旁膜病变；跟骨内、外侧压痛，提示跟骨本身的病变；跟骨两侧靠内、外踝的直下方压痛，提示距下关节病变。

（四）特殊检查

1. 双膝双髋屈曲试验

患者仰卧将双髋双膝屈曲，当屈曲不大于 90° 时，即发生疼痛，提示髋关节病变；当屈曲 90°～120° 之时疼痛，提示骶髂关节部病变；当屈曲 120° 以上时疼痛，提示腰椎或腰骶关节病变。

2. 髋关节过伸试验

患者俯卧，两下肢伸直，医者一手按压其骶后部以固定骨盆，另一手托起患侧小腿，使髋关节过伸时疼痛，提示髋关节病变。

3. 足跟叩击试验

患者仰卧，两下肢伸直，医者用一手将患肢抬起，另一

hits his or her foot heel with the other palm. Pain in the hip joint indicates a positive result of the test and pathologic change of the hip joint.

1.5.3.4.4   Figure "4" shaped test

The patient lies on his back with the normal lower limb straight and the lateral ankle of the diseased limb placed on the normal limb over the knee. And the doctor presses the anterior superior iliac spine of the normal limb with one hand and presses the diseased knee downward with the other hand (forming a "4" shape). If pain in the test is too severe for the test to be continued at that time, it indicates pathologic change in the hip joint. If the pain does not hold back the test, it suggests occurrence of disease in the sacro-iliac articulation.

1.5.3.4.5   Grinding test

The patient takes a prone position, straightens the hip joints and flexes the affected knee to 90°. The doctor fixes the patient's thighs, holds the patient's affected foot with both his hands, squeezes the patient's knee joint and rotates his shank. If pain is caused, it indicates meniscus injury. Conversely, raise the shank to get the space of the knee joint widened, and then rotate it. If pain is caused, it suggests injury of the collateral ligaments.

1.5.3.4.6   Rotation test of the knee joint

The patient lies on his back. The doctor supports the patient's knee with one hand and holds the ankle with the other hand to have the knee joint do passive flexing and extending movements. If the patient's shank feels pain when it adducts and rotates outward and stretches straight, it indicates meniscus injury of the medial side. When the shank abducts, rotates inward and stretches, and feels pain, it indicates meniscus injury of the lateral side.

手以掌击其足跟,若髋关节处疼痛为阳性,提示髋关节病变。

4."4"字试验

患者仰卧,健侧下肢伸直,患肢外踝置于健肢的膝关节上部,医者一手压住健侧髂前上棘,一手下压患膝(形如"4"字),此时若疼痛不能完成试验的,提示髋关节部病变,但若疼痛,而能完成试验的,提示为骶髂关节部病变。

5. 研磨试验

患者俯卧,髋关节伸直,患膝屈曲至 90°,医者将其大腿固定,用双手握住患足,挤压膝关节并旋转小腿,引起疼痛者为阳性,提示半月板损伤;反之,将小腿提起,使膝关节间隙增宽,并旋转小腿,如引起疼痛,提示侧副韧带损伤。

6. 膝关节旋转试验

患者仰卧,医者一手扶膝部,另一手握踝,将膝关节作被动屈伸活动,当小腿内收外旋伸直时疼痛,提示内侧半月板损伤;当小腿外展内旋伸直时疼痛,提示外侧半月板损伤。

1.5.3.4.7　Drawer test

The patient is in a supine position, flexes his knee to 90°and relaxes the muscles. The doctor holds the patient's upper shank, pushes and pulls it forward and backward repeatedly. If the patient feels pain and has a dislocating sensation like a drawer getting off from its groove when the doctor does forward pushing, it indicates pathologic change of the anterior cruciate ligament. If pain feels and dislocating sensation of a drawer is gained in the patient on backward pulling of his upper shank, there must be the pathogenic problem of the posterior cruciate ligament.

1.5.3.4.8　Internal and external rotation test of the foot

The examiner fixes the patient's shank with one hand and holds his foot with the other hand, and then turns his ankle joint inward and outward to an extreme extent. If pain is felt in the same aspect, it indicates the possibility of fracture of the inner or outer ankle. If pain feels in the opposite side, it indicates paraligament injury.

1.6　Therapeutic Principles and Reinforcement and Reduction of Tuina

1.6.1　Therapeutic Principles of Tuina

Therapeutic principles are also called therapeutic laws. They are the general directive therapeutic rules drawn for clinical cases under the guidance of the fundamental theory of holism and differentiation of syndromes to decide treatment in TCM. Therapeutic principles are different from concrete therapeutic methods in that the latter is always decided by the former and based on a definite therapeutic principle. From the viewpoint of the relationship between body resistance or vital qi and pathogenic

7. 抽屉试验

患者仰卧,屈膝至 90°,肌肉放松,医生握小腿上端将其向前和向后反复推拉,如向前时疼痛并有抽屉滑脱感,提示前交叉韧带病变;如向后时疼痛并有抽屉滑脱感,提示后交叉韧带病变。

8. 足内、外翻试验

检查者一手固定小腿,另一手握足,将踝关节极度内翻或外翻,如同侧疼痛,提示有内或外踝骨折可能;如对侧痛多提示副韧带损伤。

第六节　治疗原则与推拿补泻

一、治疗原则

治疗原则又称治疗法则,是在中医整体观念和辨证论治基本精神指导下,对临床病证制订的具有普遍指导意义的治疗规律。治疗原则和具体的治疗方法不同,任何具体的治疗方法,总是由治疗原则所规定,并从属于一定治疗原则的。比如,各种病证从邪正

factors, for example, all kinds of diseases can be assorted into struggles between body resistance and pathogenic factors and changes of vicissitudes. Therefore, Strengthening body resistance to ward off pathogenic factors is a therapeutic principle, under guidance of which nourishing the kidney, strengthening the spleen and invigorating yang, etc. are concrete methods of strengthening body resistance, while diaphoresis, catharsis, etc. are concrete methods of eliminating pathogenic factors.

Diseases are manifested by quite different signs and symptoms. Pathological changes are very complicated. Cases vary from each other in degree of seriousness and emergency. Pathological changes and transformations are also different in different individuals, different places and at different times. Therefore, it is very important for a doctor to get hold of the primary cause of a disease from its complicated and changeable phenomena and do an active and correct treatment.

There are mainly the following principles in tuina treatment.

1.6.1.1 Treatment aiming at the primary cause of disease

Searching for the primary cause of a disease in treatment is one of the fundamental principles of differentiation of syndromes to decide treatment in Chinese Tuina. Searching for the primary cause refers to understanding the nature and the principal contradiction of a disease and conducting treatment aimed at the basic etiopathogenesis.

Ben or the origin or the root or primary cause of a disease is opposite to *Biao* or superficiality in relationship. They are a pair of opposite concepts and have several implications, which can be used to illustrate the principal and secondary relations of various contradictions in the course of pathological changes. As far as vital qi and

关系来讲，离不开邪正斗争，消长盛衰的变化，因此扶正祛邪为治疗原则，而在此原则指导下采取的补肾、健脾、壮阳等法，就是扶正的具体方法；发汗、通便等方法，就属于祛邪的具体方法。

由于疾病的证候表现多种多样，病理变化极为复杂，且病情又有轻重缓急的差别，不同的时间、地点，不同的个体，其病理变化和病理转化不尽相同，因此，要善于从复杂多变的疾病现象中，抓住病变本质，去进行针对性的积极治疗。

推拿治疗中一般主要有以下几方面的原则。

（一）治病求本

"治病必求其本"是中医推拿辨证施治的基本原则之一。求本，是指治病要了解疾病的本质，了解疾病的主要矛盾，针对其最根本的病因病理进行治疗。

"本"是相对"标"而言的。标本是一个相对的概念，有多种含义，可用以说明病变过程中的各种矛盾的主次关系。如从正邪双方来说，正气是本，邪气是标；从病因与症状

pathogenic factor are concerned, the former is *ben*, the primary, while the latter is *biao*, the secondary. Judging from the pathogenesis and symptoms of a disease, the former is *ben*, the primary, whereas the latter is *biao*, the secondary. As for location of pathological changes the viscera are *ben*, the primary and the superficiality is *biao*, the secondary. As regards the sequence of a disease the original or preceding diseases are *ben*, the primary, while the newly developed or accompanying ones are *biao*, the secondary.

Occurrence and development of any diseases are always manifested through some signs and symptoms, but they are only the phenomena of a disease, do not always reflect the nature of a disease and sometimes are even some false manifestations. Only based on a full understanding of all aspects of a disease, including its various symptoms and signs, through comprehensive analysis can a doctor grasp the nature of a disease beyond the phenomena, find out its primary cause and determine a correct corresponding therapeutic method. Take pain in the lumbus and the limbs for example, which can be caused by malposition of the vertebra, rheumatism in the lumbus and leg, strain of the lumbar muscles and many other problems. Instead of simple expectant treatment of arresting pain, therapeutic methods such as correction of malposition of the vertebra, expelling wind and activating blood, relaxing tendon and activating the meridians can be adopted respectively after finding out the basic pathological changes by means of general and comprehensive analysis. Only by doing so, can a desirable result be attained, and that's the real significance of treatment aiming at the primary cause of a disease.

1.6.1.2 Strengthening vital qi to eliminate pathogenic factors

The course of a disease, in a sense, is that of the

来说,病因是本,症状是标;从病变部位来说,内脏是本,体表是标;从疾病先后来说,旧病是本,新病是标,原发病是本,继发病是标等。

任何疾病的发生、发展,总是通过若干症状显示出来的,但这些症状只是疾病的现象,并不都反应疾病的本质,有的甚至是假象,只有在充分地了解疾病的各个方面,包括症状表现在内的全部情况的前提下,通过综合分析,才能透过现象看到本质,找出病之所在,确定相应的治疗方法。比如腰腿痛,可由椎骨错位、腰腿风湿、腰肌劳损等多种原因引起,治疗时就不能简单地采取对症止痛的方法,而应通过全面地综合分析,找出最基本的病理变化,分别用纠正椎骨错位、活血祛风、舒筋通络等方法进行治疗,才能取得满意的疗效。这就是"治病必求于本"的意义所在。

(二) 扶正祛邪

疾病的过程,在一定意义

struggle between the vital qi and pathogenic factors. In the struggle, if pathogenic factors predominate over vital qi, diseases will develop; otherwise if vital qi surpasses pathogenic factors, diseases will be subdued. So in treatment of diseases it should be done to support vital qi, eliminate pathogenic factors, change the ratio of strength between vital qi and pathogenic factors so as to make diseases change for better. Strengthening vital qi to eliminate pathogenic factors is also a fundamental principle guiding clinical tuina therapy.

An excess syndrome results when the invading pathogenic factors are exuberant, and exhaustion of vital essence brings about deficiency syndrome. Wax or wane of pathogenic factors and vital qi determine asthenia and sthenia of pathological changes. Asthenia syndrome requires reinforcement while sthenia syndrome requires reduction. Invigorating deficiency and purging excess is the concrete application of the principle of strengthening vital qi to eliminate pathogenic factors. Strengthening vital qi is a reinforcing method, which is indicated in asthenia syndromes, and eliminating pathogenic factors is a reducing method, which is applied to sthenia syndromes. Strengthening vital qi and eliminating pathogenic factors interplay of each other and supplement each other though they are two different therapeutic approaches with different implications. Strengthening vital qi is to strengthen the healthy qi or body resistance and is helpful in resisting and driving away pathogenic factors, while eliminating pathogenic factors can get rid of invasion, disturbance of pathogenic factors and their impairment of healthy qi, so it is helpful in retaining and restoring vital qi.

In clinical application of the principle of strengthening vital qi to eliminate pathogenic factors, it is advisable to make careful observations and analysis of the conditions

上,可以说是正气与邪气矛盾双方互相斗争的过程,邪胜于正则病进,正胜于邪则病退。因而治疗疾病,就是要扶助正气,祛除邪气,改变邪正双方的力量对比,使之向有利于健康的方向转化,所以扶正祛邪也是指导推拿临床治疗的一条基本原则。

"邪气盛则实,精气夺则虚",邪正盛衰决定病变的虚实。"虚则补之,实则泻之",补虚泻实是扶正祛邪这一原则的具体应用。扶正即是补法,用于虚证;祛邪即是泻法,用于实证。祛邪与扶正,虽然是具有不同内容的两种治疗方法,但它们也是相互为用,相辅相成的。扶正,使正气加强,有助于抗御和驱逐病邪;而祛邪则祛除了病邪的侵犯、干扰和对正气的损伤,有利于保存正气和正气的恢复。

在临床运用扶正祛邪原则时,要认真细致地观察和分析正邪双方相互消长盛衰的

of mutual growth and declination, wax and wane between vital qi and pathogenic factors and determine the primary and secondary relations and the order of priority. That is to determine which is put at the first place, strengthening vital qi or eliminating pathogenic factors. Or strengthening vital qi and eliminating pathogenic factors are combined with each other, or strengthening vital qi is done before eliminating pathogenic factors or vice versa. In combination of strengthening vital qi and eliminating pathogenic facotrs, the principle of strengthening vital qi without retaining pathogenic factors and eliminating pathogenic factors with vital qi unaffected should be followed.

1.6.1.3   Regulating yin and yang

The primary cause of occurrence of disease lies in the breakup of the relative equilibrium between yin and yang, i. e. the normal relationship of growth and declination between yin and yang is replaced by wax and wane of yin and yang. So regulation of yin and yang is also one of the basic principles guiding clinical tuina therapy.

Relative excessiveness of yin or yang refers to the excessive and redundant state of yin or yang pathogenic factors. Excess of yang leads to disorder of yin, and excess of yin results in disorder of yang. In treatment, an approach of lessening the excess or reduction method is used.

Relative deficiency of yin or yang means the deficient state of yin or yang in vital qi, which appears in the form of yin deficiency or yang deficiency. When yin is in a state of deficiency and unable to inhibit yang, asthenia heat syndrome will occur, manifested as hypofunction of yin and hyperfunction of yang. When yang is in a deficient state and unable to inhibit yin, asthenia-cold syndrome will appear, manifested as yang deficiency and yin excess. In syndrome of yin deficiency leading to hyperfunction of

情况,根据正邪在矛盾斗争中所占地位,决定扶正与祛邪的主次、先后。或以扶正为主,或以祛邪为主,或是扶正与祛邪并举,或是先扶正后祛邪,或是先祛邪后扶正。在扶正祛邪并用时,应以扶正而不留邪、祛邪而不伤正为原则。

(三) 调整阴阳

疾病的发生,从根本上说是阴阳的相对平衡遭到破坏,即阴阳的偏盛偏衰代替了正常的阴阳消长。所以调整阴阳,也是推拿临床治疗的基本原则之一。

阴阳偏盛:即阴或阳邪的过盛有余。阳盛则阴病,阴盛则阳病,治疗时应采用"损其有余",也就是泻的方法。

阴阳偏衰,即正气中阴或阳的虚损不足,或为阴虚,或为阳虚。阴虚则不能制阳,常表现为阴虚阳亢的虚热证;阳虚则不能制阴,多表现为阳虚阴盛的虚寒证。阴虚而致阳亢者,应滋阴(即补阴)以制阳;阳虚而致阴寒者,应温阳(即补阳)以制阴。若阴阳两

yang, treatment of tonifying yin should be applied to inhibit yang. And for syndrome of yang deficiency bringing about cold syndrome of yin, warming yang to inhibit yin is used. If yin and yang are both in deficiency, invigorating yin and yang is applicable.

1.6.1.4　Treatment of diseases in accordance with seasonal, environmental and individual conditions

This therapeutic principle means that in treatment of a disease an appropriate therapeutic remedy should be adopted according to different seasonal and local conditions, physique, sex and age of an individual. This is because occurrence and development of a disease are affected by many factors, such as seasons, climate, geographic-environment, especially by constitutional factors of an individual. Therefore, in treating a disease, all factors contributing to it must be taken into consideration, a concrete analysis of concrete conditions must be made and different conditions are dealt with in different ways, thereby working out a proper therapeutic method.

In clinical practice of tuina, special attention should be paid to the principle of treating diseases in accordance with individual conditions, by which different treatments are selected according to age, sex, physique, different living modes of patients. In general, if a patient has a strong physique, the location of manipulation is on the lumbus, buttock and limbs and the pathological changes take place in the deeper areas, manipulations with strong stimulations are performed. When a patient has weak physique or is an infant, the location of manipulation is on the head, face, chest and abdomen, or pathological changes are in the superficial areas, the degree of stimulations should be small. Other factors such as the occupation, working conditions of a patient which may be concerned

虚,则应阴阳双补。

（四）因时、因地、因人制宜

因时、因地、因人制宜,是指治疗疾病时要根据季节、地区以及人体的体质、年龄等不同而制定相应的治疗方法。这是由于疾病的发生、发展,是受多方面因素影响的,如时令气候,地理环境等,尤其是患者个人的体质因素,对疾病的影响更大。因此,在治疗疾病时,必须考虑各个方面的因素,具体情况具体分析,区别对待,酌情施治。

在推拿临床中,更须注意因人制宜。根据病人年龄、性别、体质、生活习惯等不同特点,选择不同的治疗方法。一般情况下,如患者体质强,操作部位在腰臀四肢,病变部位在深层等,手法刺激量大;患者体质弱,小儿患者,操作部位在头面胸腹,病变部位在浅层等,手法刺激量较小。其他如患者的职业、工作条件等亦与某些疾病的发生有关,在诊治时也应注意。

with the occurrence of some disease should also be taken into account in treatment.

1.6.2 Reinforcement and Reduction of Tuina

That asthenia syndrome requires reinforcement while sthenia syndrome requires reduction is one of the basic therapeutic principles of TCM. Reinforcement is to make up for the deficiency of vital qi. All kinds of treatment, which can supplement the materials lacked in the human body and strengthen the function of a certain tissue, are known as reinforcement. Reduction refers to purging or getting rid of pathogenic factors from the body. Therapeutic methods, which have the direct action of eliminating pathogenic factors in the body or inhibiting the hyperfunction of a certain tissue or organ are called reduction.

Reinforcement and reduction of tuina is produced by stimulations of manipulations. Manipulations are applied to certain parts of the body, which bring about some corresponding changes of qi, blood, fluids, the meridians and viscera, which can reinforce asthenic conditions, reduce sthenic conditions and regulate qi and blood with the result of curing diseases, preserving health and building up human constitution. Therefore, reinforcement and reduction of tuina can be obtained only by combining patient's concrete conditions with strength and directions of manipulations, their directions along or against the meridians, properties of stimulations and parts being treated. Commonly used reinforcing and reducing methods of tuina are as follows.

1.6.2.1 Reinforcing and reducing methods with light or heavy manipulations

Reinforcing method is manipulations producing mild stimulations. The manipulation is gentle, quick and long-term operation, such as light kneading and pressing,

二、推拿补泻

"虚则补之,实则泻之"是中医治疗的基本大法之一,"补"乃补正气的不足,凡能补充人体物质的不足或增强人体组织某一功能的治疗方法,即称之为"补"。"泻"乃泻除邪气,凡是有直接祛除体内病邪作用或抑制组织器官功能亢进的治疗方法,即称之为"泻"。

推拿中的补泻作用乃是手法刺激在人体某一部位,使人体气血津液、经络、脏腑产生相应的变化,补虚泻实,调和人体的气血,达到治病保健强身的目的。因此,推拿的补泻必须根据病人的具体情况,与手法的轻重、方向、经络的顺逆、刺激性质及治疗的部位结合,才能体现出来。具体常用的补泻方法有以下几种。

(一)轻重补泻法

补法是较轻刺激的手法,手法柔和、轻快,时间长,如轻揉、轻按能疏通气血,扶正补

which can promote flow of qi and blood, strengthen vital qi and reinforce asthenia. Reducing method is manipulations producing strong stimulations. This manipulation is heavy, strong and short-term performance with exertion of force changing from mild to heavy, such as heavy pressing and kneading, which can arrest pain and activate blood circulation so as to disperse stagnated blood and mass and relieve swelling to stop pain.

Modern medical research maintains that manipulations with light and weak stimulations can activate and excite physiological function and promote secretion of the glands. For example, for indigestion due to splenogastric asthenia, application of light, mild pushing and grasping manipulations with one-finger to acupoints Pishu (BL 20), Weishu (BL 21), Zhongwan (CV 12), and Qihai (CV 6), etc. with long-term, rhythmic stimulations can invigorate the spleen and stomach with good results. Heavy and strong stimulations of manipulation inhibit physiological function and reduce secretion of the glands. For instance, in the case of gastrointestinal spasm, digital-pressing and pressing manipulations with strong stimulations performed for short time on the corresponding spots on the back of acupoints Weishu (BL 21), Dachangshu (BL 25), etc. can relieve the spasm.

The above examples indicate that strong stimulation means reduction, while mild stimulation means reinforcement. However, the force of reinforcing and reducing functions produced by powerful or mild stimulations of manipulations varies with the constitution of individuals, threshold value of receiving stimulation of different stimulated parts. In clinic, it is marked off by the stronger or milder extent of aching and distending sensations caused in a patient, which, of course, is only an approximate value.

虚。泻法是较重刺激的手法，手法重而强，用力由轻入重，作用时间短，如重按、重揉，能止痛活血，以疏散凝滞结聚，消肿止痛。

现代医学研究认为，轻、弱的手法刺激能活跃兴奋生理功能，增进腺体分泌，例如：脾胃虚弱的消化不良，则在脾俞、胃俞、中脘、气海等穴位上用轻柔的一指禅推拿进行较长时间的节律性刺激，可取得健运脾胃的良好效果。重、强的手法刺激能抑制生理功能，减少腺体分泌，例如：胃肠痉挛时，则在背部相应的胃俞、大肠俞等穴位上采用点、按等较强烈的手法作短时间的刺激，痉挛即可缓解。

从以上看来，重刺激为"泻"，轻刺激为"补"，但这种因手法刺激的轻、重所引起的补、泻作用，其补泻的力量分界，是随各人的体质和各个不同刺激部位接受刺激的阈值而异，在临床上则是以患者有较强烈的酸胀感和较轻微的酸胀感来分别的，当然这仅是一个近似值。

1.6.2.2 Reinforcing and reducing methods with manipulations of right or left rotation

There are lots of records about the relationship between direction of tuina and reinforcing and reducing action in medical literature through the ages. It is said in the book *Xiao'er Anmojing* that nipping the point Pitu (spleen-earth), flexing the finger and rotating it leftward have the effect of reinforcement. And it is also said in the book *Youke Tuina Mishu* that left rotation means reinforcement, while right rotation is reduction. Though these statements are quoted from works on infant tuina, clinic practice confirms that they are applicable to adults too. The practical operation of this method is to manipulate on a certain part or point with the finger, palm or thenar eminance. Generally speaking, rotating clockwise produces reinforcing effect, and rotating counter-clockwise has reducing action. In abdomen tuina, if the direction of manipulation and the moving direction of the part being treated are both clockwise, which has marked effect of catharsis, this manipulation is known as reducing method. If the direction of manipulation is counter-clockwise and the moving direction of the part being treated is clockwise, which improves the digestive function of the stomach and intestine and has the effect of invigorating the spleen and stomach, this manipulation is referred to as reinforcing method.

1.6.2.3 Reinforcing and reducing methods with manipulation along or against the meridians

Tuina therapy and acupuncture, though they respectively have their own characters and functions, technologically, are somewhat the same in reinforcing and reducing principles. It says in *Neijing* that manipulation against the meridians for elimination means reduction, while manipulation along the meridians for strengthening effect

（二）左右旋转补泻法

关于方向与补泻的关系，历代文献中有较多的记载，如明代《小儿按摩经》上说："掐脾土、曲指左转为补"，《幼科推拿秘书》上说："左转补兮右转泻"。这些论述，虽引自小儿推拿著作，但临床证实成人临床治疗中亦很适用。这种方法具体操作是以指、掌或鱼际在某一施术部位或穴位施以手法。一般来说，顺时针方向旋转为补法，逆时针方向旋转为泻法，而在腹部摩动时，手法操作的方向与治疗部位移动的方向均为顺时针方向时，有明显通便泻下的作用为泻法；若手法操作的方向为逆时针，而在治疗部位移动方向为顺时针，则可使胃肠的消化功能明显增强，起到健脾和胃的作用，此即为补法。

（三）顺逆经补泻法

推拿治疗和针灸一样，从技术上来说，虽然各有各的特色，各有各的价值，但就其补泻原则而论有些是一致的，《内经》中有"……迎而夺之者，泻也，追而济之者，补也。"

means reinforcement. In tuina clinic, for cases in need of promoting smooth flow of qi and blood to supplement vital qi, tuina should be performed along the route of the meridians. For instance, some gynecological diseases, differentiated as asthenia syndrome, are treated by selecting some acupoints from the lower sections of the three foot yin meridians connecting with the diseases and applying long-time, gentle, quick manipulations along the direction of the meridians. They can also be treated by doing tuina manipulations along the meridians to promote abundance and smooth flow of qi and blood so as to restore the normal functional activities of some debilitated tissues and organs. This is a reinforcing manipulation operated along the direction of qi and also an invigorating therapy. For cases needing promotion of qi circulation and purgation, tuina should be performed against the direction of the meridians. For example, cases differentiated as sthenia-heat syndrome, tuina with heavy or pushing manipulation is performed upward on some points against the direction of the governor vessel, which is related to the disease, to get rid of pathogenic heat in the body. This is a method of reducing excess.

1.6.2.4 Reinforcing and reducing methods with to-and-fro manipulation

This is a most commonly used method in clinical tuina, which refers to doing various to-and-fro manipulations on points or parts of the body to promote circulation of qi and blood and regulation between yin and yang.

Apart from their heaviness and directions, reinforcement and reduction of tuina manipulation are also closely related to concrete stimulated areas or points. Therefore, in treatment selection of proper treated parts or points according to diseases is also very essential for gaining good

推拿临床中,需通而补者,应顺其经脉的走向进行推拿,如辨为虚证的妇科病,在与患病有关的足三阴经经脉下段,顺着经脉方向,选取穴位进行长时间的轻快手法,或顺其经脉施以推拿的手法,以促使气血旺盛通畅,使虚衰的组织器官恢复正常的功能活动,这就是随其气去而济之的手法,是一种补虚的方法。需行而泻之者,应逆其经脉的走向进行推拿,如辨为实证热病,可在与患病有关的督脉上,逆着经脉的方向,在经或穴上进行重手法按摩或推法,以祛除体内的热邪病气,这是一种泻实的方法。

(四)平补平泻法

这是推拿临床上最常用的一种方法,即在穴位或部位上操作时,以各种手法往返操作,以促使机体气血流通、阴阳和调,即为平补平泻法。

推拿手法的补泻,除了和手法的轻重、方向等有关外,还和具体的刺激部位(穴位)有密切关系,因此,治疗时还应根据疾病选择适当的治疗

results in reinforcement and reduction of tuina.

部位(穴位),这亦是取得推拿
补泻良好作用的关键。

1.7 Indications, Contraindications and Points for Attention in Tuina

第七节 推拿的适应证、禁忌证和注意事项

Chinese tuina is an external therapy with systematic unique rules under the guidance of the theories of yin-yang, five elements, zang-fu, meridians, qi, blood and body fluid in TCM. It conducts diagnosis, examination and treatment of diseases by employing the four diagnostic methods of inspection, auscultation and ofaction, inquiring and palpation and in combination with modern medical knowledge in anatomy, physiology and biochemistry of the human body. Here is a brief introduction of indications, contraindications and points for attention in tuina.

中国推拿是以中医的阴阳五行、脏腑经络、气血津液等理论为基础,采用望、闻、问、切四诊及辨证施治等方法,又结合现代医学的人体解剖及生理、生化知识来诊查疾病的有系统的独特规律的外治方法。本节简要介绍推拿的宜忌和注意事项。

1.7.1 Indications

一、适应证

Tuina therapy has extensive indications in many kinds of diseases involving osteonosus and traumatism, internal, gynecological, pediatric, eye, ear, nose and throat, and neurological departments. Nowadays, its indication has expanded into the areas of reducing weight, cosmetology, therapeutic health care, etc.

推拿适应证广泛,涉及到骨伤、内、妇、儿、五官、神经等各科疾病,目前且扩大到减肥、美容及保健医疗等方面。

1.7.2 Contraindications

二、禁忌证

There have been some induction and summary of contraindications in tuina from the past dynasties. Here are mainly some diseases or injuries, which tuina therapy must not be applied to.

（1）Areas with open soft tissue injuries and wounded portions, which are bleeding.

（2）All kinds of fracture in the early stage.

关于推拿的禁忌证,历代亦有归纳和总结,主要有以下一些方面。

（1）开放性软组织损伤和正在出血的外伤部位。

（2）各种类型骨折的

初期。

(3) Local areas injured by dermatosis.

　　（3）皮肤病病变损害的局部。

(4) Diseases with hemorrhagic tendency such as going down of blood coagulation mechanism and hemophilia, and acute stage of visceral hemorrhage such as hemorrhage of the upper digestive tract, splenic rupture.

　　（4）有出血性倾向的疾病,如凝血机制减退、血友病等和内脏器官出血的急性期,如上消化道出血、脾破裂等。

(5) Acute infectious diseases such as virus hepatitis, pulmonary tuberculosis, bacillary dysentery.

　　（5）急性传染性疾病,如病毒性肝炎、肺结核、菌痢等。

(6) Critical diseases of the heart, brain, liver, kidney and other viscera.

　　（6）危重的心、脑、肝、肾等脏器疾病。

(7) Women during menstruation and pregnancy, whose abdomen and lumbaosacral portion tuina manipulations producing strong stimulations should not be applied to.

　　（7）妇女怀孕期和月经期,不宜在其腹部和腰骶部使用过重刺激的推拿手法。

1.7.3　Cautions

Apart from the above contraindications, the following points should also be paid attention to in tuina practice.

(1) Tuina doctors should trim their fingernails regularly and keep their hands clean and warm in winter. While operating, they should not wear rings. In the operating, a therapeutic towel should be used to prevent injuring patient's skin or muscles.

(2) In the course of tuina, the massagists should observe and inquire about the reaction of the patient all the time and regulate the force of the manipulations so as to obtain good result of tuina by performing even, mild and persistent manipulation.

(3) In tuina treatment, syncope should be avoided for those who are hungry or have just finished violent sports. Once sensations such as dizziness, dim eyesight, severe palpitation with deficient perspiration occur to the patient, manipulations should be stopped immediately.

三、注意事项

　　除以上禁忌外,推拿工作中还应注意以下一些事项。

　　（1）推拿医生应经常修剪指甲,保持手部清洁,冬季保持手部温暖,施术时不戴戒指,操作时在病人身上敷以治疗巾,以免损伤其肌肤。

　　（2）推拿过程中,要随时观察和询问患者的反应,适时地调整手法力度,做到均匀、柔和,持久有力,切实地提高推拿的疗效。

　　（3）患者饥饿时及剧烈运动后,推拿时应防止其晕厥。若一旦患者出现头晕、眼花心慌、出虚汗等感觉时,应立即停止手法操作,让患者平卧,

Meanwhile have the patient lie down, drink some warm sugar water and press and knead acupoints Hegu (LI 4), Neiguan (PC 6), Zusanli (ST 36) and so on.

(4) Generally, treatment is given to chronic diseases every other day, while for acute cases daily treatment is often applied. Uncomfortable sensation caused by heavy manipulations may relieve spontaneously in 1 to 3 days. And the doctor should also modify his or her manipulation to adapt to the case's conditions.

喝一些温和的糖水, 并可以按揉合谷、内关、足三里等穴。

(4) 一般慢性病症隔日治疗 1 次; 急性病证, 多采用每日治疗, 若因手法过重治疗后不适者, 一般 1～3 天后多能自行缓解, 医者亦应变换手法, 以适应病情需要。

2 Commonly Used Tuina Manipulations

第二章 常用手法

Tuina manipulations are the direct means of tuina therapy. There are many kinds of operating skills and various forms of movements in tuina, which include butting with the head, tramping under the foot as well as continuous manipulations conducted with the finger, palm, wrist and elbow. They are directly applied to the body surface and stimulate the body by means of exerting force to treat and prevent diseases. Since most of the manipulations are done with hands, so they are generally called manual manipulations or hand manipulations.

Tuina manipulations should be persistent, forceful, even and gentle: Persistence means that manipulations should be continued for a considerable period of time. Forcefulness means that manipulations should be performed with adequate force. Evenness means that manipulations should be rhythmical with appropriate speed and steady force. Gentleness refers to light but not superficial, heavy but not unsmooth operations with natural and smooth shift of movements, which should by no means be performed roughly and violently. The above four points are organically related to one another. To skillfully command various manipulations it is necessary to carry out long and persistent exercise and practice. In practice, the exercises should be done orderly and step by step, following a process from being inexperienced to skillful, to perfect and to able to apply with proficiency. One should try to attain the realm of "once in clinic, manipulations applied outside with wonderful result produced inside, man-

推拿手法是推拿治疗的直接手段,其操作技巧、动作形式有多种,包括用手指、手掌、手腕和肘部等的连续操作以及如头顶、脚踩等直接施于患者体表,通过功力达到刺激机体而产生防治疾病的作用,因绝大多数操作还是以手进行的,故统称为手法。

推拿的手法要求持久、有力、均匀、柔和。持久是指手法能持续运用一定时间;有力是指手法必须具有一定的力量;均匀是指手法动作要有节奏,速度不能时快时慢,压力不可时轻时重;柔和是指手法要"轻而不浮,重而不滞",用力不可生硬粗暴,不可用蛮力,变换手法动作要自然。以上四点是有机联系的,要熟练掌握各种手法,必须坚持不懈地练习和实践。在练习过程中,要循序渐进,由生而熟,熟能生巧,及至得心应手,运用自如,以达到"一旦临证,机触于外,巧生于内,手随心转,法从手出"的效果。

ual techniques closely following the train of thought and good remedies coming from excellent manipulations. "

In order to exert better curative action in practical application, tuina manipulations should carry out TCM principles of differentiating syndrome to decide treatment, which refers to applying different hand manipulations to different syndromes. People may be divided into the old and the young, constitution into weak and strong, syndrome into asthenia and sthenia, size of the operated parts into large and small and muscles into thick and thin. So selection of manipulations and application of force should be adapted to the above different conditions. Any excess or deficiency in manipulation will affect preventive and curative results or even cause some side effects.

Chinese tuina has a long history and dates back to the ancient times. Its manipulations are as many as several hundreds. There are even some compound manipulations formed by combining two of them and used in compatibility such as pressing and rubbing, palm-twisting and kneading, pinching and grasping. In infant tuina, manipulations are also combined with massaged areas or points and actions, which makes manipulations even more distinctive and their names more figurative. Among the names are Longruhukou (Dragon Getting into the Mouth of Tiger), Dama Guohe (Whipping Horse to Cross River) and Shuidi Laoyue (Fishing the Moon from the Bottom of Water). These compound manipulations are even more helpful to improving therapeutic efficacy.

推拿手法在实际应用中，要发挥更好的治疗作用，必须贯彻中医辨证施治的精神，不同病证，要施行不同的手法。人有老少，体有强弱，证有虚实，作用部位有大有小，肌肉有厚有薄。因此，手法的选择和力量的运用都必须与之相适应，过之或不及都会影响防治效果，甚至还可产生一定的副作用。

由于中国推拿的源远流长，其手法之多，数以百计，更有把两种手法结合起来，配伍应用而组成复合手法的，如按摩、搓揉、捏拿等。另外，小儿推拿中，手法更具特色，与推拿操作的部位（穴位）、动作等结合，名称形象化，如龙入虎口、打马过河、水底捞月等，这些复合手法，更加有助于提高推拿的临床疗效。

2.1　Manipulations for Adult Tuina

2.1.1　Pushing Manipulation with One-finger (Yizhichan Tuifa)

OPERATING METHOD

Exert force on a certain site or point with the tip or the whorl surface or the radial hump of the thumb. Meanwhile relax the wrist area, drop the shoulder, hang down the elbow and suspend the wrist. Having the elbow joint slightly lower than the wrist and using the elbow as a pivot, sway the forearm initiatively and make it drive the wrist to sway and the thumb joint to do flexion and extension. While the wrist is swaying, its ulnar side should be lower than the radial side, so as to make the force act on the treated area. Pressing force, frequency and swaying range should be even with nimble action. The frequency is 120 – 160 times per minute.

In operating, clench a hollow fist with the thumb covering the fist hole, relax the muscles of the upper limb. Exert force naturally with the tip or the thumb, avoiding pressing downward violently. After the tip or whorl surface of the thumb are able to fix at a certain site, begin practicing swaying the wrist and do slow, straight, to-and-fro movements, which is the so-called movement of forcefully pushing and slowly moving (Fig. 19).

CLINICAL APPLICATION

This technique has the characteristics of small touched area and great penetrating force, so it can be used for points all over the body. In clinic, it is often applied to the head, face, chest, abdomen and limbs. Diseases such as headache, stomachache, abdominal pain, aching pain in the joints, tendons and bones are often treated with this

第一节　成人手法

一、一指禅推法

【操作方法】

用大拇指指端、螺纹面或偏锋着力于一定的部位或穴位上,腕部放松,沉肩、垂肘、悬腕,肘关节略低于手腕,以肘部为支点,前臂作主动摆动,带动腕部摆动和拇指关节屈伸活动。腕部摆动时,尺侧要低于桡侧,使产生的"力"持续地作用于治疗部位上。压力、频率、摆动幅度要均匀,动作要灵活。手法频率每分钟120～160次。

练习时,手握空拳,上肢肌肉放松,拇指端自然着力,不可用蛮力下压,拇指要盖住拳眼。在拇指端或拇指螺纹面能吸定的基础上,再练习在腕部摆动时,拇指端作缓慢直线往返移动,即所谓紧推慢移(图19)。

【临床应用】

本法接触面积小,但深透度大,可适用于全身各部穴位。临床常用于头面、胸腹及四肢等处。对头痛、胃痛、腹痛及关节筋骨酸痛等疾患常用本法治疗。具有舒筋活络,

technique, which has the effect of relaxing tendons and activating the meridians, regulating ying and wei systems, eliminating blood stasis and food retention and strengthening the spleen and stomach.

调和营卫，祛瘀消积，健脾和胃的功能。

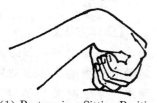

(1) Posture in a Sitting Position
(1) 坐位姿势

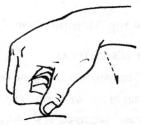

(2) Suspending, Cupping a Hollow Fist, Exerting Force Naturally with the Thumb
(2) 悬腕、手握空拳、拇指自然着力

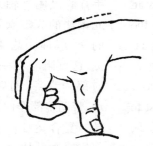

(3) The Wrist Swaying Outward
(3) 腕部向外摆动

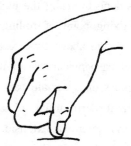

(4) The Wrist Swaying Inward
(4) 腕部向内摆动

Fig. 19 Pushing Manipulations with one-finger
图 19   一指禅推法

NOTES   Twining Manipulation or Quick Pushing Manipulation (Chanfa)

When the frequency of Pushing Manipulation with One-finger increases up to 220 - 250 times per minute, the manipulation is called Twining Manipulation or Quick Pushing Manipulation (Chanfa). Have the tip or the radial hump of the thumb exert force on a certain spot to reduce the touched area and decrease the amplitude of swaying and pressure on the body surface to increase the frequency up to the given times a minute. This technique can be

【附】 缠法

一指禅推法的频率提高到每分钟 220～250 次，称缠法。用大拇指指端或偏锋着力于一定部位以减小接触面，同时减小摆动幅度，降低对体表的压力，以提高一指禅推法的频率，使频率达到每分钟规定的次数。本法只

gradually commanded only on the basis of mastering pushing manipulation with one-finger skillfully. And it is commonly used to treat sthenia-heat syndrome, furuncle and carbuncle and other external problems.

2.1.2　Rolling Manipulation（Gunfa）

OPERATING METHOD

Rolling Manipulation is a complex movement of flexing, extending of the wrist joint and rotating of the forearm. Flexion and extension of the wrist joint is completed by using the dorsum aspect of the 2nd to 4th metacarpophalangeal joints as an axis, while rotating movement of the forearm is done by using the ulnar dorsum side as an axis. So the fixing point of rolling manipulation is the crossing point of the above two axes, or the dorsum aspect of the metacarpophalangeal joint of the little finger. Have the point fix on a certain part, use the elbow as a pivot, sway the forearm initiatively and bring the wrist to do a complex movement of extension and flexion and the forearm to rotate too. The fixing point should be close to the body surface; hauling, turning and leaping movements should be avoided; pressing force, frequency and swaying range should be even and the movements should be coordinative and rhythmic. In the operation, the shoulder and arm should try to relax, and the elbow bends in an angle of 120°(Fig. 20).

CLINICAL APPLICATION

Rolling manipulation can produce great pressure and has a large touching area, so it is suitable for parts and regions with thick muscles such as the shoulder, back, lumbus and buttocks. This manipulation is often used to treat aching pain caused by pathogenic wind and dampness, numbness and paralysis in the limbs and dyskinesia. The

有在熟练掌握一指禅推法的基础上，才能逐步掌握。缠法有较强的消散作用，临床常用于实热证及痈疖等外科病证的治疗。

二、㨰法

【操作方法】

㨰法是由腕关节的伸屈运动和前臂的旋转运动复合而成。伸屈腕关节是以第2到第4掌指关节背侧为轴来完成的；前臂的旋转运动是以手背的尺侧为轴来完成。因此㨰法的吸定点是上述两轴的交点，即小指掌指关节背侧，这点附着在一定部位，以肘部为支点，前臂作主动摆动，带动腕部作伸屈和前臂旋转的复合运动。手法吸定的部位要紧贴体表，不能拖动、转动或跳动。压力、频率、摆动幅度要均匀，动作要协调而有节律。操作时要注意肩、臂尽可能放松，肘关节微屈约120°(图20)。

【临床应用】

㨰法压力大，接触面也较大，适用于肩背、腰臀及四肢等肌肉较丰厚的部位。对风湿酸痛、麻木不仁、肢体瘫痪、运动功能障碍等疾患常用本法治疗。具有舒筋活血，滑利

rolling manipulation has the function of relaxing tendons and activating blood, smoothing joints, relieving spasm of muscles and ligaments, improving the moving ability of muscles and ligaments, promoting circulation of blood and removing fatigue of muscles.

关节,缓解肌肉、韧带痉挛,增强肌肉、韧带活动能力,促进血液循环及消除肌肉疲劳等作用。

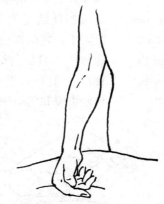

(1) The Body Position on Practicing
Rolling Manipulation
(1) 滚法训练时的体位

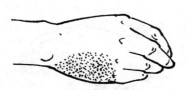

(2) Attracting Portion and
Touching Portion
(2) 滚法吸定部位和接触部位

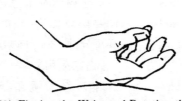

(3) Flexing the Wrist and Rotating the
Forearm Backward
(3) 屈腕和前臂施后

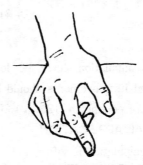

(4) Extending the Wrist and Rotating the
Forearm Forward
(4) 伸腕和前臂旋前

Fig. 20   Rolling Manipulation
图 20   滚法

2.1.3   Kneading Manipulation（Roufa)

Kneading manipulation includes palm kneading and finger kneading.

三、揉法

揉法分掌揉和指揉两种。

OPERATING METHOD

Palm kneading manipulation is performed by fixing the major thenar or the palmar base on a certain part or point, relaxing the wrist, using the elbow as a pivot, swaying the forearm initiatively and bringing the wrist to sway slowly and softly.

Finger kneading manipulation is done by fixing the whorl surfaces of the fingers on a certain spot or point, relaxing the wrist, using the elbow as a pivot, having the forearm make initiative swaying movement and bringing the wrist, palm and finger to sway slowly and softly (Fig. 21).

【操作方法】

掌揉法是用手掌大鱼际或掌根吸定于一定部位或穴位上,腕部放松,以肘部为支点,前臂作主动摆动,带动腕部作轻柔缓和的摆动。

指揉法是用手指螺纹面吸定于一定的部位或穴位上,腕部放松,以肘部为支点,前臂作主动摆动,带动腕和掌指作轻柔缓和摆动(图21)。

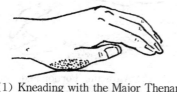

(1) Kneading with the Major Thenar
(1) 鱼际揉

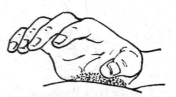

(2) Kneading with Palm Base
(2) 掌根揉

Fig. 21　Kneading Manipulations
图 21　揉法

This manipulation should be done gently with less pressure, and its movements should be coordinative and rhythmic at a frequency of 120 to 160 times per minute.

CLINICAL APPLICATION

This manipulation is soft and slow with mild stimulation and suitable for points all over the body. It is often used to treat epigastric pain, stuffiness in the chest, pain in the hypochondriac region, constipation, diarrhea and other gastrointestinal diseases as well as swelling and pain caused by injury. It has the effect of soothing the chest depression and regulating flow of qi, removing food retention, promoting circulation of blood to remove blood stasis and subduing swelling to relieve pain.

本法操作时压力要轻柔,动作要协调而有节律。一般速度每分钟120～160次。

【临床应用】

本法轻柔缓和,刺激量小,适用于全身各部。常用于脘腹痛、胸闷胁痛、便秘、泄泻等肠胃疾患,以及因外伤引起的红肿疼痛等症。具有宽胸理气、消积导滞、活血祛瘀、消肿止痛等作用。

2.1.4 Circular Rubbing Manipulation（Mofa）

This manipulation is divided into palm rubbing manipulation and finger rubbing manipulation.

OPERATING METHOD

Palm rubbing manipulation is performed by fixing the palm surface on a certain part, using the wrist joint as the center, having the palm, wrist together with the forearm making rhythmic and circular movements.

Finger rubbing manipulation is done by fixing the index, middle and ring fingers on a certain part, using the wrist joint as the center and having the palm, fingers and wrist making rhythmic and circular movements (Fig. 22).

四、摩法

本法分掌摩和指摩两种。

【操作方法】

掌摩法是用掌面附着于一定部位上，以腕关节为中心，连同前臂作节律性的环旋运动。

指摩法是用食、中、无名指面附着于一定的部位上，以腕关节为中心，连同掌、指作节律性的环旋运动（图22）。

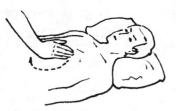

(1) Rubbing with the Palm
（1）掌摩法

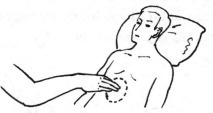

(2) Rubbing with the Fingers
（2）指摩法

Fig. 22 Circular Rubbing Manipulations
图22 摩法

In operation, the elbow joint should flex and extend naturally, the wrist relaxes and the palm and fingers are straightened naturally. Action should be slow and coordinative. The frequency is about 120 circles per minute.

CLINICAL APPLICATION

This manipulation produces light, mild and moderate stimulations, and is a commonly used manipulation on the chest, abdomen and hypochondriac regions. It is often used to treat epigastric pain and distension, dyspepsia, qi stagnation and internal injury of the chest and hypochondrium. The manipulation has the effect of regulating the stomach

本法操作时肘关节自然屈曲，腕部放松，指掌自然伸直，动作要缓和而协调。频率每分钟120次左右。

【临床应用】

本法刺激轻柔缓和，是胸腹、胁肋部常用手法。对脘腹疼痛、食积胀满、气滞及胸胁屏伤等病症常用本法治疗。具有和中理气、消积导滞、调节肠胃蠕动等作用。

to smooth qi, removing food retention to promote digestion and regulating peristalsis of the stomach and intestine.

2.1.5 To-and-fro Rubbing Manipulation (Cafa)

OPERATING METHOD

Place the major thenar, the palmar base or the minor thenar on a certain part of the body surface and do to-and-fro rubbing movements straight. In operating, straighten the wrist joint to get the forearm approximately at the same level with the hand and extend the fingers naturally and get the whole palm and all the fingers on the treated area of the patient. The shoulder joint acts as the pivot, the upper arm moves and drives the palm to make to-and-fro or up-and-down movements. The pressure under the palm should not be too strong, but the pushing range should be appropriately large enough (Fig. 23).

五、擦法

【操作方法】

用手掌的大鱼际、掌根或小鱼际附着在一定部位,进行直线来回摩擦。擦法操作时腕关节伸直,使前臂与手接近相平。手指自然伸开,整个指掌要贴在患者体表的治疗部位,以肩关节为支点,上臂主动带动手掌做前后或上下往返移动,向掌下的压力不宜太大,但推动的幅度要大(图23)。

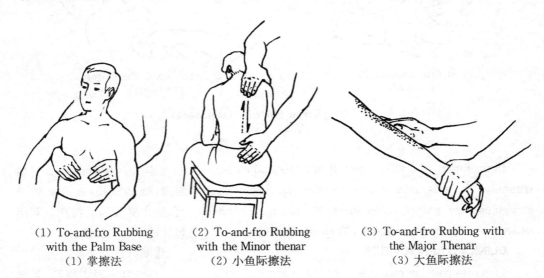

(1) To-and-fro Rubbing with the Palm Base
(1) 掌擦法

(2) To-and-fro Rubbing with the Minor thenar
(2) 小鱼际擦法

(3) To-and-fro Rubbing with the Major Thenar
(3) 大鱼际擦法

Fig. 23　To-and-for Rubbing Manipulations
图23　擦法

While this manipulation is operated, the exertion of force should be steady and action should be even and

本法操作时用力要稳,动作要均匀连续;呼吸自然,不

uninterrupted. Breathe naturally without holding breath. The frequency is about $100-120$ times per minute.

CLINICAL APPLICATION

This manipulation produces mild and warm stimulation and has the effect of warming and activating the meridians, promoting circulation of qi and blood, eliminating swelling and stopping pain and strengthening the spleen and stomach. The method is often used to treat visceral asthenia impairment and syndromes caused by dysfunction of qi and blood. It is especially effective in activating blood and eliminating blood stasis. To-and-fro rubbing manipulation with palm is commonly used on the chest, abdomen and hypochondriac regions. To-and-fro rubbing manipulation with the hypothenar is used on the shoulder, back, buttocks and lower limbs. To-and-fro rubbing manipulation with the major thenar is applicable to the chest, abdomen, back and four limbs.

While using this method, attention should be paid to the following points: exposing the treated areas and applying proper amount of lubricating oil or medicated ointment both to prevent injuring the skin and to increase curative effect through permeation of medicine.

2.1.6 Pushing Manipulation（Tuifa）

Pushing manipulation consists of finger pushing, palm pushing and elbow pushing.

OPERATING METHOD

Have the finger, palm or elbow exert force on a certain part and make one-way, rectilinear movements. Pushing with the finger is called finger pushing manipulation; pushing with the palm, palm pushing manipulation and pushing with the elbow, elbow pushing manipulation. In operating, the finger, palm and elbow should attach closely to the body surface, exertion of force should be

可屏气。频率每分钟 $100\sim$ 120 次。

【临床应用】

本法是一种柔和温热的刺激,具有温经通络、行气活血、消肿止痛、健脾和胃等作用。常用于治疗内脏虚损及气血功能失常的病证。尤以活血祛瘀的作用为更强。掌擦法多用于胸胁及腹部;小鱼际擦法多用于肩背腰臀及下肢部;大鱼际擦法在胸腹、腰背、四肢等部均可运用。

擦法使用时要注意:治疗部位要暴露,并涂适量的润滑油或配制药膏,既可防止擦破皮肤,又可通过药物的渗透以加强疗效。

六、推法

推法有指推法、掌推法和肘推法三种。

【操作方法】

用指、掌或肘部着力于一定的部位上进行单方向的直线移动。用指称指推法,用掌称掌推法,用肘称肘推法。操作时指、掌或肘要紧贴体表,用力要稳,速度要缓慢而均匀(图 24)。

steady at a slow and even speed (Fig. 24).

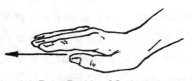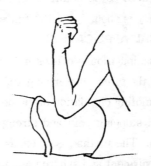

(1) Palm Pushing Manipulation
(1) 掌推法

(2) Elbow Pushing Manipulation
(2) 肘推法

Fig. 24   Pushing Manipulations
图 24   推法

CLINICAL APPLICATION

The manipulation can be applied to all parts of the body and it has an action of increasing muscular excitement, promoting blood circulation, relaxing tendon and activating the meridians.

2.1.7   Palm-twisting Manipulation (Cuofa)

OPERATING METHOD

The manipulation is performed by holding a certain part of the body with both the palms, exerting force oppositely and doing swift, two-way twisting and kneading movements repeatedly. Meanwhile, both hands move up and down. In operating, the exertion of force should be symmetric, the twisting movement should be rapid while the moving action should be slow (Fig. 25).

CLINICAL APPLICATION

Palm-twisting manipulation is applicable to the back, lumbus, hypochondrium and limbs; it is most commonly used on the upper limbs and generally used as an ending manipulation of tuina treatment. The method has an action of coordinating qi and blood and relaxing tendon and dredging the meridians.

【临床应用】

可在人体各部位使用。能增高肌肉的兴奋性,促进血液循环,并有舒筋活络的作用。

七、搓法

【操作方法】

用双手掌面夹住一定的部位,相对用力作快速搓揉,同时作上下往返移动,称搓法。操作时双手用力要对称,搓动要快,移动要慢(图25)。

【临床应用】

搓法适用于腰背、胁肋及四肢部,以上肢部最为常用,一般作为推拿治疗的结束手法。具有调和气血、舒筋通络的作用。

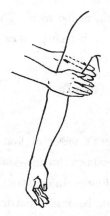

Fig. 25 Palm-twisting Manipulation
图 25　搓法

2.1.8 Wiping Manipulation（Mafa）

OPERATING METHOD

The technique is done by attaching the whorl surface of one thumb or both thumbs close to the skin and doing up-and-down or left-and-right rubbing action. In operating, exertion of force should be light but not superficial, heavy but not stuck（Fig. 26）.

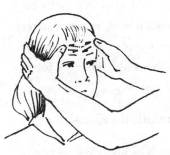

Fig. 26 Wiping Manipulation
图 26　抹法

CLINICAL APPLICATION

The manipulation is commonly applied to the head, face and nape. It is often used in compatible treatment of

八、抹法

【操作方法】

用单手或双手拇指螺纹面紧贴皮肤，作上下或左右往返移动，称为抹法。操作时用力要轻而不浮，重而不滞（图26）。

【临床应用】

本法常用于头面及颈项部。对头晕、头痛及颈项强痛

dizziness, headache, stiffness and pain in the nape. The method has an effect of tranquilization, inducing resuscitation and improving eye-sight.

2.1.9 Shaking Manipulation (Doufa)

OPERATING METHOD

Hold the distal end of the patient's upper or lower limbs with both hands and make constant, up-and-down trembling movements in a small amplitude. In operating, the range of shaking movement should be small, but the frequency should be great (Fig. 27).

等症常用本法作配合治疗。抹法有开窍镇静、醒脑明目等作用。

九、抖法

【操作方法】

用双手握住患者的上肢或下肢远端,用力作连续的小幅度的上下颤动。操作时颤动幅度要小,频率要快(图 27)。

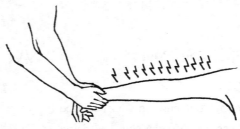

Fig. 27   Shaking Manipulation
图 27   抖法

CLINICAL APPLICATION

The technique may be used on limbs, especially on the upper limbs. In clinic, it is often used in combination with palm-twisting manipulation (Cuofa) as a finishing manipulation. It has the same therapeutic effect as palm-twisting manipulation.

2.1.10 Vibrating Manipulation (Zhenfa)

Vibrating manipulation is divided into palm vibrating manipulation and finger vibrating manipulation.

OPERATING METHOD

Vibrating manipulation is performed by placing the finger or palm on the body surface, exerting force intensively and statically with the muscles of the forearm and

【临床应用】

本法可用于四肢部,以上肢为常用。临床上常与搓法配合,作为治疗的结束手法。治疗作用与搓法相同。

十、振法

有掌振法和指振法两种。

【操作方法】

用手指或手掌着力在体表,前臂和手部的肌肉强力地静止性用力,产生振颤动作。

hand to produce vibrating movements. Exerting force with the fingers is called finger vibrating manipulation, while giving force with the palm is palm vibrating manipulation. In manipulating, force should be concentrated on the fingertips or palm, frequency should be high and force exerted should be slightly heavy (Fig. 28).

用手指着力称指振法,用手掌着力称掌振法。操作时力量要集中于指端或手掌上。振动的频率较高,着力稍重(图 28)。

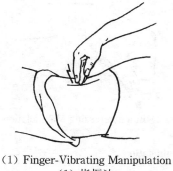

（1）Finger-Vibrating Manipulation
（1）指振法

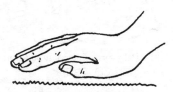

（2）Palm-Vibrating Manipulation
（2）掌振法

Fig. 28   Vibrating Manipulations
图 28   振法

CLINICAL APPLICATION

The technique is usually operated with one hand, operation with both hands is also applicable. It is suitable for all parts and points of the body and has the effect of eliminating stasis to resolve swelling, regulating the stomach to smooth qi, promoting digestion to remove food retention and regulating the function of the intestine and stomach.

【临床应用】

本法一般常用单手操作,也可双手同时操作。适用于全身各部位和穴位。具有祛瘀消肿、和中理气、消食导滞、调节肠胃功能等作用。

2.1.11   Pressing Manipulation（Anfa）

Pressing manipulation is divided into finger pressing manipulation and palm pressing manipulation.

OPERATING METHOD

Pressing the body surface with the tip of the thumb or the belly of the fingers is called finger pressing manipulation. Pressing the body surface with one palm or two palms or overlapped palms is known as palm pressing

十一、按法

有指按法和掌按法两种。

【操作方法】

用拇指端或指腹按压体表,称指按法。用单掌或双掌,也可用双掌重叠按压体表,称掌按法。按法操作时着

manipulation. While manipulating, the part exerting force should closely attach to the body surface of the patient without moving. The force exerted should be steady and increase from light to heavy. Sudden violent force should be avoided (Fig 29).

力部位要紧贴体表,不可移动,用力要由轻而重,不可用暴力猛然按压(图29)。

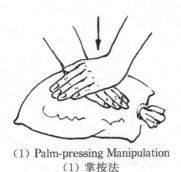

(1) Palm-pressing Manipulation　　　　(2) Finger-pressing Manipulation
　　　(1) 掌按法　　　　　　　　　　　　　　(2) 指按法

Fig. 29　Pressing Manipulations
图 29　按法

CLINICAL APPLICATION

In clinic, pressing manipulation is frequently combined with kneading manipulation to form compound pressing-kneading manipulation. Finger pressing manipulation is fit to all points of the body, while palm pressing is often used on the back and abdomen. This technique has the function of relaxing muscles, removing obstruction and activating blood circulation to relieve pain. Epigastric pain, headache, numbness and aching pain in the extremities are commonly treated with pressing manipulation.

2.1.12　Sweeping Manipulation (Saosanfa)

OPERATING METHOD

Hold lightly one side of the patient's head with one hand, place the radius aspect of the other thumb above point Taiyang (EX-HN 5) of the other side of his head. Bend slightly the other four fingers, separate them in a spread-fan shape and make them do arc-movements rota-

【临床应用】

按法在临床上常与揉法结合应用,组成"按揉"复合手法。指按法适用于全身各部穴位;掌按法常用于腰背和腹部。本法具有放松肌肉、开通闭塞、活血止痛的作用。胃脘痛、头痛、肢体酸痛麻木等病症常用本法治疗。

十二、扫散法

【操作方法】

一手轻扶住患者头部一侧,另一手以拇指桡侧面置于患者另一侧太阳穴上方。其余四指略屈曲,分开呈扇形,同时在腕关节自然摆动下随

tionally with force driven by naturally swaying of the wrist joint. Actions should be light, nimble, natural and coherent.

CLINICAL APPLICATION

Sweeping manipulation is performed with even force, mainly used for operation on the head. It has the effect of calming the liver to suppress hyperhepatic yang, dispelling wind and relieving pain, warming the meridian and dispelling pathogenic cold, tranquilization and inducing resuscitation. Headache, vertigo, hypertension, insomnia, poor memory and common cold are often treated with this technique.

2.1.13   Plucking Manipulation (Tanbofa)

OPERATING METHOD

Plucking manipulation is commonly performed by exerting force with the tip of the thumb and placing the other four fingers on the treated area. Or use the index and middle fingers to exert force and press their tips on the space between tendons or on the starting or ending point of a tendon. Pluck as if playing a string, first with light force, then heavy and at an even frequency.

CLINICAL APPLICATION

The technique is applicable to all parts of the body and has an action of relaxing tendons and meridians, loosening spasm and adhesion and activating flow of blood and relieving pain. Adhesion around the shoulder joint, sciatica, Bi-syndrome, pain and discomfort in the hypochondrium due to sprain or contusion, all kinds of pain, local spasm due to injury and adhesion are often treated with plucking manipulation.

2.1.14   Gripping Manipulation (Zhuafa)

OPERATING METHOD

Attach the fingers and palm of one hand or both hands

之稍用力作弧形绕动。动作要轻巧自如并连贯。

【临床应用】

扫散法力量均匀,主要用于头部操作,具有平肝潜阳、祛风止痛、温经散寒、镇静醒脑的作用。头痛、眩晕、高血压、失眠健忘、伤风感冒常用本法治疗。

十三、弹拨法

【操作方法】

多以拇指指端着力,其余四指附着在治疗部位;或以食指、中指着力,将着力的指端按于肌筋缝隙之间,或肌筋的起止点,由轻而重,频率均匀,如弹拨琴弦动作。

【临床应用】

本法可适用于全身各部,具有舒筋活络、松解痉挛、粘连、活血止痛的作用。对肩关节周围粘连、坐骨神经痛、痹证、扭挫岔气、各类疼痛及外伤后局部痉挛、粘连等常用本法治疗。

十四、抓法

【操作方法】

以单手或双手掌指附着

to the treated part with the five fingers slightly separating and extending naturally, squeeze and press from around to the center with force to hold the local skin and muscle in hand, and then loosen them gradually. Repeated action like that is called gripping manipulation or Zhuafa.

CLINICAL APPLICATION

The technique is commonly applied to the head, abdomen, back and other parts with thick muscles. It has the effect of dispelling wind and cold, dredging the meridians, inducing resuscitation and relieving pain. Headache, epigastric pain, aching pain and numbness of muscles are commonly treated with this manipulation.

2.1.15 Chopping Manipulation（Pifa）

OPERATING METHOD

Hold the wrist of the patient with one hand, ask him to separate the five fingers of the hand held and chop at the interdigital junctions one by one with the lateral side of the other palm.

CLINICAL APPLICATION

The technique is applicable to interdigital junctions and effective in inducing resuscitation, activating flow of blood and dredging the meridians. It is used in compatible treatment of numbness of the limbs, disharmony of qi and blood, palpitation, insomnia, depression and stuffiness in the chest and other miscellaneous diseases of internal and gynecological medicine.

2.1.16 Digital-pressing Manipulation（Dianfa）

OPERATING METHOD

Bend the middle finger or both the index and middle fingers, exert force on the treated points with the tip of the proximal interphalangeal joint, increase force and press inward. Keep the action for a properly long period

于施治部位，五指略开并自然伸直，再略用力自四周向中心挤压，合力将局部皮肤、肌肉握于掌内，然后逐渐放松，如是反复，称作抓法。

【临床应用】

本法多用于头部、腹部、背部和肌肉丰满的部位，具有祛风散寒、疏经通络、开窍止痛的功用。头痛、胃脘痛、肌肉酸痛、麻木等常用本法治疗。

十五、劈法

【操作方法】

一手握住患者腕部，嘱其五指分开，以另一手掌掌侧依次劈击其指缝。

【临床应用】

适用于两手指缝，具有醒脑开窍、活血通络等作用。对肢体麻木、气血不和、心悸失眠、抑郁胸闷及内妇科杂症可配合治疗。

十六、点法

【操作方法】

中指或食中指屈曲，指间关节端着力于施治经穴上，并加力内向按压，停留保持适当时间（图30）。

of time (Fig. 30).

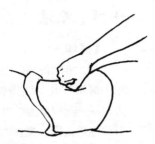 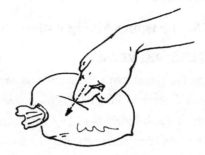

(1) Digital-pressing with the Flexed Thumb   (2) Digital-pressing with the Flexed Index Finger
        (1) 屈拇指点   (2) 屈食指点

Fig. 30   Digital-pressing Manipulations
图 30   点法

CLINICAL APPLICATION

The technique is one of digital pressing manipulations and suitable for points all over the body. It is effective in dispelling wind and cold, descending adverse qi to stop vomiting, tranquilization and easing the mind and relieving pain. Headache, dizziness, insomnia, nausea, hiccup and vomiting are often treated with this manipulation.

2.1.17   Scraping Manipulation (Guafa)

OPERATING METHOD

Scraping manipulation refers to the manipulation performed by dipping the radius side of the thumb or the pads of the index and middle fingers in water or other media, exerting force directly on certain parts or points of the body surface with them and making one-way rapid pushing movements.

CLINICAL APPLICATION

Being a manipulation with moderate stimulation, scraping manipulation has the effect of activating flow of blood and dredging the meridians, dispelling wind and cold, diaphoresis and relieving superficies and eliminating pathogenic summer-dampness. Common cold, summer

【临床应用】

适用于全身,为点按法的一种,具有祛风散寒、降逆止呕、镇静安神止痛的作用。头痛、头晕、失眠、恶心、呃逆、呕吐等症常用本法治疗。

十七、刮法

【操作方法】

用拇指桡侧面或食、中两指指面部蘸水或其他介质后,直接在体表一定部位或穴位上着力,作单方向的快速推动,称为刮法。

【临床应用】

刮法属中等刺激手法,具有活血通络、祛风散寒、发汗解表、祛除暑湿的作用。感冒、暑热、呕吐、不思饮食等病症可用本法治疗。

heat, vomiting and poor appetite can be treated with scraping manipulation.

2.1.18　Grasping Manipulation（Nafa）

OPERATING METHOD

Use the thumb with the index and middle fingers or other four fingers to lift and pinch certain operated parts or points of the body rhythmically with opposite force. In operating, exertion of force should be from light to heavy and sudden exertion should be avoided. Operation should be even, slow and coherent (Fig. 31).

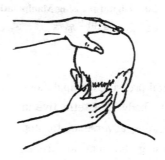

Fig. 31　Grasping Manipulation
图 31　拿法

CLINICAL APPLICATION

In clinic, the technique is often applied to the neck, nape, shoulders and limbs in combination with other manipulations. It has the effect of dispelling wind and cold, inducing resuscitation to stop pain, relaxing tendons and dredging the meridians.

2.1.19　Finger-twisting Manipulation（Nianfa）

OPERATING METHOD

Pinch a certain part of the patient and do twisting and kneading with the whorl surface of the thumb and index finger with opposite force. In operating, the manipulation should be nimble and swift, sluggish operation should be

十八、拿法

【操作方法】

用大拇指和食、中两指，或用大拇指和其余四指作相对用力，在一定的部位和穴位上进行节律性地提捏。操作时，用劲要由轻而重，不可突然用力，动作要缓和而有连贯性(图31)。

【临床应用】

临床常配合其他手法使用于颈项、肩部和四肢等部位。具有祛风散寒、开窍止痛、舒筋通络等作用。

十九、捻法

【操作方法】

用拇、食指螺纹面捏住一定部位，两指相对做搓揉动作。操作时动作要灵活、快速，用劲不可呆滞(图32)。

avoided (Fig. 32).

CLINICAL APPLICATION

The manipulation is suitable for small joints of the limbs. It has the properties of relaxing tendons, dredging the meridians and lubricating joints, and is often combined with other manipulations to treat aching pain, swelling and stiffness of interphalangeal joints.

【临床应用】

本法一般适用于四肢小关节。具有理筋通络,滑利关节的作用,常配合其他手法治疗指(趾)间关节的酸痛、肿胀或屈伸不利等症。

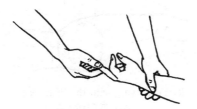

Fig. 32   Finger-twisting Manipulation
图 32   捻法

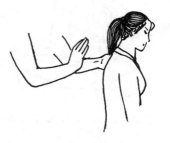

Fig. 33   Patting Manipulation
图 33   拍法

2.1.20   Patting Manipulation (Paifa)

OPERATING METHOD

While performing the manipulation, close the fingers naturally, bend the joints of the finger and palm slightly and pat the affected area steadily and rhythmically (Fig. 33).

CLINICAL APPLICATION

Patting manipulation is applicable to the shoulder, back, buttocks and lower limbs. Rheumatic aching pain, bradyesthesia in local areas and muscular spasm are treated with this manipulation in combination with others. The technique has the effect of relaxing tendons and dredging the meridians, and promoting circulation of qi and blood.

2.1.21   Percussing Manipulation (Jifa)

Percussing manipulation refers to the manipulation performed by hitting or beating the body surface rhythmi-

二十、拍法

【操作方法】

操作时手指自然并拢,掌指关节微屈,平稳而有节奏地拍打患部(图33)。

【临床应用】

拍法适用于背肩、腰臀及下肢部。对风湿酸痛、局部感觉迟钝或肌肉痉挛等症常用本法配合其他手法治疗,具有舒筋通络,行气活血的作用。

二十一、击法

用拳背、掌根、掌侧小鱼际、指尖并以腕关节带动,有

cally with the back of a fist, the palmar base, the minor thenar of the ulnar palm and the fingertip driven by the wrist joint (Fig. 34).

节奏地叩击体表,称为击法（图34）。

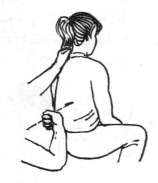

(1) Percussing with the Fist Back
(1) 拳背击

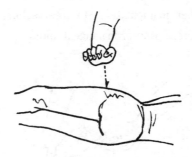

(2) Percussing with the Palm Base
(2) 掌根击

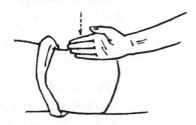

(3) Percussing with the Lateral Side of the Palm
(3) 侧击

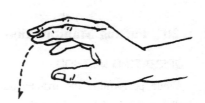

(4) Percussing with the Fingertip
(4) 指尖击

Fig. 34　Percussing Manipulations
图 34　击法

OPERATING METHOD

（1）Fist percussing manipulation. Make a hollow fist, straighten the wrist and hit the body surface with the dorsum of the fist evenly.

（2）Palm percussing manipulation. Loosen the fingers naturally, straighten the wrist and percuss the body surface with the palmar base.

（3）Lateral-palm percussing manipulation or Hypo thenar Percussing Manipulation. Stretch the fingers naturally, bend the wrist slightly backward and beat the body

【操作方法】

（1）拳击法。手握空拳,腕伸直,用拳背平击体表。

（2）掌击法。手指自然松开,腕伸直,用掌根部叩击体表。

（3）侧击法（又称小鱼际击）。手指自然伸直,腕略背屈,用单手或双手小鱼际部击

surface with the minor thenar of one palm or both.

（4）Fingertip Percussing Manipulation. Beat the body surface with the fingertips as if rain drops.

（5）Stick Percussing Manipulation. Beat the body surface with a stick made of mulberry twigs.

When percussing manipulation is operated，exertion of force should be quick with a short duration，percussing movement on the body surface is made vertically，at an even and rhythmic speed. Any dragging and whipping movement should be avoided.

CLINICAL APPLICATION

Fist percussion is often used on the back；palm percussion on the vertex of the head, lumbus, buttocks and limbs；lateral-palm percussion on the lumbus，back and limbs；fingertip percussion on the head，face，chest and abdomen；stick percussion on the vertex of the head，lumbus，back and limbs. The manipulation has an action of relaxing tendons and dredging the meridians and regulating qi and blood. It is often used in compatible treatment of rheumatic arthralgia，bradyesthesia in local areas，muscular spasm or headache.

NOTE Process of Mulberry Stick

Choose twelve mulberry twigs in a diameter of 0. 5 cm，strip the bark and dry them in the shade. Wrap each twig with mulberry paper tightly and tie with thread. Then tie all the tied twigs together，wrap them with mulberry paper tightly in several layers and tie them with thread again. Wrap with cloth finally and sew tightly. A standard mulberry stick should have proper hardness or elasticity and proper thickness，that is，4. 5 to 5 cm in diameter and 40 cm in length.

2. 1. 22   Rotating Manipulation（Yaofa）

A manipulation to make a joint do passive，circulatory

打体表。

（4）指尖击法。用指端轻轻打击体表，如雨点下落。

（5）棒击法。用桑枝棒击打体表。

击法用劲要快速而短暂，垂直叩击体表，在叩击体表时不能有拖抽动作，速度要均匀而有节奏。

【临床应用】

拳击法常用于腰背部；掌击法常用于头顶、腰臀及四肢部；侧击法常用于腰背及四肢部；指尖击法常用于头面、胸腹部；棒击法常用于头顶、腰背及四肢部。本法具有舒筋通络、调和气血的作用，对风湿痹痛，局部感觉迟钝，肌肉痉挛或头痛等症，常用本法配合治疗。

【附】 桑枝棒制法

用细桑枝十二根（粗约0.5厘米左右），去皮阴干，每根用桑皮纸卷紧，并用线绕扎，然后把桑枝合起来先用线扎紧，再用桑皮纸层层卷紧并用线绕好。外面用布裹紧缝好即成。要求软硬适中（即具有弹性），粗细合用（即用手握之合适，约4.5～5厘米），长约40厘米。

二十二、摇法

使关节作被动的环转活

movement is called rotating manipulation (Fig. 35).

动,称摇法(图 35)。

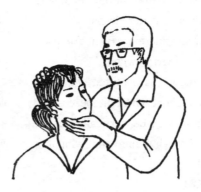

(1) Neck-rotating Manipulation
(1) 颈项部摇法

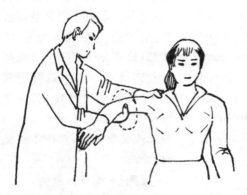

(2) Rotating Manipulation by Supporting the Elbow
(2) 托肘摇法

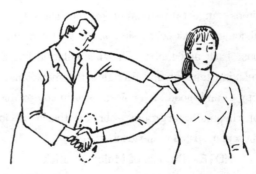

(3) Rotating Manipulation by Holding the Hand
(3) 握手摇法

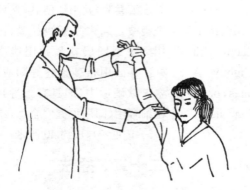

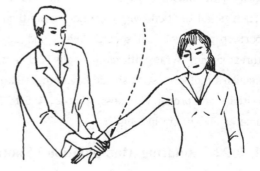

(4) Rotating Manipulation in a Great Amplitude
(4) 大幅度摇法

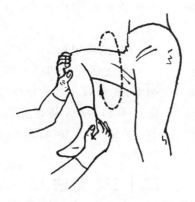

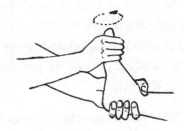

（5）Manipulation of Rotating the Hip Joint　　　（6）Manipulation of Rotating the Ankle Joint
（5）髋关节摇法　　　　　　　　　　　　　（6）踝关节摇法

Fig. 35　Rotating Manipulations
图 35　摇法

OPERATING METHOD

（1）Neck-rotating manipulation. The doctor holds the patient's head posterior to vertex with one hand, and holds the lower jaw with the other hand to make left-and-right rotational movements.

（2）Shoulder joint-rotating manipulation. Hold the patient's shoulder with one hand, and hold the wrist or support the elbow of the patient with the other hand to make rotational movements.

（3）Hip joint-rotating manipulation. The patient is in a supine position and flexes the hip and knee joints. The doctor holds the patient's foot heel with one hand and supports his knee joint with the other hand and makes rotational movements of the hip joint.

（4）Ankle-rotating manipulation. The doctor supports the patient's foot heel with one hand and holds his big toe with the other hand to make rotational movements of the ankle joint.

Movements of rotating manipulation should be moderate and mild with steady force. Direction and amplitude

【操作方法】

（1）颈项部摇法。用一手扶住患者头顶后部,另一手托住下颏,作左右环转摇动。

（2）肩关节摇法。用一手扶住患者肩部,另一手握住腕部或托住肘部,作环转摇动。

（3）髋关节摇法。患者仰卧位,髋膝屈曲。医者一手托住患者足跟,另一手扶住膝部,作髋关节环转摇动。

（4）踝关节摇法。一手托住患者足跟,另一手握住大踇趾部,作踝关节环转摇动。

摇法动作要缓和,用力要稳,摇动方向及幅度须在患者

of rotation should vary from small to large and be within the permissible physiological limit.

CLINICAL APPLICATION

The technique is applicable to the joints of the limbs, nape, and lumbus, etc. and effective for stiffness and impairment of flexing and extending movements of joints. It has the action of lubricating joints and improving their function of activity.

2. 1. 23 Back-carrying Manipulation（Beifa）

OPERATING METHOD

The doctor and the patient stand back to back. The doctor loops the patient's elbows with his own, bends his waist, flexes his knees and sticks his buttocks to carry the patient up on his back and suspend the patient's feet in order to draw and stretch the patient's lumbar spinal vertebrae. Then the doctor quickly stretches his knees and sticks his buttocks and meanwhile, exerts force with his buttocks to quiver or shake the patient's loin. In manipulating, the quiver of the buttocks should be coordinated with the flexion and extension of both knees（Fig. 36）.

生理许可范围内进行,由小到大。

【临床应用】

本法适用于四肢关节及颈项、腰部等。对关节强硬、屈伸不利等症,具有滑利关节,增强关节活动功能的作用。

二十三、背法

【操作方法】

医者和患者背靠背站立,医生两肘套住患者肘弯部,然后弯腰屈膝挺臀,将患者反背起,使其双脚离地,以牵伸患者腰脊柱,再作快速伸膝挺臀动作,同时以臀部着力颤动或摇动患者腰部。操作时臀部的颤动要和两膝的屈伸动作协调(图36)。

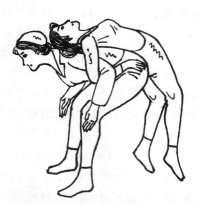

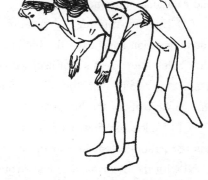

(1) Back-carrying by Bending the Waist, Flexing the Knees and Sticking the Hips
(1) 弯腰屈膝挺臀

(2) Back-carrying by Straightening the Knees and Quivering the Hips
(2) 伸膝臀部颤动

Fig. 36 Back-carrying Manipulations
图36 背法

CLINICAL APPLICATION

Back-carrying manipulation has the function of producing hyperextension of the patient's lumbar spinal vertebrae and lumbar extensor muscles on both sides so as to promote the reduction of the displaced facet joints and help to relieve symptoms caused by the protruded lumbar intervertebral disc. This manipulation is often used in compatible treatment of pain, lumbar sprain and protrusion of lumbar intervertebral disc.

2. 1. 24   Pulling Manipulation（Banfa）

Pulling manipulation refers to a manipulation performed by pulling the body with force in one or opposite directions with both hands (Fig. 37).

OPERATING METHOD

(1) Manipulation of pulling the neck. This maneuver includes two skills in the operation.

a. Manipulation of obliquely pulling the neck. The patient bends his or her head slightly forward. The doctor supports the posterior part of one side of patient's head with one hand and supports the opposite lower jaw with the other hand, rotates the patient's head sideward to the most extent, and then pulls it in the opposite direction with both hands exerting force simultaneously.

【临床应用】

本法可使腰脊柱及其两侧伸肌过伸,促使扭错之小关节复位,并有助于缓解腰椎间盘突出症的症状。对腰部扭闪疼痛及腰椎间盘突出症等常用本法配合治疗。

二十四、扳法

用双手作相反方向或同一方向用力扳动肢体称为扳法(图37)。

【操作方法】

(1) 颈项部扳法,操作时有两种方法。

① 颈项部斜扳法:患者头部略向前屈。医生一手抵住患者头侧后部,另一手抵住对侧下颏部,使头向一侧旋转至最大限度时,两手同时用力作相反方向的扳动。

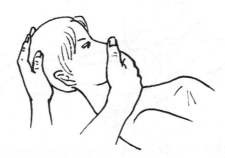

(1) Manipulation of Pulling the Rotated and Localized Neck
(1) 颈项部旋转定位扳法

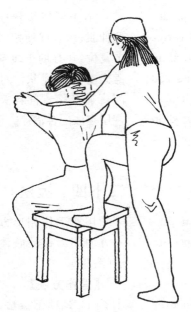

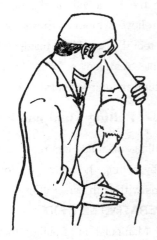

（2）Pulling Manipulation of the Counter-
reduced Thoracic Vertebrae

（2）胸椎对抗复位法

（3）Pulling Manipulation of
the Expanded Chest

（3）扩胸牵引扳法

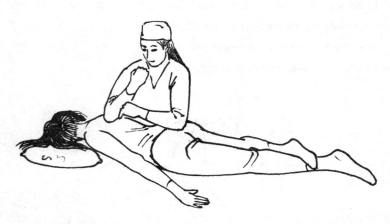

（4）Obliquely Pulling Manipulation of the Lumbar Region

（4）腰部斜扳法

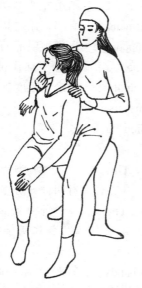
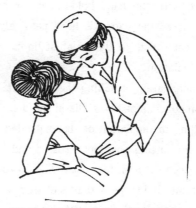

(5) Rotationally Pulling Manipulation
with the Lumbus Straight
（5）直腰旋转扳法

(6) Rotationally Pulling Manipulation
with the Lumbus Bent
（6）弯腰旋转扳法

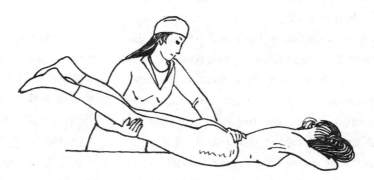

(7) Pulling Manipulation of the Retroflexed Lumbus
（7）腰部后伸扳法

Fig. 37 Pulling Manipulations
图 37 扳法

b. Manipulation of pulling the rotated and localized neck. The patient takes a sitting position and bends his or her head forward to a required angle. The doctor stands behind the patient, supports his or her lower jaw with one elbow and uses the hand to hold the patient's occiput. If

② 旋转定位扳法：患者坐位，颈前屈到某一需要的角度后，医生在其背后，用一肘部托住其下颏部，手则扶住其枕部（向右扳则用右手，向左扳

pulling is done rightward, the doctor should use his right hand to do the above movement; vice versa, the left hand is used. The other hand of the doctor is used to support the patient's shoulder. Exert force to pull the patient's nape upward with the hand holding his or her occiput. Meanwhile, have the patient's head passively rotate toward the affected side to the greatest limit, and then do pulling manipulation.

(2) Manipulation of pulling the chest and back. This manipulation consists of two skills in the operation.

a. Pulling manipulation of the expanded chest. The patient takes a sitting position, crosses and buckles both hands and places them on the nape. The doctor stands behind the patient, holds the patient's elbows with his hands and sustains the patient's back with one knee. Ask the patient to do ventriflexion and retroflexion in coordination with deep breath. The doctor performs manipulation of expanding the chest and traction.

b. Pulling manipulation of the counter-reduced thoracic vertebrae. The patient takes a sitting position, crosses and buckles both hands and places them on the nape. The doctor is behind the patient, inserts both hands from the patient's armpits to between the upper arm and forearm and holds the lower part of the forearm, and at the same time the doctor sustains the patient's spinal column with one knee. Asking the patient to bend slightly forward, the doctor does pulling manipulation forcefully backward and upward with both hands simultaneously.

(3) Manipulation of pulling the lumbar region. In operating, the manipulation commonly has obliquely pulling skill, waist-rotation pulling skill and waist-retroflexion pulling skill.

a. Obliquely pulling manipulation of the lumbar region. The patient lies on his side. The doctor props the

则用左手），另一手扶住患者肩部。托扶其头部的手用力，先作颈项部向上牵引，同时把患者头部作被动向患侧旋转至最大限度后，再作扳法。

（2）胸背部扳法，操作时有两种方法。

① 扩胸牵引扳法：患者坐位，令其两手交叉扣住，置于项部。医生两手托住患者两肘部，并用一侧膝部顶住患者背部，嘱患者自行俯仰，并配合深呼吸，作扩胸牵引扳动。

② 胸椎对抗复位法：患者坐位，令其两手交叉扣住，置于项部。医生在其后面，用两手从患者腋部伸入其上臂之前，前臂之后，并握住其前臂下段，同时医生用一侧膝部顶住患部脊柱。嘱患者身体略向前倾，医生两手同时作向后上方用力扳动。

（3）腰部扳法。本法操作时，常用的有斜扳法、旋转扳法、后伸扳法等三种。

① 腰部斜扳法：患者侧卧位，医生用一手抵住患者肩前

anterior aspect of the patient's shoulder with one hand and sustains the buttock with the other hand, or props the posterior aspect of the patient's shoulder with one hand and sustains the anterior superior iliac crest with the other hand. After rotating the lumbus to the maximal extent, pull in opposite directions with both hands exerting force simultaneously.

b. Pulling manipulation of the rotated lumbus. There are two kinds of operations. One is rotationally pulling skill with the lumbus straight, the other is rotationally pulling skill with the lumbus bent.

Rotationally pulling skill with the lumbus straight. The patient takes a sitting position. The doctor holds the patient's leg with both legs, sustains the rear aspect of the shoulder near the doctor with one hand and inserts the other hand from the patient's armpit of the other side and supports the anterior part of the shoulder. Pull in opposite directions with both hands exerting force simultaneously.

Rotationally pulling skill with the lumbus bent. The patient takes a sitting position and bends forward to a required angle. The assistant helps to fix the patient's lower limbs and pelves. The doctor presses the spinous process to be pulled with the thumb of one hand. If rotation of the spine is to the left, the right hand is used. The doctor uses the other hand to hold the patient's nape to make his lumbus turn to the affected side when it has been in bending forward position. If rotation is to the left, the doctor uses his left hand. When the rotation of the lumbus get its greatest limit, pull it toward its lateral curvature of the healthy side.

c. Pulling manipulation of the retroflexed lumbus. The patient takes a prone position. The doctor supports the patient's knees with one hand and raises them slowly, and presses the other hand firmly on the patient's affected

部,另一手抵住臀部,或一手抵住患者肩后部,另一手抵住髂前上棘部。把腰被动旋转至最大限度后,两手同时用力作相反方向扳动。

② 腰部旋转扳法:有两种操作方法。

直腰旋转扳法:患者坐位,医生用腿夹住患者下肢,一手抵住患者近医生侧的肩后部,另一手以患者另一侧腋下伸入抵住肩前部,两手同时用力作相反方向扳动。

弯腰旋转扳法:患者坐位。腰前屈到某一需要角度后,一助手帮助固定患者下肢及骨盆。医生用一手拇指按住需扳动的脊椎的棘突(向左旋转时用右手),另一手勾住患者项背部(向左旋转时用左手),使其腰部在前屈位时再向患侧旋转。旋转至最大限度时,再使其腰部向健侧侧弯方向扳动。

③ 腰部后伸扳法:患者俯卧位。医生一手托住患者两膝部,缓缓向上提起,另一手紧压在腰部患处,当腰后伸到

lumbar region. When the patient's lumbus flexes back-ward to the maximal limit, the doctor exert force in oppo-site directions with both hands simultaneously.

In manipulation, the doctor should operate resolutely and rapidly with steady force. The coordination of both hands is needed. The range of pulling should not exceed the limit of the normal physiological movements of all joints.

CLINICAL APPLICATION

Pulling manipulation is often used in combination with other manipulations in clinic to gain a result of supplemen-ting each other. It is commonly applied to the spinal col-umn and joints of the limbs. Malposition and dysfunction of joints are often treated with this manipulation, for it has the function of relaxing tendons and dredging the me-ridians, lubricating joints, replacing and reducing dis-placed anatomic sites.

2.1.25　Traction Manipulation（Bashenfa）

Traction means pulling and extending. A manipula-tion operated by fixing one end of a joint or limb or the body and pulling and drawing the other end is called trac-tion manipulation (Fig. 38).

OPERATING METHOD

(1) Manipulation of traction of the head and neck. The patient sits straight. The doctor stands behind the pa-tient, supports the inferior aspect of the patient's occipital bone with his or her thumbs, holds the inferior aspects of the angles of the lower jaws on both sides with the palmar bases and presses the patient's shoulders with his or her forearms. The doctor pulls with great force upward with both hands and presses downward with both forearms in opposite directions simultaneously.

(2) Manipulation of traction of the shoulder joint. The patient takes a sitting position and the doctor holds

最大限度时，两手同时用力作相反方向扳动。

扳法操作时动作必须果断而快速，用力要稳，两手动作配合要协调，扳动幅度一般不能超过各关节的生理活动范围。

【临床应用】

本法临床常和其他手法配合使用，起到相辅相成的作用。常用于脊柱及四肢关节。对关节错位或关节功能障碍等病症，常用本法治疗，有舒筋通络，滑利关节，纠正解剖位置的失常等作用。

二十五、拔伸法

拔伸即牵拉、牵引的意思。固定肢体或关节的一端，牵拉另一端的方法，称为拔伸法（图 38）。

【操作方法】

（1）头颈部拔伸法。患者正坐，医生站在患者背后，用双手拇指顶在枕骨下方，掌根托住两侧下颌角的下方，并用两前臂压住患者两肩，两手用力向上，两前臂下压，同时作相反方向用力。

（2）肩关节拔伸法。患者坐势。医生用双手握住其腕

the patient's wrist or elbow with both hands and pulls gradually with force. Ask the patient to move his or her body to the opposite side, or ask the assistant to help fix the patient's body to counteract the pulling force.

部或肘部,逐渐用力牵拉,嘱患者身体向另一侧倾斜(或有一助手帮助固定患者身体),与牵拉之力对抗。

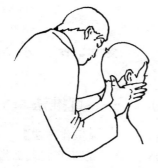

(1) Traction of the Head and Neck
(1) 头颈部拔伸

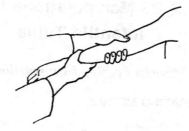

(2) Traction of the Shoulder Joint
(2) 肩关节拔伸

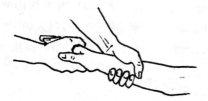

(3) Traction of the Wrist Joint
(3) 腕关节拔伸

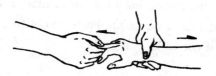

(4) Traction of the Interphalangeal Joint
(4) 指间关节拔伸

Fig. 38   Traction Manipulations
图 38   拔伸法

(3) Manipulation of traction of the wrist joint. Hold the lower end of the patient's forearm with one hand, hold his or her hand with the other hand to do opposite traction with force simultaneously

(4) Manipulation of traction of the interphalangeal joint. Hold the proximal end of the joint to be pulled with one hand and hold the distal end of the joint with the other hand to do opposite traction with force simultaneously.

In the application of this manipulation, exertion of force should be even and lasting, while the operation

(3) 腕关节拔伸法。医生一手握住患者前臂下端,另一手握住其手部,两手同时作相反方向用力,逐渐牵拉。

(4) 指间关节拔伸法。用一手捏住被拔伸关节的近侧端,另一手捏住其远侧端,两手同时作反方向用力牵引。

本法操作时用力要均匀而持久,动作要缓和。

should be moderate.

CLINICAL APPLICATION

This manipulation is often used for malposition of joints, injury of tendons, etc. It has the effect of reduction for sprained muscles and tendons and displaced joints.

2.2   Manipulations for Infantile Tuina

2.2.1   Straight Pushing Manipulation (Zhituifa)

OPERATING METHOD

A manipulation performed by pushing one way straightly on the point with the radial aspect of the thumb or the pads of the index and middle fingers is called straight pushing manipulation. In operating, the surface of the finger exerting force should attach firmly to the operated area or the point. Force should be exerted steadily, but not stickily (Fig. 39).

【临床应用】

本法常用于关节错位、伤筋等。对扭错的肌腱和移位的关节有整复作用。

第二节   小儿手法

一、直推法

【操作方法】

以拇指桡侧面指面,或用食、中二指指面,在穴位上做单方向直线推动,称为直推法。操作时,着力指面要与施术部位(穴位)贴紧,用力既要着实,但亦不可滞涩(图 39)。

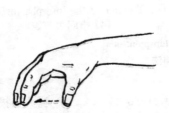

(1) Straight Pushing Manipulation   (2) Straight Pushing Manipulation with
　　　with the Thumb　　　　　　　　　the Index and Middle Fingers
　　　(1) 拇指直推　　　　　　　　　　　(2) 食、中指直推
Fig. 39   Straight Pushing Manipulations
图 39   直推法

CLINICAL APPLICATION

This is one of the most commonly used manipulations of infantile tuina. The manipulation is applicable to linear points all over the body such as Kaitianmen, Tuitianzhugu. The

【临床应用】

本法是小儿推拿最常用手法之一,适用全身所有的"线状穴",如开天门、推天柱

manipulation is also suitable for points of regional form such as pushing Pitu and Feijing. Operation between points is mainly of reducing method. But reinforcing or reducing effect induced by pushing on certain points are concerned with directions, which in clinic should be determined by the pushed parts and points.

骨等；也适用于"面状穴"，如推脾土、推肺经等，多属泻法。但在某些穴位上推动时补泻尚与方向有关，临床上应据部位和穴位而定。

2.2.2 Rotationally Pushing Manipulation （Xuantuifa）

OPERATING METHOD

Make the clockwise rotational movements on the point with the pad of the thumb at a great speed and with steady force (Fig. 40).

CLINICAL APPLICATION

The technique has invigorating effect, and is applicable to points on the fingers such as reinforcing Pitu, Weijing and Shenjing (the spleen, stomach and kidney meridians).

二、旋推法

【操作方法】

以拇指指面在穴位上做顺时针方向的旋转移动，速度稍快，用力要均匀（图40）。

【临床应用】

以此法操作有补益作用，多适用于指部穴位，如补脾土、补胃经、补肾经等。

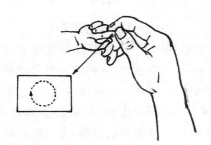

Fig. 40 Rotationally Pushing Manipulation
图 40   旋推法

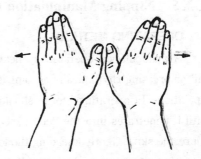

Fig. 41 Separating Manipulation
图 41   分法

2.2.3 Separating Manipulation （Fenfa）

OPERATING METHOD

Push from a point to both its sides with the radius aspect or the whorl surface of the thumbs or the pads of the

三、分法

【操作方法】

用两手拇指桡侧或螺纹面，或用食、中指二指面，自穴

index and middle fingers. In the operation, exertion of force by both hands should be even and coordinative and the movement should be along a straight line (Fig. 41).

CLINICAL APPLICATION

The manipulation is chiefly suitable for points on the head, face, chest, abdomen and back regions.

2.2.4　Joining Manipulation (Hefa)

OPERATING METHOD

Push from two sides of a point to its center with the whorl surface of both thumbs. The operation is opposite to that of separating manipulation. This manipulation is also called Hefa (Meeting manipulation).

CLINICAL APPLICATION

This manipulation is mainly operated on the hand, for example, pushing hand yin and yang points, which has the effect of regulating yin and yang and balancing the function of zang and fu organs.

2.2.5　Nipping Manipulation (Qiafa)

OPERATING METHOD

A manipulation operated by heavily stabbing with a nail or pressing rhythmically a point is called nipping manipulation. In operating, force should be gradually given until it penetrates into the deep part, and be sure not to injure the skin. Gently kneading the local area is often applied after nipping to relieve the irritated sensation. The manipulation is often used in combination with kneading manipulation and called nipping-kneading manipulation (Fig 42).

CLINICAL APPLICATION

Nipping manipulation is one of the manipulations inducing strong stimulations in infantile tuina, which is applicable to points on the face and four extremities such as

位向两侧分推。操作时,双手用力要均匀一致或配合协调,移动轨迹要保持直行(图41)。

【临床应用】

分推法主要适用于头面部、胸腹部与背部。

四、合法

【操作方法】

用两拇指螺纹面自穴两旁向穴中推动合拢,动作方法和分法相反,本法又称为和法。

【临床应用】

本法多在手部操作,如推手阴阳穴,有调和阴阳、平衡脏腑功能的作用。

五、掐法

【操作方法】

用指甲重刺或有节律地按穴位,称掐法。操作时要逐渐用力达深透为止,注意不要损伤皮肤,掐后轻揉局部,以缓解不适之感,常与揉法配合应用,称掐揉法(图42)。

【临床应用】

掐法是小儿推拿中强刺激手法之一,适用于面部及四肢腧穴,如水沟、素髎、内关、

Shuigou (GV 26), Suliao (GV 25), Neiguan (PC 6), Lao long. The method is commonly used for acute problems such as convulsion, loss of consciousness for its action of inducing resuscitation and restoring consciousness and relieving spasm.

老龙等穴位,多用于急性病症,如惊风、昏迷等,有醒脑开窍,解痉止搐的作用。

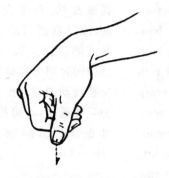

Fig. 42   Nipping Manipulation
图 42   拍法

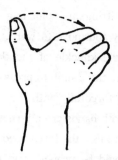

Fig. 43   Arc-pushing Manipulation
图 43   运法

2. 2. 6   Arc-pushing Manipulation (Yunfa)

OPERATING METHOD

A manipulation operated by pushing and rubbing on certain points in an arc or rotary route with the thumb or the tip of the middle finger is called arc-pushing manipulation. In manipulating, light and slow motion is advisable without involving the deep muscular tissues. The frequency is better at 80 to 100 times per minute (Fig. 43).

CLINICAL APPLICATION

The manipulation is light, mild and moderate in nature and often applied to operation on certain specific points on the hand such as Yunbagua. It has the effect of promoting qi circulation to activate blood and regulating meridian qi. Common cold, fever, indigestion and abdominal distension and borborygmus are often treated with this manipulation.

六、运法

【操作方法】

以拇指或中指指端在一定穴位上由此往彼作弧形或环形推摩,称运法,此法操作时,宜轻不宜重,宜缓不宜急,要在体表旋绕摩擦推动,不带动深层肌肉组织,频率一般以每分钟 80 ～120 次为宜(图 43)。

【临床应用】

本法轻柔缓和,多用于手掌的特定穴位上操作,如运八卦等,有行血活血,通调经气的作用,感冒、发热、消化不良、腹胀肠鸣等常以此法治疗。

2.2.7　Pinching Manipulation（Niefa）

OPERATING METHOD

Support the skin with the radial aspect of the thumb, press forward with the index and middle fingers. Then grasp and lift the skin up with the three fingers simultaneously. Do the lifting and pinching operation with both hands alternately and move forward. Or use the radial aspect of the middle knuckle of the flexed index finger to support the skin, the thumb to press forward. Then grasp and lift the skin forcefully with the two fingers and move forward while both hands are alternately doing the manipulation. In operating, the force used for pinching and lifting the skin should be proper, and twisting and rotating operation must be avoided. Pinching, lifting and then loosening the skin should be done one after another along a straight way（Fig. 44）.

七、捏法

【操作方法】

用拇指桡侧顶住皮肤，食、中指前按，三指同时用力提拿皮肤，双手交替捻动向前，或以食指弯曲，用食指中节桡侧顶住皮肤，拇指前按，两指同时用力提拿皮肤，双手交替捻动向前。操作时捏、提力量要适当，不可拧转，随捏、随提、随放，向前直线前进（图44）。

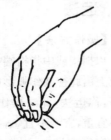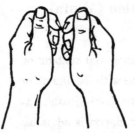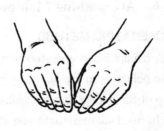

(1) Pinching Manipulation
(1) 捏法

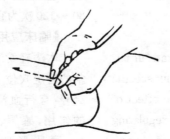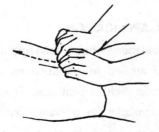

(2) Manipulation of Pinching the Spine
(2) 捏脊法

Fig. 44　Pinching Manipulations
图44　捏法

CLINICAL APPLICATION

This manipulation is also called manipulation of lifting the spine or manipulation of pinching the spine. It is, therefore, commonly applied to the spine and the areas lateral to it. The technique has the effect of promoting digestion to eliminate stagnation, strengthening the spleen and stomach, regulating the spleen and stomach to dissipate dampness and promote qi circulation to activate blood. Epigastric distension and fullness, indigestion, anorexia and chronic diarrhea can be treated with the manipulation.

2. 2. 8　Squeezing Manipulation（Jifa）

OPERATING METHOD

Grip the skin around a point and lift it gently with both the thumbs and index fingers. Then squeeze the point in opposite direction with force to cause pain in the local area around the point. The operation of gripping, squeezing each point should be less than ten times.

CLINICAL APPLICATION

The method is suitable for all parts of the body. It is mostly used on Taiyang (EX-HN 5), Yintang (EX-HN 3), Fengchi (GB 20) and other acupoints on the head, and is also used on Jianjing (GB 21) and acupoints on the chest, abdomen and back. The method has the effect of dispersing wind to relieve the exterior, diaphoresis to reduce fever and removing blood stasis to eliminate mass. Common cold, headache, summer heat, vomiting, nausea, liver stagnation and blood stasis can be treated with this manipulation.

2. 2. 9　Pounding Manipulation（Daofa）

OPERATING METHOD

The manipulation is performed by striking certain

【临床应用】

本法又称提脊法或捏脊法,故多适用在脊柱或旁开两侧部分,有消积导滞、健运脾胃、和中化湿、行气活血的作用,脘腹胀满、消化不良、不思饮食、慢性腹泻等病症可用此法治疗。

八、挤法

【操作方法】

用两手拇、食指同时将穴位周围的皮肤夹持并轻轻提起,再相对用力挤压穴位,以使穴位点处局部产生疼痛;操作时,夹持挤压每穴不超过10次。

【临床应用】

适用于全身,多用于头部的太阳、印堂、风池等穴位,以及肩井、胸腹及背部,有疏风解表、发汗祛热、祛瘀散结等功效,感冒、头痛、暑热、呕吐、恶心、郁结瘀血可用本法治疗。

九、捣法

【操作方法】

用中指指端或食指、中指

points or areas rhythmically with the tip of the middle finger or the process of the proximal interphalangeal joints of the flexed index and middle fingers. In operating, the wrist joint is used as the moving center and the striking should be elastic.

CLINICAL APPLICATION

The manipulation is suitable for all points of the body, especially those on the palm, the spinal column and the back such as pounding Xiaotianxin. It has the action of removing obstruction, expelling pathogenic cold, relieving pain and tranquilizing the mind. The manipulation is commonly used in treating convulsion, fever, restlessness with fear and spasm of limbs, etc.

2.2.10　Flicking Manipulation（Tanfa）

OPERATING METHOD

The manipulation is done by flicking and hitting the affected area or points quickly and continuously with the nail of one or more fingers. In operating, the pad of the thumb presses firmly the nail of the operating finger to make its interphalangeal joint do rapid flexing and extending movements so as for the nail surface to flick quickly and continuously the treated area and acupoint. The force exerted should be even, and the frequency is 80 to 120 times per minute (Fig. 45).

屈曲后的近侧指间关节突起部为着力点，在一定的穴位或部位上做有节律的点击。操作时，要以腕关节为活动中心，点击要有弹性。

【临床应用】

适用于全身各部穴位，尤以手掌、脊背部为多，如捣小天心等，具有开导闭塞、祛寒止痛、镇惊安神的作用。常用于治疗惊风、发热、惊惕不安、四肢抽搐等症。

十、弹法

【操作方法】

以一个或多个手指的指甲面快速、连续地弹击治疗部位或穴位。操作时即用指腹紧压住施术手指的指甲，使其指间关节做快速的屈伸运动时以指甲面迅速连续弹击治疗部位或穴位。弹击时用力要均匀，频率每分钟 80 ～120 次（图 45）。

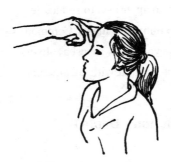

Fig. 45　Flicking Manipulation
图 45　弹法

CLINICAL APPLICATION

The manipulation is applicable to points all over the body, especially to those on the head, face, neck, chest and abdomen. It has the function of inducing resuscitation and restoring consciousness, tranquilizing the mind and promoting circulation of qi and blood. The method is often used in compatible treatment of stiffness of the nape, headache, cough, asthma, abdominal distension, diarrhea and constipation, etc.

2.2.11 Manipulation of Dragon Getting into the Mouth of a Tiger (Longruhukou)

OPERATING METHOD

Support the dorsum of the infant patient's hand with one hand, insert the index finger of the other hand into its Hukou (the junction part of the thumb and index finger), and then push or press or press and knead the infant's Banmen point (on the major thenar) with the thumb (Fig. 46).

【临床应用】

本法适用于全身各部,尤以头面、颈项、胸腹部最为常用,具有开窍醒脑、镇静安神、行气活血的作用,项强、头痛、喘咳、腹胀、腹泻、便秘等病症常用本法配合治疗。

十一、龙入虎口

【操作方法】

一手托患儿掌背,另一手食指叉入虎口(大拇指与食指交叉处)用大拇指或推或按或按揉患儿板门穴(大鱼际处)(图 46)。

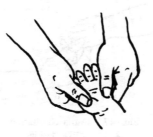

Fig. 46 Longruhukou
图 46 龙入虎口

CLINICAL APPLICATION

The manipulation is a compound manipulation of infant tuina, whose name is given vividly in the way of the operation. It has the effect of clearing away heat and eliminating dampness and descending adverse qi and stopping diarrhea. Exogenous fever, fever due to food reten-

【临床应用】

本法为小儿复式操作手法,名称以形象而定,具有清热利湿,降逆止泻的作用,外感发热或食积热重、呕吐、腹泻、四肢瘈跳等症均可用本法

tion, vomiting, diarrhea, and subsultus of the limbs, etc. can be treated with this manipulation.

治疗。

2. 2. 12　Manipulation of Beating the Horse to Cross the Heaven River (Dama Guo-tianhe)

十二、打马过天河

OPERATING METHOD

Hold the infant patient's fingers with the left hand, flick and beat with the index and middle fingers or the index, middle and ring fingers of the right hand dipped in cool water from acupoint Zongjin, along Tianhe (the Heaven River) to Quze (PC 3). In flicking operation, the force exerted should be even and proper and the up-and-down movements should be rhythmic. Meanwhile, puffs of breath are given along with the manipulation (Fig. 47).

【操作方法】

用左手托拿住患儿手指，用右手食、中指或食、中、无名三指指面蘸凉水由总筋穴起，沿天河弹打至曲泽穴止，弹打时用力均匀、适当，一起一落并有节律，同时可一面用口吹气随之（图 47）。

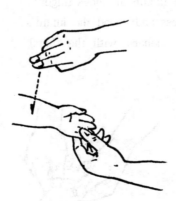

Fig. 47　Dama Guotianhe
图 47　打马过天河

CLINICAL APPLICATION

The manipulation is mainly applied to point Tianhe-shui, for it is indicated in pyretic syndromes. The manipulation has the function of clearing away pathogenic heat, expelling toxin and purging fire to relieve dysphoria. Cold, fever, headache with aversion to wind, slight sweating, sore throat and excess fever and high fever caused

【临床应用】

本法主要用在天河水穴，因天河水穴主治热证等，故打马过天河手法具有清热解毒，泻火除烦的作用，感冒发热、头痛恶风、汗微出、咽痛等外感风热及其他病证导致的实

by exogenous pathogenic wind-heat and other syndromes can be treated with this manipulation.

热、高热等症，可用本法治疗。

2. 2. 13 Manipulation of Fishing the Moon from the Bottom of Water (Shuidilaoyue)

十三、水底捞月

OPERATING METHOD

The doctor uses his or her left hand to support the infant patient's four fingers, having the palm facing upward. Dip the right hand in cool water and drop some on the infant's point Neilaogong. Arc-push and push from the infant's little finger base through Zhangxiaohengwen, Xiaotianxin to Neilaogong with the pad of the middle finger dipped in cool water. The pushing action should be coherent and gentle, and puffs of breath are given simultaneously (Fig. 48).

【操作方法】

用左手托起小儿施术手四指，掌心向上，右手蘸凉水滴于小儿内劳宫处，用中指指腹沾凉水由小指根推运起，经掌小横纹、小天心至内劳宫，推运时动作连贯柔和，边推运边吹凉气（图 48）。

CLINICAL APPLICATION

The manipulation is a specific compound manipulation of infantile tuina, which has the function of clearing away heat, cooling blood, tranquilizing the mind to relieve dysphoria. In clinic, fever, dysphoria, coma and delirium are often treated with the method.

【临床应用】

本法为小儿推拿特定复式操作法，具有清热凉血宁心除烦的作用，临证中发热烦躁，神昏谵语等病症可用本法治疗。

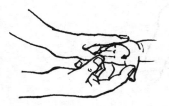

Fig. 48 Shuidilaoyue
图 48 水底捞月

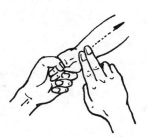

Fig. 49 Qing Tianheshui
图 49 清天河水

2. 2. 14 Manipulation of Clearing Water of the Heaven River (Qing Tianheshui)

十四、清天河水

OPERATING METHOD

Push with the whorl surface of the index and middle

【操作方法】

用食、中两指螺纹面自腕

fingers from the wrist to acupoint Hongchi 〔Quze (PC 3)〕 with lissom and coherent movement (Fig. 49).

CLINICAL APPLICATION

This manipulation is slightly cool in nature and the manipulation is more moderate than that of Beating the Horse to Cross the Heaven River (Damaguotianhe). It has the function of clearing away heat, expelling toxin, relieving dysphoria and purging fire, and is very effective in treating exogenous wind-heat syndrome manifested as common cold with fever, headache, aversion to wind, slight sweating. It is also used together with pushing Cuanzhu (BL 2) and Kangong, kneading Taiyang (EX-HN 5), etc.

2.2.15 Manipulation of Twisting and Rubbing like Plucking the String (Anxuan Cuomo)

OPERATING METHOD

Stand behind the infant patient, twist and rub with both palms the infant's hypochondriac areas under the armpits downward with gentle and coherent movement (Fig. 50).

推向洪池(曲泽穴)。动作轻快连续(图 49)。

【临床应用】

清天河水性微凉,较打马过天河操作手法平和,具有清热解毒、除烦泻火的作用。对于感冒发热、头痛、恶风、汗微出、咽痛等外感风热者,有较好治疗作用,也常与推攒竹、推坎宫,揉太阳等合用。

十五、按弦搓摩

【操作方法】

站于小儿身后,用双手掌在小儿两腋下胁肋处,自上而下搓摩,动作柔和连续(图 50)。

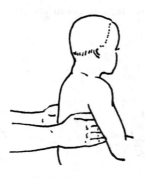

Fig. 50　Anxuan Cuomo
图 50　按弦搓摩

CLINICAL APPLICATION

The manipulation is mainly used on the lumbar side and the hypochondriac regions. The operation may be illustrated as plucking the string of a musical instrument. It has the effect of regulating qi to dissipate phlegm, guiding

【临床应用】

本法主要用于腰侧胁肋部,形象说明动作如抚琴操弦状,具有理气化痰、顺气生血的作用,咳嗽、哮喘、痰积、胸

qi downward and promoting blood generation. Cough, asthma, phlegm stagnation and chest stuffiness can be treated with the technique.

闷可用此法治疗。

2.2.16 Manipulation of an Old Man Pulling a Fishnet (Laohan Banzeng)

十六、老汉扳罾

OPERATING METHOD

Nip the infant's thumb base with the left thumb, nip and pinch point Pitu and shake its thumb with the right hand. While nipping, force is slightly exerted, but sticky and heavy sensation should not be produced and shaking should be coherent, light and soft (Fig. 51).

【操作方法】

用左手拇指掐住小儿拇指根处,右手掐捏脾土穴并摇动小儿拇指,掐时稍用力但不滞重,摇动连续轻柔(图51)。

CLINICAL APPLICATION

The method is a compound manipulation and has the function of invigorating the spleen and stomach, promoting digestion to eliminate food retention. Infantile diseases such as indigestion, milk vomiting, foul and viscid feces, abdominal distension and dyspepsia can be treated with this method.

【临床应用】

本法为复式操作手法,具有健运脾胃、消导食积的作用。婴幼儿消化不良、呕吐奶块、大便臭秽粘滞、腹胀食积等病症可用本法治疗。

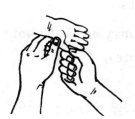

Fig. 51 Laohan Banzeng
图 51 老汉扳罾

2.2.17 Manipulation of Carrying Earth into Water (Yuntu Rushui)

十七、运土入水

OPERATING METHOD

Hold the infant's four fingers with the left hand and have the palm facing upward. Push and arc-push with the right thumb from point Pitu at the thumb base of the

【操作方法】

用左手拿住小儿四指,掌心向上,右手拇指指端由小儿拇指根部脾土穴推运起,经小

infant through Xiaotianxin, Zhangxiaohengwen to Shen-shui at the little fingertip. The movement should be heavy but not sticky, light but not superficial (Fig. 52).

天心、掌小横纹到小指端肾水穴,推运时重而不滞,轻而不浮(图 52)。

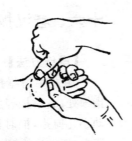

Fig. 52 Yuntu Rushui
图 52 运土入水

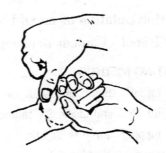

Fig. 53 Yunshui Rutu
图 53 运水入土

CLINICAL APPLICATION

The method is a compound manipulation and involves four areas or points from the beginning to the end. It has the function of normalizing the lower energizer, nourishing the kidney, clearing away heat and promoting diuresis and can be used to treat frequent and hot urination, lower abdominal distension and fullness.

2.2.18 Manipulation of Carrying Water into Earth (Yunshui Rutu)

OPERATING METHOD

Hold the infant's palm and have it facing upward, push and arc-push with the tip of the right thumb from point Shenshui at the little finger along the palm root to Pitu at the end of the thumb or to the thumb base. Pushing movement should be proper in heaviness and lightness (Fig. 53).

CLINICAL APPLICATION

The method is a compound manipulation, and has the function of strengthening the spleen to help transformation and transportation, moistening dryness to relieve constipation. Diarrhea, dysentery, indigestion, food re-

【临床应用】

本法为复式手法,起止并经过计 4 个部位(穴位),具有通利下焦、滋肾清热、通淋利水的作用,小便赤涩、频数,小腹胀满等病症可用本法治疗。

十八、运水入土

【操作方法】

用一手托拿住小儿手掌,掌心向上,右手拇指指端由小儿小指肾水穴部沿掌根推运向大指端脾土或指根,推运时亦要重轻相宜(图 53)。

【临床应用】

本法为复式手法,具有健脾助运,润燥通便的作用,腹泻、痢疾、消化不良、食积、便秘等,可用本法治疗。

tention and constipation, etc. can be treated with the method.

2.2.19 Manipulation of Opening up Xuanji (Kaixuanji)

OPERATING METHOD

Push separately with both hands from point Xuanji (CV 21)on the chest downward along the intercostal space toward both sides of the body to acupoint Jiuwei (CV 15), straight push on downward to the umbilicus region. Then rub right and left on the umbilicus and abdomen, and finally push from the center of the umbilicus down to the lower abdomen.

CLINICAL APPLICATION

The method belongs to a compound manipulation. It has the function of removing obstruction, descending adverse qi to stop vomiting, promoting digestion and regulating the stomach, relieving convulsion and stopping pain. Short breath, phlegm stagnation, vomiting, diarrhea and convulsion can be treated with this method.

2.2.20 Finishing Manipulation (Zongshoufa)

OPERATING METHOD

Press and knead the area around Jianjing (GB 21) of the infant with the left thumb or index and middle fingers, hold its fingers on the same side with the right hand, flex and extend its elbow and wrist and shake its upper arm. The movement should be coordinative and coherent. Exertion of force should be even and moderate.

CLINICAL APPLICATION

The methed is a compound manipulation. It is often used when tuina on an infant ends. The manipulation has the function of warming the meridians, expelling cold, promoting circulation of qi and blood and regulating the

十九、开璇玑

【操作方法】

双手先从胸部璇玑穴开始,沿胸肋间隙自上而下向左右两旁分推,至鸠尾穴处向下直推脐部,然后再在脐腹部左右摩擦,最后从脐中推下小腹。

【临床应用】

本法为复式手法,具有开通闭塞,降逆止呕,消食和胃,镇惊止痛的作用。气急、痰闭吐泻、惊风可用本法治疗。

二十、总收法

【操作方法】

用左手拇指或食、中指按揉小儿肩井穴部,右手拿住其同侧手指,曲伸肘腕并摇动其上肢。动作协调连贯,用力均匀,和缓。

【临床应用】

本法为复式手法,多用于小儿推拿结束时,具有温经散寒、疏通气血、调节整体的作用。久病体虚、气血失调、上

function of the whole body. Weakness due to long-standing illness, disturbance of qi and blood and arthralgia in the upper extremity can also be treated with this method.

肢痹痛亦可用此法治疗。

2.3　Approaches of Manipulation Practice

第三节　手法的 练习方法

In order to command techniques of tuina manipulations skillfully and obtain persistent strength, it is necessary to conduct hard, attentive and serious exercises. Some manipulations, especially those with complicated and more difficult skills such as rolling must be practised repeatedly for a long period.

要熟练掌握推拿手法技巧和持续的力量,必须进行认真刻苦的练习,尤其对一些比较复杂而难度较高的手法,如㨰法等,更应长期反复练习。

Practice of manipulation chiefly refers to training in skills of manipulation and strength of the finger, wrist and arm. It is generally divided into two stages: the first, basic training on the sand sack, and the second, operating practice on the human body after sand sack practice has laid some foundation. While conducting exercises of manipulation, no matter what they are, on a sand sack or on the human body, the student should have his mind concentrated on and be devoted to them wholeheartedly. Especially when doing practice on the human body, one should fathom the implications of gentleness, evenness, persistence and forcefulness of manipulations again and again. Only by painstaking training can one attain the objective of having everything under one's perfect control and gain a better effectiveness.

手法练习的内容,主要是动作技巧和指力、腕力、臂力的锻炼。一般在学习时,先分两个阶段进行:第一阶段,在沙袋上进行基本训练;第二阶段,待沙袋练习有一定基础后,再转入人体的操作练习。进行手法练习时,无论是沙袋还是人体,均要集中思想,专心致志,尤其在人体上操作练习时,要反复揣摩"柔和、均匀、持久、有力"的手法要求,只有刻苦练习,才能达到"手随心转,法从手出"的得心应手程度和功效。

2.3.1　Practice on Sand Sack

一、沙袋练习法

Prepare a sack 26 cm long and 16 cm wide, fill it with sand or rice (it will be better to mix some broken sponge in to make the sack more elastic.), and then stitch the sack mouth. Coat the sack with a clean cloth bag

备布袋一只,约长 26 厘米、宽 16 厘米,内装黄沙或大米(掺入一部分碎海绵更佳,使其具有弹性),将袋口缝合,

which is washed easily. At the beginning of practice, the sack may be tied tight and later loosened gradually. According to difficult degrees and essential points of movement of manipulations, one should have more practice on pushing manipulation with one-finger, rolling, kneading, grasping, pressing and rubbing manipulations first. Through the practice, the technique of movement and nimbleness of the principal manipulations can be mastered and the strength of the finger and wrist can also be built up. Either sitting or standing postures may be taken in practice. Manipulations of pushing with one-finger, kneading, pressing, rubbing, and arc-pushing, etc. should be practiced in a sitting posture, while manipulations of rolling and grasping in a standing posture. In practicing rolling manipulation, both the right and left hands should be trained alternately, while for other manipulations, practice is mainly conducted with the right hand.

2.3.2 Practice on the Human Body

Practice on the human body is in fact a transition to application of tuina manipulations. So it should be conducted on every part of the human body in combination with the general routine operations in clinical treatment and according to the indications of manipulations as much as possible. In practice, attention is paid not only to operation of a single manipulation, but also to coordination of several manipulations such as pressing and kneading, nipping and grasping. Meanwhile, one should experience and observe carefully morphologic change and structure of the human body, activities of joints, elasticity and tension of muscles, tendons and other soft tissues, and exert different force and range in massage. A brief introduction to commonly used manipulations on different human parts and operating procedures will be given as follows.

外套一干净布袋,便于换洗。开始练习时,袋可扎得紧些,以后逐渐放松。根据手法的动作要领和难度,重点练习一指禅推法、㨰法、揉法、拿法、按法、摩法等。通过练习,重点掌握主要手法的动作技巧和灵活度,同时也可增强指力和腕力。练习姿势可采取坐势和站势。坐势练习手法有一指禅推法、揉法、按法和摩法等;站势练习手法主要是㨰法和拿法。练习㨰法时,要求左、右手交替进行,其他手法则以右手为主。

二、人体练习法

人体操作练习,是实际应用推拿手法的过渡,所以尽可能结合临床治疗的一般操作常规,按手法的适应证在人体各部位进行练习。练习中,不但要注意单一手法的操作,而且要注意各种手法的配合运用,如按揉、捏拿等。同时还应细心体会,根据人体的形态、结构、关节活动功能以及肌肉、肌腱等软组织的弹性、张力等情况,施以不同的力量和幅度。下面简要介绍人体各部常用的手法和操作程序。

2.3.2.1 Operating Procedures of Tuina on the Head and Face

The patient is in a sitting or supine position, and the doctor takes a standing or sitting posture.

(1) Pushing manipulation with one-finger

a. Operate to and fro twice or three times from Yintang (EX-HN 3) to Shenting (GV 24).

b. Operate to and fro on both the right and left sides twice or three times respectively from Cuanzhu (BL 2) to Yangbai (GB 14) to Taiyang (EX-HN 5) and to Touwei (ST 8).

c. Do "∞" type operation twice or three times from Jingming (BL 1) along the left orbit to the right orbit, from inside to outside and from top to bottom, combined with wiping the area around the orbit.

d. Operate to and fro on both the right and left sides twice or three times respectively from Jingming (BL 1) to Yingxiang (LI 20) to Dicang (ST 4) to Xiaguan (ST 7) to Jiache (ST 6) and to Chengjiang (CV 24).

e. Operate to and fro twice or three times from Yintang (EX-HN 3) to Shenting (GV 24) and to Baihui (GV 20) or push Baihui (GV 20).

(2) Press and knead the acupoints on the head and face with the thumb or major thenar, each point for 1 - 3 minutes.

(3) Grasp the five meridians. Fix the patient's forehead with one hand. Grasp the governor vessel on the head, the foot -taiyang meridians and the foot -shaoyang meridians on both sides with the separated five fingers of the other hand 5 - 10 times from the face to the back of the head and stop at Fengchi (GB 20).

(4) Sweeping manipulation. Fix one side of the patient's head with one hand, put the five fingers of the other hand on the other side of his head and perform the

（一）头面部推拿操作程序

患者坐位或仰卧位,医者取站势或坐势。

（1）一指禅推法

① 自印堂 → 神庭穴,往返 2～3 次。

② 自攒竹 → 阳白 → 太阳 → 头维穴,往返 2～3 次,左右同。

③ 自睛明穴沿眼眶周围,由内向外,从上到下,自左眼向右眼,呈"∞"字形操作 2～3 遍,配合抹眼眶周围。

④ 自睛明 → 迎香 → 地仓 → 下关 → 颊车 → 承浆等穴,往返操作 2～3 遍,左右同。

⑤ 自印堂 → 神庭 → 百会穴(或推百会穴),往返操作 2～3 次。

（2）拇指按揉或大鱼际按揉头面部诸穴,每穴 1～3 分钟。

（3）拿五经。一手固定前额,一手五指分拿头部督脉和双侧足太阳、足少阳经,从前向后推拿,止于风池穴,操作 5～10 次。

（4）扫散法。一手固定头侧,另一手五指分置另一头侧,沿耳上向两边头侧部操作

operation on both sides 3-5 times along the part above the ear.

(5) Wipe the head and face. Wipe with the major thenar of both hands 3 - 5 times from the forehead separately to Taiyang (EX-HN 5) to mastoidea, and then to Fengchi (GB 20) on both sides of the patient's head.

2.3.2.2 Operating Procedures of Tuina on the Nape and Back

The patient takes a sitting or prone position and the masseur stands behind or on one side of the patient.

(1) Push with one-finger manipulation 3 - 5 times from the inferior part of the occipital bone through Fengfu (GV 16) to Dazhui (GV 14).

(2) Stick the lateral hump of the thumb to Fengchi (GB 20) and operate in a gesture of double-flying butterflies (Hudie Shuangfeishi) for 3 - 5 minutes.

(3) Straight push the acupoint Qiaogong 5 - 10 times with the thumb of one hand.

(4) Operate rolling manipulation to and fro from the inferior part of the occipital bone through Fengfu (GV 16) to Dazhui (GV 14) in combination with the patient's passive movement.

(5) Operate rolling manipulation on Jianjing (GB 21) from one side to the other side to and fro 5 - 10 times.

(6) Rotate and pull the nape moderately.

(7) Percuss and vibrate the back up and down 3 - 5 times with the dorsum of a fist.

(8) Pull and vibrate the thoracic vertebrae and thorax 3 - 5 times.

(9) Grasp the area around Jianjing (GB 1) on both sides 5 - 10 times.

2.3.2.3 Operating Procedures of Tuina on the Chest and Abdomen

The patient takes a supine posture and the massagist

（5）抹头面。两手大鱼际自前额向两侧太阳穴 → 耳后高骨 → 风池穴分抹3~5遍。

（二）项背部推拿操作程序

患者坐位或俯卧位，医者立于后侧或一侧。

（1）一指禅推自枕骨下经风府至大椎穴3~5遍。

（2）偏峰吸定风池穴，以蝴蝶双飞势操作3~5分钟。

（3）单侧手拇指向下直推桥弓穴5~10次。

（4）滚法自枕骨下经风府穴 → 大椎穴，往返操作，并配合被动运动。

（5）滚法自一侧肩井向另一侧肩井部，往返操作5~10遍。

（6）摇、扳项部适度。

（7）拳背叩震背部，上下3~5次。

（8）扳振胸椎、胸廓3~5次。

（9）拿双侧肩井部5~10次。

（三）胸腹部推拿操作程序

患者仰卧位，医者坐

sits beside him or her.

(1) Push the conception vessel from Danzhong（CV 17）to Zhongwan（CV 12）to Qihai（CV 6）to Guanyuan （CV 4）, or other acupoints to and fro 5 - 10 times with pushing manipulation with one finger.

(2) Push and rub Zhongwan（CV 12）and Tianshu （ST 25）for 1 - 3 minutes respectively.

(3) Rub the abdomen rotationally with the whole palm clockwise and counterclockwise, each for 3 - 5 minutes.

(4) Rub transversely the area from the infraclavicular part gradually to Danzhong（CV 17）, Rugen（ST 18）and Jiuwei（CV 15）with the whole palm with to-and-fro rubbing manipulation. Or push and rub with the palm side from Tiantu（CV 22）along the front middle line downward twice or three times.

(5) Push separately the chest and hypochondrium areas with both hands until they become hot.

(6) Vibrate the gastroabdominal regions with one palm or overlapped palmar bases for 1 - 3 minutes with vibrating manipulation, which is performed by putting the finger or palm on the body surface or point and doing even, rhythmic and up-and-down vibrating movement. Or Digitally-vibrate Zhongwan（CV 12）, Qihai（CV 6）or other points with the middle finger each for 1 minute.

(7) Palm-twist the hypochondriac region, which is done by pressing from both sides of the trunk and twisting back and forth with both palms up and down 5 - 10 times.

2.3.2.4 Operating Procedures of Tuina on the Shoulder and Arm

The patient takes a sitting or lying position and the massagist stands beside the diseased side.

(1) Push the area round the shoulder joint with pushing manipulation with one finger for 3 - 5 minutes.

一侧。

（1）推任脉,一指禅推法自膻中 → 中脘 → 气海 → 关元等穴,往返5～10次。

（2）推摩中脘、天枢穴各1～3分钟。

（3）全掌环转摩腹部,逆、顺时针各3～5分钟。

（4）擦法以全掌自锁骨下横擦渐至膻中、乳根、鸠尾部,或以掌侧自天突穴沿正中线向下推擦2～3遍。

（5）双手分推胸胁部,以热为度。

（6）以振颤法（以指或掌置按于体表或穴位上,做均匀而有节奏的上下振颤动作,称为振颤法）单掌或叠掌振脘腹1～3分钟,或中指点振中脘、气海穴各1分钟。

（7）搓双胁、双掌夹搓两胁肋,上下往返5～10次。

（四）肩及上肢部推拿操作程序

患者坐位或卧位,医者立于患侧。

（1）一指禅推法,推肩关节周围3～5分钟。

(2) Push from Jianyu (LI 15) to Binao (LI 14) to Quchi (LI 11) to Shousanli (LI 10) to Hegu (LI 4) to and fro 3 - 5 times with pushing manipulation with one finger.

(3) Rolling manipulation

a. Roll the anterior border of the shoulder joint with rolling manipulation, combined with passive inward and outward rotation of the shoulder joint for 3 - 5 minutes.

b. Roll the lateral border of the shoulder joint with rolling manipulation, combined with raising and adduction of the shoulder joint for 3 - 5 minutes.

c. Roll the posterior border of the shoulder joint with rolling manipulation, combined with retroflexion and inward rotation of the shoulder joint for 3 - 5 minutes.

(4) Rotate the shoulder joint by holding the elbow or in the great amplitude 5 - 10 times.

(5) Palm-twist the shoulder joint for 1 - 3 minutes.

(6) Palm-twist the upper limb up and down 5 - 10 times.

(7) Finger-twist and pull-extend all the interphalangeal joints once respectively.

(8) Shake the upper limb moderately.

2.3.2.5 Operating Procedures of Tuina on the Lumbus and Lower Limb

The patient takes a prone or supine position and the massagist stands beside him or her.

(1) Operate rolling manipulation along the sacrospinal muscles on both sides of the back and the lumbus to lumbosacral areas to and fro 5 - 10 times.

(2) Operate rolling manipulation on each leg from Huantiao (GB 30) to Weizhong (BL 40) to Chengshan (BL 57) and other acupoints to and fro 5 - 10 times.

(3) Press and knead Jiaji acupoints to and fro 3 - 5 times.

(4) Rub directly the spinal column and the sacrospinal

（2）一指禅推法,自肩髃 → 臂臑 → 曲池 → 手三里 → 合谷等穴,往返 3～5 遍。

（3）㨰法

① 㨰肩关节前缘,配合肩关节内、外旋被动运动 3～5 分钟。

② 㨰肩关节外缘,配合肩关节上举、内收运动 3～5 分钟。

③ 㨰肩关节后缘,配合肩关节后伸、内旋运动 3～5 分钟。

（4）摇肩关节(托肘摇、大摇)5～10 次。

（5）搓肩关节 1～3 分钟。

（6）搓上肢,自上而下往返 5～10 次。

（7）捻、拔伸各指关节 1 遍。

（8）抖上肢适度。

（五）腰及下肢部推拿操作程序

患者俯卧或仰卧,医者立一侧。

（1）施㨰法沿背腰两侧骶棘肌至腰骶部,往返操作 5～10 遍。

（2）施㨰法沿环跳 → 委中 → 承山等穴,左右往返操作5～10 遍。

（3）按揉夹脊穴,往返3～5 遍。

（4）直擦脊柱、两侧骶棘

muscles on both sides of the trunk until they become hot.

(5) Operate rolling manipulation on each leg from Biguan (ST 31) to Futu (ST 32) to Zusanli (ST 36) to Juegu (GB39) to and fro twice or three times.

(6) Operate rolling manipulation along the medial aspect from the thigh to the shank to and fro twice or three times.

(7) Press and knead the knee joints 3 - 5 times.

(8) Percuss the areas from the thigh to the shank to and fro 3 - 5 times.

(9) Operate oblique pulling manipulation or fixed-location waist-twisting once on the lumbar region.

肌,以热为度。

(5) 施擦法自髀关 → 伏兔 → 足三里 → 绝骨穴,左右各往返操作2~3遍。

(6) 施擦法从大腿内侧至小腿内侧2~3遍。

(7) 按揉膝关节 3～5分钟。

(8) 叩击自大腿至小腿部,往返3~5遍。

(9) 腰部斜扳或旋转定位扳1次。

3 Auxiliary Therapy

第三章　辅助方法

In the course of treatment and health care with Chinese Tuina, according to different diseases and symptoms, some simple and effective means, such as cupping, moxibustion, finger-pressing point, massage of auricular points, massage with ointments (Gaomo) and hot compress with Chinese herbs are used as auxiliary methods. These auxiliary methods may help achieve more satisfactory therapeutic results. The following is a brief introduction of the most commonly used massage with ointments (Gaomo) and hot compress.

中国推拿的治疗和保健过程中,根据不同的病症及病情,选用一些诸如拔罐、艾灸、点穴指压、耳穴按摩、膏摩、中草药热敷等简便有效的方法做为辅助疗法,这样更能取得满意的疗效。现就最常用的膏摩和热敷法做一简介。

3.1 Massage Therapy with Ointment —— Gaomo

第一节　膏摩

Gaomo or massage with ointments is actually a general term of techniques in which some ointments applied to the treated areas of the body surface before performing some manipulations, especially pushing, to-and-fro rubbing, palm-twisting, kneading and circular rubbing, in the course of massage. The ointments are prepared in the forms of cream, oil solution, or tincture from some Chinese herbal medicines and other substances with curative and preventive effects. Gaomo functions in two aspects. Firstly, these preparations act as lubricators to protect the skin from injury in tuina therapy. Secondly, the medical components of preparations will permeate into the body during manipulation, and become an active factor to prevent and treat diseases. Gaomo prescriptions started to be

膏摩,就是根据病情,采用对证的中草药等具有防治疾病作用的物质制成膏剂或油剂及酊剂等,在推拿过程中尤其是推、擦、搓、揉、摩等一些手法时,敷抹在施术体表,然后再进行操作。这种方法有两个作用:首先是这些制剂在推拿过程中起到润滑保护皮肤的作用,再者制剂中的药物等成分可随手法渗透体内,成为一个积极防治疾病的因素。膏摩成方从古就有记载,类型很多。但目前推拿临床

recorded in ancient times with various kinds and types. At present, however, only those easily-prepared, effective medicines and substances are usually adopted as components of ordinary Gaomo prescriptions in clinic, which are also called Tuina media, and applied selectively in treatment according to the specific symptoms or diseases.

3.1.1 Chinese Holly Ointment

Preparation: Mix the holly oil (methyl salicylate) with vaseline evenly in the proportion of one to five.

Actions: Relieving swelling to stop pain and dispersing pathogenic wind and cold.

Indications: All kinds of swelling or pain caused by traumatic injury and cold pain syndrome of old wounds.

3.1.2 Sesame Oil (or Other Vegetable Oils)

Actions: Expelling pathogenic wind, clearing away heat, regulating blood circulation and restoring qi.

Indications: Consumptive deficiency due to long-term illness, poor constitution of the aged, infant or child.

3.1.3 Juice of Shallot and Ginger

Preparations: Cut an equal quantity of fresh shallot without leaves and ginger into pieces, pestle them and soak them in 95% alcohol in the proportion of one to three. Leave the mixture for 3 - 5 days, and get the juice for use.

Actions: Activating yang and relieving the exterior, warming the middle energizer and promoting circulation of qi.

Indications: Common cold, headache or other symp-

上,通常采用以下几种易备、有效的药或物质,作为基本膏摩剂的组成,这些基本膏摩剂又通称为推拿介质,治疗时可根据具体的病症灵活选用。

一、冬青油膏

配制:以冬绿油(水杨酸甲酯)与凡士林按 1：5 混合调匀而成。

功效:消肿止痛,祛风散寒。

适用:一切跌打损伤的肿胀、疼痛,以及陈旧性损伤的寒性痛证等。

二、麻油(也可用其他植物油代替)

功效:祛风清热,和血补虚。

适用:久病虚损或年老体弱、婴幼儿等。

三、葱姜汁

配制:取葱白、鲜生姜等量切碎、捣烂,按 1：3 比例浸入 95% 酒精中,停放 3～5 日后,取汁液应用。

功效:通阳解表、温中行气。

适用:风寒引起的感冒、

toms caused by pathogenic wind and cold, pain in the stomach and abdomen due to cold and qi stagnation, etc.

3.1.4   Egg White

Preparation: Make a small opening on a fresh chicken's or duck's egg, hang it on a container, and get the egg white for use.

Actions: Eliminating vexation, clearing away heat, removing food retention and promoting digestion.

Indications: The advanced stage of febrile or lingering diseases, feverish sensation in the palm and sole, irritability, insomnia, belching, and acid regurgitation.

3.1.5   White Liquor

Preparation: Cereal liquor or medicated liquor with high concentration.

Actions: Warming and dredging the meridians, activating blood circulation and relieving pain.

Indications: Lingering pain of injury, numbness, contracture in the hand or foot, soreness, lassitude and weakness in the lumbus and knee, etc.

3.1.6   Talcum（Either Medicated Talcum or Talcum Powder）

Actions: Drying, eliminating dampness and lubricating the skin.

Indications: Infant or patient with delicate skin and manipulations in hot summer.

3.1.7   Mint Water

Preparation: Soak fresh mint leaves (or dried leaves in double quantity) in proper amount of boiling water,

头痛等症,以及因寒凝气滞而致的脘腹疼痛等。

四、鸡蛋清

配制:将生鸡蛋(鸭蛋亦可)一端磕一小孔后,悬置于容器上,取渗出蛋清应用。

功效:除烦去热、消导积滞。

适用:热病、久病后期,手足心热,烦躁失眠,嗳气吐酸等病症。

五、白酒

配制:浓度较高的粮食白酒或药酒。

功效:温通经络,活血止痛。

适用:损伤疼痛日久或麻木不仁,手足拘挛,腰膝酸软无力及瘀肿等病症。

六、滑石粉(医用滑石粉或爽身粉等均可)

功效:干燥除湿,润滑皮肤。

适用:婴幼儿及皮肤娇嫩者,以及在炎热夏季手法操作时应用。

七、薄荷水

配制:取鲜薄荷叶(可用干薄荷叶替代,但量需加倍),

cover the container and leave it for one day, and then filter the remains out and get the juice for use.

Actions: Cooling, relieving the exterior and clearing away summer heat.

Indications: All kinds of febrile diseases, such as fever, regional redness and swelling, pyretic pain. It can also be used for some disorders in summer.

Besides above-mentioned media, some other ready-made products can also be selected, such as Wanhuayou or carthamin oil for traumatic injury.

3.2　Medicated Hot Compress Therapy

Medicated hot compress refers to fumigating, washing, ironing or to-and-fro rubbing the affected sites of patients' body surface in different ways with different Chinese medicines under the guidance of the basic theory of TCM. This therapy is an external treatment, and has the advantages of quick effects, simple methods, easy learning, convenient promotion, safe application and less side effects. Therefore, this method is not only applied in departments of surgery, orthopaedics and traumatology, dermatology and the eye, ear, nose and throat diseases, but also in internal medicine, gynecology, pediatrics often with satisfactory results. It is another auxiliary treatment in massotherapy.

Medicated hot compress has a long history and can trace back to the ancient time. In the book *Wushierbingfang* (*Fifty two Medical Prescriptions*), unearthed in Mawangdui, external treatments were recorded such as warming and ironing, massage with ointment, washing externally. In *Neijing*, the earliest extant Chinese medi-

浸泡于适量的开水中,容器加盖停放 1 日后,去渣取汁液应用。

功效:清凉解表,祛暑除热。

适用:一切热病如发热或局部红肿热痛诸症,以及夏日治疗时应用。

除以上介绍的介质外,尚可采用成品,如跌打万花油、红花油等。

第二节　热敷疗法

热敷疗法是以中医基础理论为指导,用不同的中药按照不同的用药方法薰洗熨擦患者的机体病变部位,以达到治疗目的的一种外治方法。它具有作用迅速、方法简便、易学易用、容易推广、使用安全、毒副作用少等优点。此疗法不仅适应于外、骨伤、皮肤、五官等科疾病,而且对内、妇、儿科病症也有显著疗效,是推拿按摩中又一个很好的辅助疗法。

本疗法源远流长,起源很早,马王堆出土的《五十二病方》就有"温熨"、"药摩"、"外洗"等外治方法的记述。中国医学现存最早的经典著作《内经》中就有用蜀椒、干姜、桂心

cal classics, there was a record about a preparation from Shujiao (Pericarpium Zanthoxyli) found in Sichuan, China, Ganjiang (Rhizoma Zingiberis) and Gui Xin (Cortex Cinnamomi) soaked in liquor to iron cold arthralgia. Actually, this method has been generally practiced throughout Chinese history.

3.2.1 Actions of Medicated Hot Compress

Medicated hot compress is based upon the Zang-fu theory and the theory of the meridians in TCM. The zang and fu organs are essential to the physiological function of the human body, and they control the normal life activities. The meridians are the passages of circulation of qi and blood, and the link associating the exterior and the interior, connecting the upper and the lower of the human body as well. Therefore, diseases, no matter they are caused by exogenous or endogenous factors, all occur only through attack at the body surface, the meridians and the zang and fu organs first. Medicated hot compress is to apply medicines close to the skin after heated, get them travel through the meridians to the viscera, then distribute all over the body to regulate the meridians and balance yin and yang. It also has the function of warming and activating the meridians, promoting blood circulation to remove blood stasis and relieving pain. Here its therapeutic principles are summarized in the following aspects.

3.2.1.1 Local Stimulation

In medicated hot compress, medicines with stimulating effects are used to dilate local blood vessels, promote blood circulation and improve the supply of nutrients of the surrounding tissues so as to play the role of relieving swelling and subduing inflammation. For example, the application of warm and hot drugs in hot compress may produce the same stimulating effect as moxibustion does,

渍酒以熨寒痹的记载。这一疗法素为历代医家普遍使用。

一、热敷作用

热敷疗法是以中医脏腑经络学说的理论为依据的。脏腑是人体生理功能的核心，又是生命活动的主宰,经络是气血运行的通道,又是沟通表里,联系上下的纽带。所以不论外邪和内邪,都要通过作用于人体体表、脏腑和经络而致病。热敷疗法是以药物加热后外敷或浸渍作用于皮肤,促使药性(力)由经入脏,输布全身以达到调节经脉、平衡阴阳的目的,并具有温通经络、活血化瘀、止痛的作用。因此,本疗法的治疗原理可概括为以下几方面。

(一)局部的刺激作用

选用具有一定刺激性作用的药物,使局部血管扩张,促进血液循环,改善周围组织的营养,从而起到消炎退肿的作用。如运用温热药物对局部的刺激,有类似灸法的效应,即具有温经通络、行气活

which can achieve the result of warming and dredging the meridians, activating circulation of qi and blood, dispersing cold and expelling dampness. Moreover, nerve reflex caused by medicines acted on some local areas can stimulate the auto-regulation of the human body and promote the formation of some antibodys, which improves the immunologic function of the body. In general, through its local stimulation medicated hot compress attains the object of regulating the function of zang and fu organs, and preventing and treating diseases.

3.2.1.2 Direct Action of Medicines

Through the administration of fumigating, washing, ironing and to-and-fro rubbing, medicines can directly contact the foci and play the role of clearing away heat, detumescence by detoxification, expelling wind and arresting itching, drawing out of the pus and removing the slough.

3.2.1.3 Regulating and balancing action of the meridians

Applied to the body surface, effective part of medicines with different property and actions is absorbed. Then through blood vessels and the meridians, the effective part passes to the zang and fu organs, activates meridian qi to distribute all over the body or directly reach the foci. By all the means, medicines function to replenish deficiency and purge excess, regulate yin and yang to treat diseases.

3.2.1.4 Absorption of the Skin

This therapy relies upon the unity of osmosis of the medicines and absorption of the skin to make medicines get into the human body. Then through the regulation, balance and distribution of the meridians and zang and fu organs, medicines treat the general or local diseases. Or by directly acting on the foci of the skin, they take effect

血、祛湿散寒的效果。另外通过药物作用于局部而引起的神经反射作用来激发机体的自身调节作用，促使某些抗体的形成，借以提高机体的免疫功能。总之，通过局部的刺激作用来达到调整脏腑功能和防治疾病、恢复健康的目的。

（二）药物的直接作用

药物通过薰洗熨擦的给药方法，能直接作用于患处或病灶，起到清热解毒消肿、祛风止痒、拔毒祛腐等作用。

（三）经络的调衡作用

在体表给药，通过经络血脉或信息传递，通过不同药性与功效的药物的透皮吸收，由经脉而入脏腑，激发经气输布全身，或直达病所，借以产生补虚泻实、协调阴阳等经络调控作用。

（四）皮肤的吸收作用

本疗法是以药物的渗透性和皮肤的吸收功能的统一而进入体内，再通过经络、脏腑的调衡、输布作用，或直接作用于皮肤的病灶上而起到全身或局部的治疗作用。

to treat diseases.

3.2.2   Most Commonly Used Methods in Medicated Hot Compress

3.2.2.1   Warm Ironing Method

It is also called dry fomenting method. That is done by grinding all medical substances into thick powder, parching them hot in a pan (or parching with some adjuvants like white liquor, vinegar), or steaming them hot without touching water, then putting them into a white cloth bag. If steaming method is used, it is better to place the medicines into a bag first before steam. Finally get out the medicine bag, iron and rub specific regions or affected areas when it is hot. Warm ironing method may be used to treat algesthesia syndrome and cold syndrome. In operation, however, attention should be paid to an appropriate temperature of the medicine bag to avoid scald of skin.

3.2.2.2   External Washing Method

Select some medicines according to syndrome differentiation, and boil them in a proper quantity of clean water. When the temperature of the medicated liquid is lowered down and appropriate for operation, namely when it doesn't scald the hand, soak towels or the hand completely in it and rub and wash the whole body or merely some local areas. The method has the effect of warming the meridians, dispelling pathogenic cold, activating blood circulation and removing blood stasis.

3.2.2.3   Macerating Method（Jinzifa）

It is also called wet fomenting method. "Jin" in Chinese means to immerse the affected part such as the limb in medicated liquid for 20 - 30 minutes. "Zi" is to apply the squeezed hot towel soaked in a medicated liquid to the affected part after it has been given an external washing

二、热敷常用方法

（一）温熨法

温熨法，又称干热敷，将所有药物研成粗末，放入锅内炒热（或加白酒、醋等佐料拌炒）或隔水蒸热后，装入一白布袋中（如系蒸热，宜先装袋后再蒸），取药袋趁势熨摩特定部位或患部，可用来治疗痛证、寒证。使用时要注意药温适度，防止烫伤皮肤。

（二）外洗法

选用一些针对病情的（辨证用药）药物加清水（适量）煎煮沸后，待药温适宜时（以不烫伤手为度）用手或毛巾浸透后擦洗全身或局部。本法具有温经散寒、活血化瘀的作用。

（三）浸渍法

浸渍法，又称湿热敷。浸，就是将患部（如四肢）浸泡在药液中，一般 20～30 分钟为宜。渍，就是外洗后，再用毛巾浸药液，稍拧干趁热敷于

method to enhance therapeutic effects. Meanwhile patting is preferred additionally.

3.2.3　Commonly Used Chinese Medicines in Medicated Hot Compress

3.2.3.1　Medicines for activating blood circulation to remove blood stasis

Danggui (*Radix Angelicae Sinensis*), Ruxiang (*Olibanum*), Moyao (*Myrrha*), Chuanxiong (*Rhizoma Chuanxiong*), Jixueteng (*Caulis Spatholobi*), Taoren (*Semen Persicae*), Honghua (*Flos Carthami*), Niuxi (*Radix Achyranthis Bidentatae*), Jiangxiang (*Ligni Dalbergiae Odoriferae*), Sumu (*Lignum Sappan*), Xuejie (*Sanguis Draconis*), etc.

3.2.3.2　Medicines for Dispelling Wind and Eliminating Dampness

Duhuo (*Radix Angelicae Pubescentis*), Weilingxian (*Radix Clematidis*), Fangji (*Radix Stephaniae Tetrandrae*), Qinjiao (*Radix Gentianae Macrophyllae*), Mugua (*Fructus Chaenomelis*), Xuchangqing (*Radix Cynanchi Paniculati*), Haitongpi (*Cortex Erythrinae*), Xungufeng (*Herba Aristolochiae Mollissimae*), Haifengteng (*Caulis Piperis Kadsurae*), Qiannianjian (*Rhizoama Homalomenae*), Yousongjie (*Lignum Pini Nodi*), Shenjincao (*Herba Lycopodti*), Rendongteng (*Caulis Lonicerae*), Banxia (*Rhizoma Pinelliae*), Tiannanxing (*Rhizoma Arisaematis*), etc.

3.2.3.3　Medicines for Expelling Cold and Relieving Pain

Guizhi (*Ramulus Cinnamomi*), Mahuang (*Herba Ephedrae*), Shengjiang (*Rhizoma Zingiberis Recens*), Jingjie (*Herba Schizonepetae*), Fangfeng (*Radix Saposhnikoviae*), Qianghuo (*Rhizoma Seu Radix Notopterygii*), Fuzi (*Radix Aconiti Lateralis Preparata*),

患处，以利加强疗效，同时也可以施以拍打手法。

三、热敷常用中药

（一）活血化瘀类

当归、乳香、没药、川芎、鸡血藤、桃仁、红花、牛膝、降香、苏木、血竭等。

（二）祛风除湿类

独活、威灵仙、防己、秦艽、木瓜、徐长卿、海桐皮、寻骨风、海风藤、千年健、油松节、伸筋草、忍冬藤、半夏、天南星等。

（三）散寒止痛类

桂枝、麻黄、生姜、荆芥、防风、羌活、附子、干姜、肉桂、吴茱萸、花椒、丁香等。

Ganjiang（*Rhizoma Zingiberis*），Rougui（*Cortex Cinnamomi*），Wuzhuyu（*Fructus Evodiae*），Huajiao（*Pericarpium Zanthoxyli*），Dingxiang（*Flos Caryophylli*），etc.

3.2.3.4　Medicines for Promoting Circulation of Qi and Dredging the Meridians

　　Muxiang（*Herba Equiseti Hiemalis*），Xiangfu（*Rhizoma Cyperi*），Chenxiang（*Lignum Aquilariae Resinatum*），Tanxiang（*Lignum Santall Albi*），Jupi（*Pericarpium Citri Reticulatae*），Sangzhi（*Ramulus Mori*），Lulutong（*Fructus Liquidambaris*），Quanxie（*Scorpion*），Wugong（*Scolopendra*），Dilong（*Lumbricus*），etc.

　　In composing a prescription of medicated hot compress，two to four medicines are chosen from each group above. Usually，one formula consists of 12 – 14 medicines of 10 – 30 g each. Here's one set prescription for example. Honghua（*Flos Carthami*）10 g，Jixueteng（*Caulis Spatholobi*）30 g，Shenjincao（*Herba Lycopodti*）15 g，Yousongjie（*Lignum Pini Nodi*）10 g，Zuandifeng（*Radix Rubi Obcordati*）10 g，Qiannianjian（*Rhizoama Homalomenae*）15 g，Luoshiteng（*Caulis Trachelospermi*）15 g，Wujiapi（*Cortex Acanthopanacis*）10 g，Xuanmugua（*Fructus Chaenomelis-mugua*）10 g，Ruxiang（*Olibanum*）10 g，Moyao（*Myrrha*）10 g，Weilingxian（*Radix Clematidis*）30 g，Sangzhi（*Ramulus Mori*）30 g，Guizhi（*Ramulus Cinnamomi*）20 g，Ganjiang（*Rhizoma Zingiberis*）20 g.

　　In practice，soak the medicines of the above prescription in cold water for 30 – 40 minutes，boil them first on strong fire until boiling and then on slow one for 20 – 30 minutes to get about 500 ml of medicated liquid，which is stored in a bottle for later use. Put the remains of the medicines into a bag of 20 cm long and 30 cm wide，and

（四）行气通经类

　　木香、香附、沉香、檀香、橘皮、桑枝、路路通、全蝎、蜈蚣、地龙等。

　　热敷方组成时，可在以上各类药物中，每类选取 2～4 味。一副方药大约 12～14 味药物组成，每味药用量可以 10～30 克，如下例方：红花 10克，鸡血藤 30 克，伸筋草 15克，油松节 10 克，钻地风 10克，千年健 15 克，络石藤 15克，五加皮 10 克，宣木瓜 10克，乳香 10 克，没药 10 克，威灵仙 30 克，桑枝 30 克，桂枝 20 克，干姜 20 克。具体运用时，即将上药先以凉水浸泡 30～40 分钟，用火煎沸后，再以小火煎煮 20～30 分钟，倒出药液约 500 毫升，以瓶贮存备用，药渣以一20 cm×30 cm 布袋装好，扎口，趁热在布袋上喷洒高浓度白酒少许，再以干毛巾包裹敷患部，药袋凉后，可隔物在锅内蒸热，如上

tie the mouth of the bag. When the bag is still hot, spray some liquor of high concentration to it and wrap it with a dry towel. Apply the hot medicine bag to the affected part. When the bag becomes cool, heat it in a pan without touching water. Spray some liquor of the same kind again and wrap it with a dry towel. The bag may be used repeatedly for twice or three times. After the operation, keep the bag in a shade, or wrap it with a plastic bag and put it in a refrigerator. When hot compress is performed again, spray some stored medicated liquor on the bag to get it wet. Then steam it and spray some liquor to it for use. In this way, the medicine of this prescription may be used for 5 - 7 days. In addition, take 30 -50 ml of the stored medicated liquid each time to mix with 1,000 ml hot water. The medicated solution may be used to wash the affected part, which is especially suitable for the hand and foot.

3.2.4 Commonly Used Set Prescriptions for Medicated Hot Compress

3.2.4.1 The clinical set prescription of celebrated physicians of TCM

Composition: Danggui (*Radix Angelicae Sinensis*), Qianghuo (*Rhizoma seu Radix Notopterygii*), Honghua (*Flos Carthami*), Baizhi (*Radix Angelicae Dahuricae*), Fangfeng (*Radix Saposhinokoviae*), Zhiruxiang (*Olibanum Preparata*), Zhimoyao (*Myrrha Preparata*), Gusuibu (*Rhizoma Drynariae*), Xuduan (*Radix Dipsaci*), Xuanmugua (*Fructus Chaenomeloes*), Tougucao (*Herba Impatientis*), Chuanjiao (*Pericarpium Zanthoxyli*), etc. with proper quantity each.

Modification: For problems in the hand, add Guizhi (*Ramulus Cinnamomi*) and Yuliren (*Semen Pruni*). For problems in the foot, add Huangbai (*Cortex Phello-

述喷洒白酒,干毛巾包裹重复使用 2～3 次,用后药袋置阴凉处或以塑料袋封好置冰箱内,再用时先以原贮存药汁少许洒在布袋上,使其湿润后,蒸热洒酒再行运用。如此,每袋药可用 5～7 天。另外,贮存之药汁,亦可每次以 30～50 ml 入 1 000 ml 热水中浸洗患部,此法手足部较为适合。

四、热敷疗法常用成方

(一)名中医临床经验方

当归、羌活、红花、白芷、防风、制乳香、制没药、骨碎补、续断、宣木瓜、透骨草、川椒等各适量。

加减法:手部加桂枝、郁李仁;足部加黄柏、茄根;腿部加牛膝、虎杖;腰部加杜仲、桑

dendri) and Qiegen (*Radix Solanum Melongena*). For problems in the leg, add Niuxi (*Radix Achyranthis Bidentatae*) and Huzhang (*Rhizoma Polygoni Cuspidati*). For problems in the lumbus, add Duzhong (*Cortex Eucommiae*) and Sangjisheng (*Herba Taxilli*). For problems in the chest, add Yujin (*Radix Curcumae*) and Yinchen (*Herba Artemisiae Scopariae*). For problems in the left costal region, add Zhizi (*Fructus Gardeniae*) and Jiangxiang (*Ligni Dalbergiae Odoriferae*). For problems in the right costal region, add Chenpi (*Pericarpium Citri Peticulatae*) and Zhike (*Fructus Aurantii Immaturus*). For problems in the scapular region, add Chuanxiong(*Rhizoma Chuanxiong*) and Shengjianghuang (*Rhizoma Curcuma Longa*). For fracture, add Zhechong (*Eupolyphaga seu Steleophaga*) and Zirantong (*Cuprum, natural copper*). For patients with wind-cold syndrome, add Houpo (*Cortex Magnoliae Officinalis*) and Rougui (*Cortex Cinnamomi*). If it is for the purpose of regulating circulation of qi, add Jupi (*Pericarpium Citri Reticulatae*) and Muxiang (*Radix Aucklandiae*). If it is to regulate blood circulation, add Sanqi (*Radix Notoginseng*) and Jixueteng (*Caulis Spatholobi*). If it is to relax tendons, add Weilingxian (*Radix Clematidis*), Sigualuo (*Retinervus Luffae Fructus*), Sangzhi (*Ramulus Mori*) and Lulutong (*Fructus Liquidambaris*).

Actions: Promoting blood circulation to remove blood stasis, warming and dredging the meridians, alleviating swelling and relieving pain, relaxing tendons and setting of fracture. The prescription is used for fracture, dislocation and injury of tendons and Bi-syndrome in all parts of the body.

Administration: ① Foment, fumigate and wash the affected area with the medicated liquid twice a day for

寄生;胸部加郁金、茵陈;左肋部加栀子、降香;右肋部加陈皮、枳壳;肩部加川芎、生姜黄;骨折加䗪虫、自然铜。兼风寒加厚朴、肉桂;理气加橘皮、木香;理血加三七、鸡血藤;舒筋加威灵仙、丝瓜络、桑枝、路路通。

功效:活血散瘀、温通经络、消肿止痛、舒筋接骨,用于全身各部位的骨折、脱位,伤筋及痹证。

用法:① 药液热敷薰洗,每日 2 次,重复用数日。② 上

several days repeatedly. ② Grind the medicines into thick powder, mix the powder up with 30 g of salt and 30 g of white liquor evenly, put them into a bag. After parching or steaming preparation, apply the medicines to the affected part twice a day. After being used, leave the bag in fresh air and spray some white liquor on it. One bag can be used for 4 - 7 days.

3.2.4.2　Formula for Washing Injured Limbs

Composition：Sangzhi (*Ramulus Mori*), Guizhi (*Ramulus Cinnamomi*), Shenjincao (*Herba Lycopodti*), Tougucao (*Herba Impatientis*), Niuxi (*Radix Achyranthis Bidentatae*), Mugua (*Fructus Chaenomelis*), Ruxiang (*Olibanum*), Moyao (*Myrrha*), Honghua (*Flos Carthami*), Qianghuo (*Rhizoma seu Radix Notopterygii*), Duhuo (*Radix Angelicae Pubescentis*), Luodeda (*Herba Centellae*), Buguzhi (*Fructus Psoraleae*), Yinyanghuo (*Herba Epimedii*), Beixie (*Rhizoma Dioscoreae Hypogiaucae*), etc. each with a proper quantity.

Actions：Warming and dredging the meridians, promoting blood circulation and expelling pathogenic wind. The recipe is mainly used for contracture and aching pain in tendons after fracture, dislocation and sprain of the limbs.

Administration：This recipe can be decocted for washing injured limbs or for taking orally.

3.2.4.3　Formula for Hot Compress of Injury in the Early Stage

Composition：Haitongpi (*Cortex Erythrinae*) 6 g, Tougucao (*Herba Impatientis*) 6 g, Ruxiang (*Olibanum*) 6 g, Moyao (*Myrrha*) 6 g, Danggui (*Radix Angelicae Sinensis*) 5 g, Chuanjiao (*Pericarpium Zanthoxyli*) 10 g, Chuanxiong (*Rhizoma Chuanxiong*) 3 g, Honghua (*Flos Carthami*) 3 g, Weilingxian (*Radix*

药研为粗末,加入青盐、白酒30克调匀,装入布袋,炒或蒸后敷于患部,每日2次,用后置通风处,在药袋上洒少许白酒,每袋可用4～7天。

(二)四肢损伤洗方

桑枝、桂枝、伸筋草、透骨草、牛膝、木瓜、乳香、没药、红花、羌活、独活、落得打、补骨脂、淫羊藿、萆薢等各适量。

功效：温经通络、活血祛风。用于四肢骨折、脱位、扭挫伤后筋络挛缩酸痛。

用法：上药煎液外洗伤处,亦可内服。

(三)损伤早期热敷方

海桐皮6克,透骨草6克,乳香6克,没药6克,当归5克,川椒10克,川芎3克,红花3克,威灵仙3克,甘草3克,防风3克,白芷2克。

Clematidis）3 g, Gancao （*Radix Glycyrrhizae*）3 g, Fangfeng （*Radix Saposhinokoviae*）3 g and Baizhi （*Radix Angelicae Dahuricae*）2 g.

Action：Activating the collaterals to relieve pain. It is used for injury of muscles and other soft tissues in the early stage.

Administration：This recipe can be decocted to take orally, or used for fumigating, washing and fomenting preparation.

3.2.4.4   Formula for Hot Compress of Injury in the Middle and the Late Stages

Composition：Danggui （*Radix Angelicae Sinensis*）10 g, Moyao （*Myrrha*）10 g, Wujiapi （*Cortex Acanthopanacis*）10 g, Pixiao （*Natrii Sulfas*）10 g, Qingpi （*Pericarpium Citri Reticulatae Viride*）10 g, Chuanjiao （*Pericarpium Zanthoxyli*）10 g, Xiangfuzi （*Rhizoma Cyperi*）10 g, Dingxiang （*Flos Caryophylli*）3 g, Digupi （*Cortex Lycii*）3 g, Mudanpi （*Cortex Moutan Radicis*）6 g, Laocong （*green Onion*）3 pieces, artificial Shexiang （*Moschus*）0.3 g.

Actions：Regulating blood circulation to relieve pain and relaxing tendons. It is used for injury of muscles and other soft tissues in the middle and late stages.

Administration：This recipe can be decocted for external washing or for hot compress. artificial Shexiang （*Moschus*）may be excluded.

3.2.4.5   Formula for Hot Compress of Unhealed Old Wounds or for Washing Old Wounds

Composition：Shengcaowu （*Radix Aconiti Kusnezoffii*）9 g, Shengchuanwu （*Radix Aconiti*）9 g, Qianghuo （*Rhizoma Seu Radix Notopterygii*）15 g, Duhuo （*Radix Angelicae Pubescentis*）15 g, Sanleng （*Rhizoma Sparganii*）9 g, Ezhu （*Rhizoma Curcumae*）9 g, Zelan （*Herba Selaginellae*）9 g, Rougui （*Cortex Cinnamomi*）

功效：活络止痛,用于肌肉等软组织损伤早期。

用法：此方可以煎服,也可薰洗热敷。

（四）损伤中、后期热敷方

当归 10 克,没药 10 克,五加皮 10 克,皮硝 10 克,青皮 10 克,川椒 10 克,香附子 10 克,丁香 3 克,地骨皮 3 克,牡丹皮 6 克,老葱 3 根,人造麝香 0.3 克。

功效：和血定痛舒筋。用于肌肉等软组织伤患后期。

用法：煎水外洗热敷(可去人造麝香)。

（五）久伤不愈热敷方(旧伤洗方)

生草乌 9 克,生川乌 9 克,羌活 15 克,独活 15 克,三棱 9 克,莪术 9 克,泽兰 9 克,肉桂 9 克,当归尾 9 克,桃仁 9 克,红花 9 克,乌药 9 克,牛膝 15 克。

9 g, Dangguiwei (*Radix Angelicae Sinensis*) 9 g, Taoren (*Ramulus Cinnamomi*) 9 g, Honghua (*Flos Carthami*) 9 g, Wuyao (*Radix Linderae*) 9 g and Niuxi (*Radix Achyranthis Bidentatae*) 15 g.

Actions: Promoting blood circulation to remove blood stasis, expelling pathogenic wind to relieve pain, relaxing tendons and soothing the meridians. It is often used for pain due to prolonged unhealed wounds and blood stasis.

功效：活血祛瘀、祛风止痛，舒筋活络。用于久伤蓄瘀作痛。

Administration: The medicines are decocted in water for fumigating, washing and fomenting. Add 45 g of old vinegar to each dose. One dose a day.

用法：水煎薰洗热敷，每剂加陈醋 45 克，每日 1 剂。

3.2.4.6　Formula for Dispersing Pathogenic Wind and Cold

（六）祛风散寒方

Composition: Qianghuo (*Rhizoma Seu Radix Notopterygii*), Baizhi (*Radix Angelicae Dahuricae*), Danggui (*Radix Angelicae Sinensis*), Xixin (*Herba Asari*), Yuanhua (*Flos Genkwa*), Baishaoyao (*Radix Paeoniae Alba*), Wuzhuyu (*Fructus Evodiae*), Rougui (*Cortex Cinnamomi*). All the medicines are taken in an equal quantity, and several red-skinned shallots with the root are added.

羌活、白芷、当归、细辛、芫花、白芍药、吴茱萸、肉桂各等量，连须赤皮葱适量。

Actions: Warming the meridians and dispersing pathogenic cold, expelling wind to relieve pain. It is indicated in pain in the tendons and bone caused by rheumatic arthralgia syndrome.

功效：温经散寒、祛风止痛。治风寒湿痹证所致的筋骨疼痛。

Administration: Grind the medicines into powder. Each time take a proper quantity of the powder and add some red-skinned shallots with the root to it and pestle them into mud. Then parch the medicated mud with vinegar hot, and finally wrap them in a cloth bag. Iron the affected part with the medicine bag.

用法：药共为末，每次取适量药末，与适量的连须赤皮葱捣烂混合，醋炒热，布包，热熨患处。

3.2.4.7　Formula for Promoting Blood Circulation and Relaxing Tendons

（七）活血舒筋方

Composition: Dangguiwei (*Radix Angelicae Sinen-*

当归尾、赤芍药、片姜黄、

sis), Chishaoyao (*Radix Paeoniae Rubra*), Pianjiang-huang (*Rhizoma Wenyujin Concisa*), Shenjincao (*Herba Lycopodti*), Songjie (*Terebinthinae*), Haitongpi (*Cortex Erythrinae*), Luodeda (*Herba Centellae*), Lulutong (*Fructus Liquidambaris*), Qianghuo (*Rhizoma Seu Radix Notopterygii*), Duhuo (*Radix Angelicae Pubescentis*), Fangfeng (*Radix Saposhinokoviae*), Xuduan (*Radix Dipsaci*), Gancao (*Radix Glycyrrhizae*). For problems in the upper limb, Chuanxiong (*Rhizoma Chuangxiong*) and Guizhi (*Ramulus Cinnamomi*) are added. For problems in the lower limb, Niuxi (*Radix Achyranthis Bidentatae*) and Muxiang (*Radix Aucklandiae*) are added. For cases with severe pain, Ruxiang (*Olibanum*) and Moyao (*Myrrha*) are added.

伸筋草、松节、海桐皮、落得打、路路通、羌活、独活、防风、续断、甘草。上肢加用川芎、桂枝,下肢加用牛膝、木香,痛甚者加用乳香、没药。

Actions: Promoting blood circulation to remove blood stasis, relaxing tendons and soothing the meridians. The prescription is used for swelling and pain in the joints of the limbs and their dysfunction of movements.

功效:活血祛瘀,舒筋活络。用于四肢关节肿痛,活动功能障碍。

Administration: The medicines in this formula may be decocted to take orally, or boiled in water for fumigating, washing, and fomenting the affected parts.

用法:此方可煎服,也可水煎后热敷薰洗患处。

3.2.5 Cautions in Medicated Hot Compress

(1) Clothes should not be dirtied in operation, and the patient should avoid attack by wind and cold after treatment.

(2) The temperature of medicine should be controlled properly in accordance with the treated areas, condition and age of patients. Generally, it should be within the endurance of the hand or avoid scald. If the temperature is too high, it will damage the skin. If it is too low, the therapeutic effects will be poor. Special attention should be paid to avoiding scald in the aged patients and patients with slow sensitivity.

五、热敷注意事项

(1) 治疗中避免弄脏衣被,治疗后应避免患者受风寒侵袭。

(2) 要严格控制药温,一般又要按部位、病情、年龄等因素而异。总之以不烫手或能忍耐程度而定。药温不宜太高,太高则会烫伤皮肤,过低则又会影响疗效。对于老年人等感觉迟钝者,尤要注意烫伤。

(3) The towel should be flat and medicines should be evenly spread on the towel so as to avoid scald.

(4) Selection of medicines and formulae should be made strictly according to concrete conditions. For example, medicines with strong stimulation should avoid being applied to the head, face, lumbosacral region or other sensitive areas, otherwise blister will appear and the skin is damaged. Children have delicate skin, so this kind of medicines should be less used or not used on them at all. For pregnant women, some medicines like artificial Shexiang (Mocchus) should be forbidden in case miscarriage and other adverse effects should occur.

(5) If hypersensitivity of the skin occurs in practice, change the formulae or stop the treatment immediately. If cases of broken skin take place, an appropriate application of medicines should be selected in agreement with patients' conditions and the diseased areas.

(6) After hot compress, if necessary, patting manipulation may be used to enhance the therapeutic effect, yet other massage manipulations should not be used lest the skin be injured.

（3）毛巾平整，使药量均匀，防止烫伤。

（4）临证选方用药，视具体情况而定，如头面、腰骶部以及某些敏感部位，不宜选用刺激性太强的药物，否则会引起发泡，损伤皮肤。小儿皮肤薄，尤宜少用或不用。孕妇对某些药物如人造麝香等应忌用，以免引起流产等不良后果。

（5）若发现有皮肤过敏者，宜随时更方或停止治疗；有皮肤破损者，随病位病情选用适宜的用药方法。

（6）必要时可配合拍打手法提高疗效，但不可以在敷后使用其他推拿手法，以防损伤皮肤。

4 Clinical Treatment with Tuina

第四章 临床 治疗

4.1 Adult Diseases

In the course of Tuina therapy, the basic theory of TCM as well as the four basic diagnostic methods of inspection, listening and smelling examination, interrogation, and palpation should be comprehensively used to make accurate diagnosis and careful treatments of various diseases. The size of the consulting room should be decided in accordance with the requirement of the doctors' movement, and the consulting bed must be solid enough to ensure the safety of patients in treatment. In addition, for patients who are physically weak, highly sensitive to pain, over-hungry or over-nervous, soft and mild manipulations are supposed to be given in the course of massage. If a patient feels dizzy, giddy, or palpitant, the manipulations must be stopped immediately, and the patient should lie down to have a rest. Meanwhile, his Neiguan (PC 6) and Hegu (LI 4), etc. should be pressed. Sugar water can be recommended for the patient to prevent possible faint.

The course of tuina treatment should be determined by the condition of a disease. Generally, the treatment is given everyday or every other day, and 3 - 5 times of treatment form one course for acute diseases, 10 - 15 times for chronic diseases.

第一节 成人疾病

推拿治疗过程中,应综合运用中医学的基础知识,以望、闻、问、切四诊方法,对各种疾病细心诊察治疗。诊疗室大小应切实符合医生手法操作时运动的要求,诊疗床则更应坚固,以保证病人治疗中的安全。另外,推拿临床过程中,对于体质虚弱,疼痛过于敏感,或过于饥饿及过度紧张的患者,手法应轻柔、缓和,若患者出现头晕、眼花、心慌等感觉时,应立即停止操作,让其平卧休息并轻柔按压内关、合谷等穴,并嘱病人服用糖水,以防晕厥。

推拿治疗的疗程,应视病情而定,一般每日或隔日治疗,急性病症以3~5次为1个疗程,慢性病症以 10~15 次为1个疗程。

4.1.1 Common Cold

INTRODUCTION

Common cold occurs all the year round, while its highest incidence is seen in changeable weather and at the turning points between autumn and winter or between winter and spring. According to modern medical science, common cold is the infection of the upper respiratory tract caused by rhinovirus, with severe local symptoms and slight general symptoms as its clinical characteristics. While influenza is an acute communicable disease of the respiratory tract caused by influenza virus, it is characterized by sudden onset and marked general symptoms, and may have fulminating epidemic.

In TCM, slight common cold is called "Shangfeng", and the severe one is called "Zhongshangfeng" or "Rampant cold". TCM holds that the lung governs respiration, opens into the nose and communicates with the skin and hair. When the weather changes suddenly or the temperature is irregular or when one is sweating and being exposed to wind, if at that time the human body is of fatigue or in weak resistance, the six exogenous pathogenic factors will invade the body, first attack the lung through the mouth, nose or skin and stay in it with the result of dysfunction of the superficial defensive system, which leads to obstructed lung-qi and the occurrence of the disease.

MAIN POINTS FOR DIAGNOSIS

The main symptoms of common cold are chills, fever, headache, stuffy nose, nasal discharge, cough and so on.

1. Wind-cold Syndrome   Symptoms such as severe chills, slight fever, anhidrosis, headache, aching pain in the extremities, cough, stuffy nose, nasal discharge, pale tongue with thin and whitish fur and floating or tense

一、感冒

【概述】

感冒一年四季均有发生，但在气候变化多端，冷热交替的秋冬之际和冬春之际发病最多。现代医学认为，普通感冒是由鼻病毒等引起的上呼吸道感染，局部症状较重、全身症状较轻为其临床特点。流行性感冒是由流感病毒引起的一种急性呼吸道传染病，临床特点为起病急，全身症状明显，可有暴发性流行。

感冒轻者，中医称为伤风；重者，称为重伤风或时行感冒。认为其致病原因是当气候骤变，冷热失常，或汗出当风时，适值人体疲劳，体虚等正气低弱情况下，六淫邪气乘虚侵袭，首先犯肺，而由于肺主呼吸，系喉，开窍于鼻，外合皮毛，风邪自口鼻、皮毛而入，客于肺卫，导致表卫调节失司，肺气不宣而发病。

【诊断要点】

感冒多出现恶寒、发热、头痛、鼻塞、流涕、咳嗽等症状。

1. 风寒型   症状可见恶寒重、发热轻、无汗头痛、四肢酸痛、咳嗽、鼻塞、流清涕、舌质淡、苔薄白、脉浮或紧。

pulse can be seen.

2. Wind-heat Syndrome   Severe fever, slight aversion to wind or chills, sore and swollen throat, dry mouth, cough, thick sputum hard to expectorate, reddened tongue periphery with thin, greasy and yellowish fur and floating pulse are often seen.

BASIC MANIPULATIONS

The principle of tuina therapy: Dispersing wind and relieving the exterior, dispelling cold and clearing away heat.

(1) The patient takes a sitting or prone position, and the doctor press-kneads Feishu (BL 13) on the patient's back with the thumbs for 1 - 3 minutes; then dips slightly his palm into sesame oil or other media and pushes the patient's back and lumbus up and down along the two sides of the spine with his hypothenar eminence until a hot sensation is achieved on the back.

(2) Press-knead or push with one-finger manipulation Fengchi (GB 20) on both sides for 1 - 3 minutes.

(3) Apply rolling manipulation to the patient's shoulder and arm regions repeatedly for 3 - 5 minutes.

(4) Rub, knead and push with one-finger manipulation Yintang (EX-HN 3) and the forehead, and press Yingxiang (LI 20) for 3 - 5 minutes.

(5) Press-knead Hegu (LI 4) and Zusanli (ST 36) for 1 minute respectively.

MODIFIED MANIPULATIONS WITH SYNDROME DIFFERENTIATION

1. Wind-cold Syndrome   Besides the basic manipulations above, the following manipulations may be added according to the syndrome differentiation.

i. Grasp-knead the muscles of the upper and lower limbs, and do to-and-fro rubbing on every part with the palm 3 - 5 times.

2. 风热型　症状可见发热重、微恶风或恶寒、咽红肿、口干、咳嗽、痰粘难咯、舌边尖红、苔薄腻微黄、脉浮。

【基本治法】

根据其证型不同,推拿治疗时,多以疏风解表,散寒清热为原则。

(1) 患者坐或俯卧,医者以双手拇指在背部肺俞穴按揉1～3分钟,再以手掌蘸少许麻油或其他对症介质沿脊柱两侧以小鱼际着力上下推擦背、腰部,以热为度。

(2) 按揉或一指禅推双侧风池穴 1～3 分钟。

(3) 㨰法在肩臂部反复操作 3～5 分钟。

(4) 摩、揉、一指禅推印堂及前额部,并按迎香穴 3～5 分钟。

(5) 按揉合谷、足三里穴各 1 分钟。

【随症加减】

1. 风寒型　除以上基本治法外,可以再加:① 拿揉上下肢部肌肉并做掌擦每部位 3～5次。② 双手提拿肩井穴部位肌肉 5～10 次,手法刺激应稍重。

ii. Lift-grasp the muscles around Jianjing（GB 21）with both hands 5 – 10 times with relatively strong stimulation.

2. Wind-heat Syndrome　Besides the basic manipulations, the following manipulations may be added.

i. Press-knead Fengfu（GV 16）, Taiyang（EX-HN 5）, and Quchi（LI 11）, etc. for 1 minute respectively.

ii. Rub the back with the palm dipped into liquor for 1 – 3 minutes if there is a high fever.

iii. Lift-grasp Jianjing（GB 21）with slight stimulation.

In addition, for patients with severe cough and profuse sputum, press-knead Tiantu（CV 22）and Fenglong（ST 40）for 1 minute each. For those with stuffiness in the chest, rub Danzhong（CV 17）and the sternocostal region to and fro for 1 – 3 minutes respectively. For those with poor appetite, rub the abdomen for 5 minutes.

4.1.2　Cough and Asthma

INTRODUCTION

Cough and asthma are often seen in cold weather of winter or spring. Some symptoms of chronic bronchitis, emphysema and asthma defined in modern medicine are included in this field.

In TCM, the occurrence and development of cough and asthma are related to the invasion of exogenous pathogenic factors, such as wind, cold, summer heat, dampness, dryness, fire and the dysfunction of the lung, spleen, and kidney. When exogenous pathogenic factors attack the human body, they will stagnate in the body, and further affect the dispersing and descending function of lung qi and cause adverse rising of lung qi, which induces cough and asthma. Cough and asthma can also be induced due to spleen asthenia, which induces sputum with

2. 风热型　除同基本治法外，再可加：① 按揉风府、太阳、曲池穴等各 1 分钟。② 热重可蘸酒平擦背部 1～3 分钟。③ 提拿肩井穴部位，手法刺激应稍轻。

另外，感冒症见咳嗽痰多者加按揉天突、丰隆穴各 1 分钟。胸闷可擦膻中穴及胸肋部各 1～3 分钟。饮食不香加摩腹部 5 分钟。

二、咳喘

【概述】

咳喘多见于冬春严寒季节，现代医学所谓的慢性支气管炎及肺气肿、哮喘等病症都属其范畴。

中医学认为本病的发生和发展与外邪（如风、寒、暑、湿、燥、火等）的侵袭及肺、脾、肾三脏功能失调有关。每当外邪侵袭人体后，邪气壅滞，影响肺气宣降功能，肺气上逆而咳喘；或因脾虚生痰、痰浊贮肺；或因心肝火旺，肝火烁痰，生化痰热，壅塞肺气；或因下元亏损，肾气不足，纳气失

the stagnation of thick sputum in the lung. They may still be caused by excessive heart fire and liver fire, which generate phlegm. Turbid phlegm retards in the lung and blocks flow of lung qi. Cough and asthma can also result from renal asthenia or insufficiency of kidney qi, which cause failure of the kidney in maintaining normal function of inspiration, leading to asthenic asthma and so on.

MAIN POINTS FOR DIAGNOSIS

The common symptoms of cough and asthma are long-time repeated cough and expectoration accompanied by dyspnea, shortness of breath or chest distress.

1. Phlegm-damp Syndrome   Cough with profuse sputum, whitish sputum easy to expectorate, chest distress, pale tongue with greasy and whitish fur and floating and slippery pulse.

2. Phlegm-heat Syndrome   Cough with shortness of breath, thick and yellowish sputum, dry or sore throat, hot sensation in the mouth and nose while breathing, distress and discomfort in the chest, reddish tongue with yellowish and greasy fur and slippery pulse.

3. Asthenic Asthma Syndrome   Frequent asthma on exertion, shortness of breath, forceless speech, aversion to cold, spontaneous perspiration, fatigue of both limbs, lassitude, anorexia, pale tongue with thin fur and weak pulse.

BASIC MANIPULATIONS

The principle of tuina therapy: Facilitating flow of lung qi to relieve asthma, relieving chest stuffiness and regulating flow of qi. In clinical treatment, stress should be put on eliminating pathogenic factors for sthenia syndromes, and strengthening the vital qi for asthenia syndromes.

(1) The patient takes a sitting or prone position, the doctor chiefly performs pushing manipulation of one finger

摄而作虚喘等等。

【诊断要点】

咳喘常见症状可有长期的反复咳嗽,咯痰,伴有喘息,气短或胸闷。

1. 痰湿型 症状可见咳嗽痰多,痰白易咯,胸脘痞闷,舌质淡,苔白腻,脉濡滑。

2. 痰热型 症状可见咳喘气急,痰粘稠,色黄,咽干或痛,口鼻气热,胸闷不舒,舌质红,苔黄腻,脉滑等等。

3. 虚喘型 症状可见动辄气喘,呼吸短促,言语乏力,怯寒自汗,肢倦神疲,纳食不馨,舌淡,苔薄脉弱。

【基本治法】

推拿时对本病治疗总的原则是宣肺平喘,宽胸理气。临床治疗时,实证以祛邪为主,虚证以扶正为主。

(1)患者坐或俯卧,医者着重在背部的肺俞穴部位采

or pushing, rolling, pressing and kneading manipulation on Feishu (BL 13) of both sides of the back for 5 - 10 minutes.

(2) The patient lies on his side, and the doctor stands behind him, puts both his hands on the patient's lateral chest, does vibrating and digitally-pressing manipulations with the palms or fingers for 1 - 3 minutes.

(3) The patient lies on the back. The doctor stands in front of the patient's head, places both thumbs oppositely on both sides of Tiantu (CV 22) and the other four fingers tightly on both sides of the chest, pushes respectively outwards along the intercostal space to the middle axillary lines and downwards to the intercostal space at the level of Rugen (ST 18) for 1 - 3 minutes.

(4) Hook and digitally-press, and press-knead Tiantu (CV 22) with the overlapped index and the middle finger for 1 minute.

(5) Press-knead and pluck Zusanli (ST 36) and Feng long (ST 40) for 1 minute.

MODIFIED MANIPULATIONS WITH SYNDROME DIFFERENTIATION

1. Phlegm-damp Syndrome   Besides the basic manipulations, the following can be performed additionally.

i. Scrub horizontally the back until a hot sensation is gained, namely, the doctor feels a modest degree of hot sensation during the course of manipulation.

ii. Press-grasp Chize (LU 5) and Neiguan (PC 6) on both sides for 1 minute respectively.

iii. Grasp Jianjing (GB 21) forcefully 10 - 15 times.

iv. Digitally-press Danzhong (CV 17) and Neiguan (PC 6) for 1 minute each.

2. Phlegm-heat Syndrome   The following may be added to the basic manipulations:

i. Press-knead Fengchi (GB 20), Quchi (LI 11) and

用一指禅推或用㨰、按、揉等手法操作 5～10 分钟。

(2) 患者侧卧,医者立其后,两手掌并置其胸侧,以掌、指作颤动点按 1～3 分钟。

(3) 患者仰卧,医者立其头前,以两手拇指相对分置于天突穴两侧,两手其余四指抱定胸部两侧,沿肋间隙自内向外分推至腋中线,自上而下至乳根穴平高处肋间隙止,操作 1～3 分钟。

(4) 医者以食、中指相叠,勾点并按揉患者天突穴 1 分钟。

(5) 按揉并弹拨患者足三里、丰隆穴各 1 分钟。

【随症加减】

1. 痰湿型 基本手法再加:① 横擦背部,以热为度(即以医者在操作中感到适中的热度而言)。② 按拿双侧尺泽、内关等穴各 1 分钟。③ 重拿肩井穴部位 10～15 次。④ 点按膻中、内关穴各 1 分钟。

2. 痰热型 基本手法再加:① 按揉风池、曲池、合谷穴各 1 分钟。② 点按膻中穴

Hegu (LI 4) for 1 minute each.

   ii. Digitally-press Danzhong (CV 17) for 1 minute.

   iii. Rub and palm-twist the sternum and ribs for 1 - 3 minutes.

   iv. Grasp and knead the muscles on both sides of the spinous processes of the cervical vertebrae up and down from Dazhui (GV 14) to Tianzhu (BL 10) with the thumb, the index and middle fingers 5 - 6 times.

   3. Asthenic Asthmatic Syndrome　Besides the basic therapy, the following manipulations can also be performed:

   i. Press-knead Neiguan (PC 6), Hegu (LI 4), Shenmen (HT 7) and Quchi (LI 11) for 1 minute each.

   ii. Push with one-finger and digitally-press Guanyuan (CV 4) and Qihai (CV 6) for one minute each.

   iii. Rub the abdomen clockwise around the umbilicus first, and then gradually extend to the chest-abdominal region for 3 - 5 minutes.

   iv. Rub horizontally Shenshu (BL 23), Mingmen (GV 4) and the area from Shangliao (BL 31) to Xialiao (BL 34) until a hot sensation is gained.

4. 1. 3　Headache

INTRODUCTION

   Headache is a common symptom in clinic. According to modern medical science, it is mainly caused by some harmful factors which affect the nerves, blood vessels, and cerebral membranes. It is divided into the functional type and the organic type. TCM holds that the occurrence of headache is related to the attack of six exogenous pathogenic factors and internal injury of seven emotions. That refers to disturbance of the mind by wind-cold and wind-heat, hyperactivity of liver-yang, and deficiency of kidney which cause failure of blood to nourish the brain. All of

1分钟。③ 擦搓胸胁1～3分钟。④ 食、中、拇指三指拿揉颈椎棘突（自大椎到天柱之间）两侧肌肉，往返5～6遍。

   3. 虚喘型　基本手法再加：① 按揉内关、合谷、神门、曲池等穴各1分钟。② 一指禅推、点按关元、气海穴各1分钟。③ 顺时针摩腹，以脐为中心，圈从小到大，至胸腹3～5分钟。④ 横擦肾俞、命门、八髎穴（部），以热为度。

三、头痛

【概述】

   头痛是临床常见的一种症状。现代医学认为，头痛主要是神经、血管和脑膜受到某些不良因子的影响而引起的病症，它可分为功能性与器质性两类。中医学认为头痛的发生与外感六淫之邪及内伤七情有关，即风寒、风热侵扰清窍，肝阳上亢，肾虚精血不能上荣于脑，均可导致头痛的

them may lead to headache.

MAIN POINTS FOR DIAGNOSIS

Common symptoms of headache in clinic are headache with heavy sensation in the head, which may be localized or errant, accompanied by stuffy nose, aversion to cold, fever, reddened face and ear or pale complexion. The pain is usually significantly felt or localized in the anterior, lateral, top, or posterior parts of the head.

BASIC MANIPULATIONS

The principle of tuina therapy is dispelling wind and removing obstruction, nourishing blood and relieving pains.

(1) The patient sits. The doctor performs pushing manipulation with one finger up and down along the bladder meridians on the neck for 3 - 4 minutes, combined with pressing Fengchi (GB 20), Fengfu (GV 16) and Tianzhu (BL 10). Then grasps both Fengchi (GB 20) and the bladder meridians on the neck from top to below 4 - 5 times.

(2) The patient takes a sitting position. The doctor pushes with one finger manipulation to and fro from Yintang (EX-HN 3) along the anterior hairline to Touwei (ST 8) and Taiyang (EX-HN 5) for 3 - 4 times, meanwhile combined with pressing points Yintang (EX-HN 3), Taiyang(EX-HN 5), and Baihui (GV 20). Then grasps with five fingers from the top of the head to Fengchi (GB 20), and grasps with three fingers back and forth from the neck to Dazhui (GV 14) 4 - 5 times.

(3) The patient sits upright, and the doctor stands behind him and does lifting-grasping manipulation on Jianjing (GB 21) and the tendons around the point repeatedly with both hands 5 - 10 times.

MODIFIED MANIPULATIONS WITH SYNDROME DIFFERENTIATION

(1) Anterior headache results from pathological

发生。

【诊断要点】

头痛临床常见症状是：头痛昏重，痛有定处或无定处，伴见鼻塞、畏寒、发热、面红耳赤或面色苍白等。常分别局限于前头部、偏头部、头顶部、后头部疼痛为著。

【基本治法】

推拿治疗头痛的原则是疏风通窍，养血止痛。

（1）患者坐位，医者用一指禅推法沿项部两侧膀胱经上下往返治疗3～4分钟，配合按风池、风府、天柱等穴。再拿两侧风池，沿项部两侧膀胱经自上而下操作4～5遍。

（2）患者坐位，医者用一指禅推法，从印堂开始向上沿前额发际至头维、太阳穴，往返3～4遍，配合按印堂、太阳、百会等穴。然后用五指拿法从头顶至风池穴，改用三指拿法，拿颈项至大椎穴，往返4～5次。

（3）患者正坐，医者立其后，双手提拿肩井穴及周围大筋，反复5～10次。

【随症加减】

（1）前头痛为阳明经脉病

changes of the yangming meridian, which is mostly caused by illness in the eyes, nose and throat. It also occurs in patients with anemia. Besides the basic manipulations, the following manipulations may be added.

i. Pinch and grasp the muscles around Yintang (EX-HN 3) with the thumb and the index finger of one hand, lifting and releasing alternately for 20 times altogether.

ii. Grasp and knead Hegu (LI 4) for 1 - 3 minutes.

(2) Migraine results from pathological changes of the shaoyang meridians, which is often induced by otopathy, odontopathy and gynecopathy. The following methods may be added to the basic manipulations:

i. Rub and scratch both sides of the head with sweeping manipulation for 3 - 5 minutes.

ii. Pinch and press Dadun (LR 1) for 1 minute.

(3) Vertex headache results from pathological changes of the liver meridian of foot-jueyin and governor vessel, which is mainly caused by functional diseases of the nerves such as neurasthenia and neurosis. The following manipulations may be added as diseases require:

i. Press and knead Baihui (GV 20) with the thumb for one minute.

ii. Press-knead Taiyang (EX-HN 5) for one minute.

(4) Posterior headache results from pathological changes of the taiyang meridian, which is mainly caused by hypertension and diseases of the cervical vertebrae. The additional manipulations are as follows:

i. Rub horizontally the back of the neck with one palm until a hot sensation is gained.

ii. Press-knead and pluck Weizhong (BL 40) for 1 - 3 minutes.

(5) Overall headache is mostly induced by cerebral arteriosclerosis or concussion of the brain. The following methods may be added to the basic ones during treatment.

变,多为眼、鼻、咽喉等疾病引起,也可见于贫血的病人。基本手法再加:① 医者用单手拇、食指捏拿印堂穴处肌肉,一提一松,共做 20 次。② 拿揉合谷穴 1～3 分钟。

(2) 偏头痛为少阳经脉病变,多为耳病、牙病及妇科病引起。基本手法再加:① 医者扫散头两侧各 3～5 分钟。② 掐按大敦穴 1 分钟。

(3) 头顶痛为足厥阴肝经和督脉病变。多为神经功能性疾病,如神经衰弱、神经官能症等引起。基本手法再加:① 以拇指按揉百会穴 1 分钟。② 按揉太阳穴 1 分钟。

(4) 后头痛为太阳经脉病变,多为高血压、颈椎病等引起。基本手法再加:① 单掌横擦后颈部,以热为度。② 按揉并弹拨委中穴 1～3 分钟。

(5) 全头痛多为脑动脉硬化、脑震荡等引起,基本手法再加:① 医者用双侧手掌按

i. Press, rub, palm-twist, and lift-grasp Tongtian (BL 7) with both palms 5 – 10 times till a hot and distending sensation is achieved.

ii. Knead and palm-twist the auricles with the thumbs and index fingers of both hands, combined with pulling the auricular lobules till they become hot.

4.1.4　Insomnia

INTRODUCTION

In modern medical science, insomnia refers to shallow sleep or inability to fall asleep caused by various factors. It usually can be seen in neurasthenia caused by dysfunction of the nervous system. According to the theory of TCM, there are many inducing factors for insomnia: one is emotional factor which causes the liver qi to lose its smoothly moving state and stagnated liver qi generates fire with the result of disturbance of the mind; another is overstrain which impairs the heart and spleen resulting in excessive consumption of heart blood and failure of nourishing the mind, or weak physique and long-term illness which develops excessive consumption of kidney yin and hyperactivity of heart fire, resulting in disturbance of the mind; there is also the factor of improper diet leading to injury of the stomach and the intestine, giving rise to disharmony of stomach qi.

MAIN POINTS FOR DIAGNOSIS

1. Deficiency Syndrome   Dreamy and unsound sleep, palpitation, amnesia, fatigue and weakness, pale complexion, pale tongue with thin fur, thready and weak pulse.

2. Excess Syndrome   Difficulty in falling asleep, restlessness and irritability, fullness in the gastric region and belching, discomfort in the abdomen, constipation, greasy and thick fur, slippery and rapid pulse.

四、失眠

【概述】

现代医学认为,失眠是一种源于多种因素而致睡眠不足或睡眠不深的病症,常见于神经系统的功能失调,如神经衰弱。中医认为导致失眠的原因很多:有因情志所伤,肝失条达,气郁化火,扰动心神;有因劳倦太过,伤及心脾,心血暗耗,神失所养;有因素体虚弱或久病之后,肾阴耗伤,心火亢盛,热扰神明;亦有因饮食不节,肠胃受伤,胃气不和等。

【诊断要点】

1. 虚证　症状为多梦易醒,心悸健忘,神疲乏力,面色少华,舌质淡,苔薄,脉细弱。

2. 实证　症状多为不易入睡,烦躁易怒,脘闷嗳气,腹中不舒,大便干结,苔腻浊,脉滑数。

BASIC MANIPULATIONS

The general principle of treating insomnia with tuina is chiefly nourishing the heart and tranquilizing the mind. For deficiency syndromes, nourishing liver is added; for excess syndromes clearing away heat and regulating the stomach may be additionally used.

(1) The patient takes a prone position. The doctor applies rolling manipulation first along both sides of the spine, and then combines it with kneading and digitally-pressing Xinshu (BL 15), Jueyinshu (BL 14), Pishu (BL 20), Weishu (BL 21) and Shenshu (BL 23) for 5 minutes.

(2) The patient sits. The doctor applies pushing or kneading manipulation with one-finger from Yintang (EX-HN 3) upward to Shenting (GV 24) up and down 5 - 6 times; next from Yintang (EX-HN 3) along the brows toward Taiyang (EX-HN 5) on both sides to and fro 5 - 6 times; then pushes with one finger manipulation along the orbits repeatedly 3 - 4 times; finally, from Yintang (EX-HN 3) along both sides of nose, via Yingxiang (LI 20) and the zygoma to the areas in front of the ears 2 - 3 times. During the treatment, the acupoints of Yintang (EX-HN 3), Shenting (GV 24), Jingming (BL 1), Cuanzhu (BL 2) and Taiyang (EX-HN 5) should be laid on stress and given more operation.

(3) Apply wiping manipulation to the regions mentioned above with both hands back and forth 5 - 6 times, and meanwhile press Jingming (BL 1) and Sibai (ST 2) coordinately. Then press Fengchi (GB 20) in the occipital part with the two hands oppositely to each other for 1 minute.

(4) Apply one-minute sweeping manipulation to the regions above the ear-tips on both sides of the head, where the gallbladder meridian passes. An arch-like

【基本治法】

推拿治疗失眠总的原则是益心安神为主,虚证辅以养血柔肝,实证佐以清热和胃。

(1)患者俯卧,医者先以㨰法沿其脊柱两侧操作,且配合揉、点按心俞、厥阴俞及脾俞、胃俞、肾俞等穴操作5分钟。

(2)患者取坐位,医者先用一指禅推法或揉法,从印堂开始向上至神庭,往返5～6次;再从印堂向两侧沿眉弓至太阳穴往返5～6次;然后以一指禅推法沿眼眶周围治疗,往返3～4次;最后从印堂沿鼻两侧向下经迎香沿颧骨至两耳前,往返2～3次。治疗过程中以印堂、神庭、睛明、攒竹、太阳穴为重点。

(3)沿上述治疗部位,用双手抹法治疗,往返5～6次,抹时配合按睛明、四白穴。最后两手对按枕后风池穴1分钟。

(4)用扫散法(五指微屈,指尖随腕动而作弧形绕擦运动,多用于头侧部)在头两侧

rounding and wiping movements is performed by shaking the wrist and having it drive the slightly bent five fingers. The manipulation is usually applied to the lateral sides of the head.

(5) Manipulate from the anterior top of the head to the nape, first by using five-finger grasping manipulation, then three-finger grasping manipulation, combined with pressing-kneading Fengchi (GB 20) 3 - 5 times. Finally grasp Jianjing (GB 21) on both sides 5 - 10 times.

(6) Ask the patient to sit upright and breathe naturally with his eyes open and his mouth closed tightly. The doctor stands in front of him, and knock the fontanel with the base of the palm 3 - 5 times. The fontanel lies at the 1/3 anterior part of the line between Yintang (EX-HN 3) and Dazhui (GV 14).

MODIFIED MANIPULATIONS WITH SYNDROME DIFFERENTIATION

1. Deficiency Syndrome　Besides the basic manipulations, the following may also be used.

i. The patient sits. The doctor stands at the patient's side, holds his shoulder with one hand and rubs his chest with the other hand left and right, up and down repeatedly 5 - 10 times, and then changes into the other hand to rub his back in the same way as above 5 - 10 times.

ii. The patient sits. The doctor stands in a horse-riding stance behind the patient, places both hands under his armpits, and palm-twists this area up and down 10 - 15 times.

2. Excess Syndrome　The following manipulations may be added to the basic manipulations.

i. The patient lies on his back. The doctor sits beside him and applies pushing manipulation with one finger to Zhongwan (CV 12), Qihai (CV 6), Guanyuan (CV 4) and Tianshu (ST 25) up and down 5 - 10 times.

耳尖上方即胆经的循行部位治疗各 1 分钟。

（5）从前头顶部开始用五指拿法到颈项，转用三指拿法，配合揉按、拿风池穴 3～5 次，再拿两侧肩井穴5～10 次。

（6）医者站于患者前侧，嘱患者正坐，眼睛睁开，口紧闭，呼吸均匀，然后用掌根击囟门 3～5 次（囟门在从印堂到大椎穴连线前 1/3 的部位）。

【随症加减】

1. 虚证　基本治法再加：① 患者坐位，医者站于患者一侧，一手扶肩部，一手擦胸部，左右往返，自上而下 5～10 遍，随后换一手如上次序擦背部5～10 遍。② 患者坐位，医者马步站裆势于其后，双手放于其两腋下，自上而下搓动，反复 10～15 遍。

2. 实证　基本手法再加：① 患者仰卧，医者坐于一旁，用一指禅推法操作于中脘、气海、关元、天枢穴，自上而下往返5～10 次。② 患者仰卧，医者单掌置于脐上，以脐为圆

ii. The patient lies on his back. The doctor places one palm on his umbilicus, and does arc-rubbing-abdomen manipulation counterclockwise with a gradually-extending range for 3 - 5 minutes.

For patients with insomnia, persistent physical exercises should be recommended. If insomnia is caused by organic pathological changes, etiological treatment should be emphasized.

4.1.5 Vertigo

INTRODUCTION

Vertigo is usually known as dizziness and dim eyesight. Modern medicine holds that it is the sensory disturbance of the human body in orientating and balancing, and a symptom of many diseases, which can often be seen in anemia, hypertension, arteriosclerosis, neurosis, etc. There is another type of vertigo accompanied by tinnitus and hypoausis, called Meniere's syndrome. In the theory of TCM, many factors can lead to vertigo, such as pathogenic wind, phlegm, asthenia and fire. The pathological manifestations of vertigo could be classified as two types. One is asthenic syndrome due to deficiency of the heart and spleen, insufficiency of blood and qi, or excessive consumption of liver yin and kidney yin which can not nourish the brain. The other is sthenic syndrome caused by hyperhepatic yang and stagnation of turbid phlegm in the middle energizer which leads to failure of rising of lucid yang and obstruction of the mind.

MAIN POINTS FOR DIAGNOSIS

Common symptoms of vertigo are giddiness, blurred vision, inclination of vomiting, spinning sensation in the head like seasick in clinic.

1. Syndrome of Hyperhepatic Yang   Symptoms are

心,作逆时针摩腹,范围由小到大 3～5 分钟。

对于失眠者,鼓励坚持体育锻炼或练功。器质性病变引起的失眠,应重视病因的治疗。

五、眩晕

【概述】

眩晕通常称为头晕眼花。现代医学认为眩晕是人体对于空间关系的定向感觉障碍或平衡感觉障碍,是多种疾病的一种临床常见症状,最常见于贫血、高血压、动脉硬化、神经官能症等。还有一种眩晕,伴有耳鸣和听力减退的,称为梅尼埃病。中医认为造成眩晕的致病因素很多,风、痰、虚、火均可导致发病。病理表现有虚实两个方面:虚证为心脾亏虚,气血不足,或肝肾阴精亏损,不能上荣于脑;实证为肝阳上亢或痰浊中阻,清阳不升,清窍闭塞等。

【诊断要点】

眩晕临床常见症状是:头晕旋转,两目昏黑,泛泛欲吐,甚至昏眩欲扑,如处舟楫之中。

1. 肝阳上亢型   症状常

dizziness, tinnitus, distending pain in the head, less or dreamy sleep, restlessness and irritability, numbness in the extremities, flushed face, stuffiness in the chest, reddened tongue with yellowish fur and floating pulse.

2. Syndrome of Deficiency of Blood and Qi Symptoms are dizziness, which can be aggravated by motion, induced by overwork, pale complexion, lips and nails, palpitation, insomnia, lassitude and less speech, poor appetite, pale tongue, and thready and weak pulse.

3. Syndrome of Stagnation of Turbid Phlegm in the Middle energizer Dizziness accompanied by heavy sensation in the head and eyes, stuffiness in the chest, nausea, poor appetite and somnolence, whitish and greasy tongue fur, weak and slippery pulse.

BASIC MANIPULATIONS

The principle of tuina therapy is awakening the brain, reinforcing the deficiency and reducing the excess.

(1) Ask the patient to lie on his back, push with one finger manipulation or knead his forehead and Baihui (GV 20), and Tongziliao (GB 1) for one minute respectively.

(2) Use the closed-up index, middle, ring and small fingers, or the thumb alone to wipe the Qiaogong point on the left and right sides from above to below 10 times each. (Note: the wiping manipulation should be gentle and soft.) After the manipulation on one side is finished, do on the other side in the same way. Be sure not to move the head in case of aggravating vertigo.

(3) Hold the wrist of the patient with one hand, ask him to separate his five fingers apart, and chop-strike the metacarpal-phalangeal areas with the side of the other palm orderly 3 - 5 times. Exchange the hands and repeat the above operation.

(4) Press-knead the foot-balance region for 1 - 3 minutes, which is a clinical empirical point for treating

有眩晕耳鸣,头昏胀痛,少寐多梦,急躁易怒,四肢麻木,面赤胸闷,舌质红,苔黄,脉弦。

2. 气血亏虚型 症状可见眩晕动则加剧,劳累即发,面色㿠白,唇甲不华,心悸,失眠,神疲懒言,饮食欠馨,舌质淡,脉细弱。

3. 痰浊中阻型 症状可见眩晕时头目昏重,胸闷恶心,少食多寐,舌苔白腻,脉濡滑。

【基本治法】

推拿治疗眩晕的原则是醒脑开窍,补虚泻实。

(1) 嘱患者仰卧,以一指禅推或揉法在前额和百会、瞳子髎等穴各操作1分钟。

(2) 再以食、中、无名、小指四指并拢,或单独以拇指,自上而下抹桥弓穴左右各10次(注意操作时手法要柔和),一侧操作毕,再操作另一侧,且不要摆动头部,以免加剧眩晕发作。

(3) 一手握住患者腕部,嘱其五指分开,以另一手掌掌侧依次劈击其指掌交接处3～5遍,交换操作。

(4) 按揉临床治疗眩晕的经验穴——足平衡区(在足背

vertigo and located at the junction of the forth and fifth metatarsal bones.

MODIFIED MANIPULATIONS WITH SYNDROME DIFFERENTIATION

1. Syndrome of Hyperhepatic Yang   Besides the basic manipulations, the following ones could be performed additionally.

i. Push with one finger manipulation or press-knead Fengchi (GB 20), Tianzhu (BL 10), and Fengfu (GV 16) for one minute respectively.

ii. Press-knead Taiyang (EX-HN 5) on both sides for one minute each.

iii. Pluck acupoints Quchi (LI 11) and Yanglinquan (GB 34) 10 - 15 times each.

iv. Press-knead Taichong (LR 3) and Zulinqi (GB 41) for one minute respectively.

v. Digitally-press Danzhong (CV 17), and rub the sternocostal region for 1 - 3 minutes each.

2. Syndrome of Deficiency of Blood and Qi   Besides the basic manipulation, the doctor can also select the following methods：

i. Push with one finger manipulation or knead acupoints Guanyuan (CV 4) and Qihai (CV 6) for one minute respectively.

ii. Rub the abdomen for 3 - 5 minutes, digitally-press Zhongwan (CV 12) and Tianshu (ST 25) for one minute each.

iii. Roll and push horizontally acupoints of Jiaji (EX-B 2) for 3 - 5 minutes respectively.

3. Syndrome of Stagnation of Turbid Phlegm in the Middle Energizer   Besides the basic manipulations, the doctor may use the following manipulations.

i. Push-rub the abdominal and epigastric region clockwise and counterclockwise for 5 minutes respectively.

第四五趾骨分叉处）1～3 分钟。

【随症加减】

1. 肝阳上亢型 基本治法再加：① 一指禅推或按揉风池、天柱、风府穴各 1 分钟。② 按揉双侧太阳穴 1 分钟。③ 弹拨曲池、阳陵泉穴各10～15 次。④ 揉按太冲、足临泣穴各 1 分钟。⑤ 点膻中穴、擦胸胁部各 1～3 分钟。

2. 气血亏虚型 基本治法再加：① 一指禅推或揉关元、气海穴各 1 分钟。② 摩腹3～5 分钟，点按中脘、天枢穴各 1 分钟。③ 擦、平推夹脊穴部各 3～5 分钟。

3. 痰浊中阻型 基本治法再加：① 推摩腹部、胃脘部。手法应稍重，顺、逆时针各操作 5 分钟。② 点按中脘、天枢穴各 1 分钟。③ 按揉脾

The force applied should be relatively strong.

ii. Digitally-press Zhongwan（CV 12）and Tianshu （ST 25）for one minute respectively.

iii. Press-knead Pishu（BL 20）and Weishu（BL 21） for one minute respectively.

iv. Digitally-press Zusanli（ST 36）and Fenglong（ST 40）for one minute respectively.

4.1.6 Coronary Heart Disease

INTRODUCTION

Coronary heart disease is the simplified term of coronary atherosclerotic heart disease, and can often be seen in middle-aged and aged people. According to modern medical science, it is induced by myocardiac ischemia and hypoxia of different degree due to coronary atherosclerosis, while TCM holds that insufficiency of heart-qi, stagnation of pathogenic cold in the meridians, or internal injury by seven emotions, which cause block of qi, and obstruction of blood vessels, can all lead to the occurrence of coronary heart disease.

MAIN POINTS FOR DIAGNOSIS

Common clinical symptoms include retrosternal paroxysmal pain, which may radiate to the shoulder, the upper limb or the back, especially radiate to the left shoulder or left upper limb or even directly to the little finger and the ring finger along the medial side of the forearm. Sometimes, symptoms of cold limbs, shortness of breath and cyanosis are also present.

BASIC MANIPULATIONS

The principle of tuina treatment is activating the flow of qi and promoting blood circulation, relieving stuffiness in the chest and regulating qi.

（1）The patient takes a sitting or prone position, and the doctor presses and kneads Xinshu（BL 15）, and

俞、胃俞穴各 1 分钟。④ 点按 足三里、丰隆穴各 1 分钟。

六、冠心病

【概述】

冠心病是冠状动脉粥样 硬化性心脏病的简称，多见于 中、老年。现代医学认为由于 冠状动脉粥样硬化导致不同 程度的心肌缺血缺氧而发病。 中医则认为心气不足、寒邪凝 滞经脉，或七情内伤、气滞不 通、血脉瘀塞等均可导致 发病。

【诊断要点】

临床常见症状是：胸骨后 有阵发性疼痛，可放射至肩、 上肢或背，以左肩或左上肢由 前臂内侧直达小指与无名指 较多见。有时伴有四肢厥冷 或气短、发绀等。

【基本治法】

推拿治疗该病症的原则 是行气活血，宽胸理气。

（1）患者坐或俯卧，医者 用拇指按揉心俞穴并挤推至

squeezes and pushes from it toward Geshu (BL 17) with the thumb for 1 – 3 minutes respectively.

(2) For patients with severe angina pectoris, press additionally Zhiyang (GV 9), which is located in the midline of the back and between the seventh and the eighth thoracic spinous processes for 1 – 3 minutes.

(3) Pat the back and the shoulders of the patient with a slightly-bent palm for one minute. The manipulations should be light, gentle with appropriate force.

(4) Press-knead Neiguan (PC 6) on both sides for one minute respectively.

(5) The patient lies on his back, the doctor places the palm on the patient's superior thoracic region, and does pushing manipulation through the anterior area of the shoulder to the medial side of the upper limb 10 times and repeat the above operation on the other side of the body. Then knead-twists the cardiac region with the palm rapidly for 3 – 5 minutes.

(6) Grasp-knead the muscles in the medial aspect of the upper limb 3 – 5 times, and digitally-press Jiquan (HT 1) with the index and the middle fingers for one minute.

MODIFIED MANIPALTIONS WITH SYNDROME DIFFERENTIATION

(1) For patients with severe palpitation, chest distress and insomnia, the following manipulations may be added.

i. Digitally-press Shenmen (HT 7) and Tongli (HT 5) for one minute respectively.

ii. Press-knead Danzhong (CV 17) for 1 – 3 minutes, combined with palm-rubbing manipulation.

iii. Press-knead and scrub Yongquan (KI 1) till a hot sensation is achieved.

(2) For patients with dizziness, nausea, or poor

膈俞穴各1～3分钟。

（2）对心绞痛剧者，加按至阳穴（背部中线，第7、8胸椎棘突之间）1～3分钟。

（3）医者以空掌拍打患者肩背部1分钟，手法要轻柔适当。

（4）按揉双侧内关穴各1分钟。

（5）患者仰卧，医者用手掌置患者胸上部，经肩前至上肢内侧做推法各10次，然后以掌在心前区做快速的揉搓3～5分钟。

6. 拿揉上肢内侧肌肉3～5次，并以食、中指点按极泉穴1分钟。

【随症加减】

（1）如心慌、胸闷、失眠严重者，基本治法加：① 点按神门、通里穴各1分钟。② 按揉膻中穴1～3分钟，并配合掌摩法。③ 按揉并搓擦涌泉穴，以热为度。

（2）如头晕欲呕，食欲不

appetite, the following manipulations may be performed additionally.

i. Press-knead Zhongwan (CV 12) for one minute.

ii. Rub the abdomen clockwise and counterclockwise for 3 – 5 minutes.

iii. Press-knead Taiyang (EX-HN 5), Yintang (EX-HN 3) and Zusanli (ST 36) for one minute respectively.

(3) Since coronary heart disease often attacks at night, the patient may pat gently the anterior cardiac region 20 – 30 times, and digitally-press Jiquan (HT 1) and Neiguan (PC 6) for 1 – 3 minutes before sleep for prevention.

4.1.7 Epigastric Pain

INTRODUCTION

Epigastric pain is an illness of the digestive tract, which is manifested by pain in the epigastrium. It is also a symptom commonly seen in clinic. According to modern medical science, the problem is mainly caused by chemical and physical stimuli or inflammatory reaction of the gastric wall caused by bacteria, viruses or other factors. It also includes gastric and duodenal ulcer. TCM holds that gastric pain results from pathogenic cold invading the stomach and excessive intake of cold food which cause cold to accumulate in the stomach and yang qi to be blocked. It also results from improper diet, failure of the middle energizer in transformation and transportation, which causes damp-heat to accumulate in the stomach and qi function to stagnate. It still results from stagnation of liver-qi which transversely invades the stomach. Epigastric pain can also result from long-time stagnation of qi, stasis of blood flow, deficiency and cold in the middle energizer, and exhaustion of spleen-yang and kidney-yang.

MAIN POINTS FOR DIAGNOSIS

Epigastric pain is generally divided into two types in

振者,基本治法再加:① 按揉中脘穴 1 分钟。② 顺、逆时针摩腹 3～5 分钟。③ 按揉太阳、印堂、足三里穴各 1 分钟。

(3) 冠心病常于夜间发作,故每睡前可轻拍心前区 20～30 次,点按极泉、内关穴各 1～3 分钟,作为预防。

七、胃脘痛

【概述】

胃脘痛是以上腹部疼痛为主症的消化道疾病,也是临床常见的一个症状。现代医学认为本病症的发生多因化学、物理刺激及细菌、病毒等因素引起胃壁的炎性反应,也包括胃及十二指溃疡等。中医学认为,寒邪犯胃,过食生冷,寒积于中,阳气被遏;或饮食不节,中焦不运,内蕴湿热,气机凝滞;亦可因肝气郁结,横逆犯胃;气滞日久,血行瘀阻,中气虚寒,脾肾阳衰等都能造成胃脘疼痛的发生。

【诊断要点】

胃脘痛临床一般可分虚

clinic: the sthenia syndrome and the asthenia syndrome. The common symptoms are pain in the epigastrium accompanied by eructation with fetid odor and acid regurgitation or vomiting of watery fluid, lack of appetite, loose stools or constipation.

1. Sthenia Syndrome   Pain in the stomach and refusal of pressing, abdominal fullness and discomfort, belching with fetid odor, nausea, gastric discomfort with acid regurgitation, weak pulse, and greasy tongue fur.

2. Asthenia Syndrome   Dull pain in the stomach, preference for warmth and pressing, vomiting of watery fluid, cold extremities, deep and thready pulse and pale whitish tongue fur.

BASIC MANIPULATIONS

The principle of tuina treatment is reinforcing the spleen and regulating the stomach, regulating flow of qi and relieving pain.

(1) The patient lies on his back. The doctor sits beside him, applies pushing manipulation with one finger from Shangwan (CV 13) to Shenque (CV 8) (the center of the umbilicus) 5 - 10 times, and then presses and kneads Zhongwan (CV 12), Qihai (CV 6) and Tianshu (ST 25) for one minute each.

(2) The patient takes a prone position. The doctor applies rolling manipulation to the spinous region on his back to and fro 5 - 10 times, and meanwhile combines it with pressing-kneading points Pishu (BL 20), Weishu (BL 21), Ganshu (BL 18) and Sanjiaoshu (BL 22), etc.

(3) Press-knead Neiguan (PC 6) and Zusanli (ST 36) for one minute each.

(4) Rub-twist the hypochondriac areas on both sides for 3 - 5 minutes respectively.

(5) Press-knead Weitong points (at the upper part of the bone cleft between the second and the third metacar-

实两大类,常见症状是:胃脘部疼痛,伴见嗳腐吐酸或冷吐清水,食欲不振,大便溏薄或便秘。

1. 实证型   胃痛拒按,腹胀不适,嗳气息秽,恶心嘈杂,脉弱,苔腻。

2. 虚证型   胃痛隐隐,喜按喜暖,泛吐清水,手足不温,脉沉细,苔淡白。

【基本治法】

推拿治疗胃脘痛的原则是:健脾和胃,理气止痛。

(1) 患者仰卧位,医者坐其侧,先以一指禅推法从上脘穴推至神阙穴 5～10 次。然后按揉中脘、气海、天枢穴各 1分钟。

(2) 患者俯卧,医者以㨰法在其背脊部往返操作 5～10遍,同时配合按揉脾俞、胃俞、肝俞、三焦俞等穴位。

(3) 按揉内关穴、足三里穴各 1分钟。

(4) 搓擦患者两胁肋部3～5分钟。

(5) 按揉双侧胃痛穴(2、3掌骨缝间上端处)各 1分钟。

pal bones) on both sides for one minute respectively.

MODIFIED MANIPULATIONS WITH SYNDROME DIFFERENTIATION

1. Sthenia Syndrome   The following manipulations may be added to the basic manipulations.

i. The patient lies on his back. The doctor stretches out his two hands, presses the thumbs on Zhongwan (CV 12) and pushes toward the middle and the lower abdomen horizontally with both hands 5 - 10 times.

ii. Push horizontally and scrub vertically from the lumbar region to the sacral region until a hot sensation is gained.

iii. Circularly rub the abdomen counterclockwise for 3 - 5 minutes.

2. Asthenia Syndrome   Besides the basic manipulations the following may be added as the case requires.

i. Digitally-press Chengshan (BL 57) and Weizhong (BL 40) for one minute respectively.

ii. Circularly rub the abdomen clockwise for 3 - 5 minutes.

iii. Vibrate with the finger Zhongwan (CV 12) for 1 - 3 minutes.

iv. Scrub horizontally the lumbar-sacral region till a hot sensation is gained.

4.1.8   Gastroptosis

INTRODUCTION

Gastroptosis is a chronic disease, and is one of the commonly seen visceral ptosis. Modern medicine believes that most part of the stomach locates normally in the left hypochondrium, and the rest part in the upper abdomen. But when the abdominal muscles loosen, or the abdominal pressure becomes abnormal due to physical fatigue, childbearing and some other reasons, gastroptosis will occur.

【随症加减】

1. 实证型　基本治法再加：① 患者仰卧，医者双手分开，两拇指合按中脘穴处，双手用力向中、下腹部平推5～10遍。② 平推、直擦患者腰背至骶部，以热为度。③ 逆时针摩腹3～5分钟。

2. 虚证型　基本治法再加：① 点按承山、委中穴各1分钟。② 顺时针摩腹3～5分钟。③ 指振中脘穴1～3分钟。④ 横擦腰骶部，以热为度。

八、胃下垂

【概述】

胃下垂是一种慢性疾病，是比较常见的内脏下垂之一。现代医学认为胃的正常位置大部分在左季肋部，小部分在上腹部，但因身体虚弱、生育和各种原因，腹部肌肉松弛，不能保持正常腹压，导致胃

According to TCM, gastroptosis is mainly caused by weakness of the spleen and stomach, and sinking of the middle energizer qi. For the spleen and stomach are the foundation of acquired constitution, they govern transportation and transformation of nutrients and control the muscles. Once the spleen is weak, its function of transportation and transformation will be abnormal and the middle energizer qi will fail in lifting. Thus gastroptosis will take place.

MAIN POINTS FOR DIAGNOSIS

The main symptoms of gastroptosis are loss of appetite, dull pain in the stomach, belching, tenesmus sensation in the abdomen, which is aggravated by taking food or walking, flat upper abdomen and bulging lower abdomen, while standing, loose abdominal muscles with decreased myodynamia, marked intra-abdominal pulsation under slight palpation. In most cases, symptoms such as abdominal fullness and pain, loose stools or constipation, palpitation, hypodynamia, emaciation, and dizziness are also present.

In barium meal examination of gastro-intestinal tract, the lowest point of the lesser curvature of stomach can be seen dropped below the inter-iliac-crest line or the duodenal bulb has moved towards the left side.

BASIC MANIPULATIONS

The principle of tuina therapy: reinforcing the spleen and regulating the stomach, nourishing the middle energizer and strengthening qi.

(1) The patient lies on his back. The doctor stands by his side, gently manipulates the area of Zhongwan (CV 12) with pushing manipulation of one-finger, cooperated with kneading manipulation with the major thenar eminence for 3 - 5 minutes, and then manipulates orderly

下垂。

中医学认为本病症多因脾胃虚弱、中气下陷所致。因脾胃为后天之本，主运化、主肌肉。脾虚则运化失常，中气升举无力而发生胃部下坠。

【诊断要点】

胃下垂主要症状为食欲减退，胃部隐痛，嗳气并有胃脘部的下坠感，饭后或行走时加重，站立时，上腹部平坦，下腹部膨隆，腹部肌肉松弛、肌力降低，稍按压即可触及腹内脉动，并多伴有腹胀、腹痛，大便或稀或干，心悸，乏力，消瘦，头晕等。

胃肠钡餐造影可见胃小弯弧线最低点下降到髂嵴连线以下或十二指肠球部向左偏移。

【基本治法】

推拿治疗胃下垂的原则是健脾和胃，补中益气。

(1) 患者仰卧，医者居其侧，以一指禅推法并配合大鱼际揉法在中脘穴处和缓操作3～5分钟，然后循序往下至腹部及小腹部往返操作 5～

toward the abdomen and the lower abdomen back and forth 5 - 10 times.

(2) The patient takes a prone position. The doctor mainly presses and kneads Pishu (BL 20), Weishu (BL 21) and Sanjiaoshu (BL 22) with the fingers, combined with plucking manipulation, for 1 - 3 minutes.

(3) The patient sits or stands. The doctor stands behind him, inserts the index, the middle and the ring fingers with their dorsal side touching the skin from the medial and inferior angle of the scapulae toward its interior and superior angle to the extent of the patients tolerance for 1 - 3 minutes. Then, continue the operation with the other hand.

(4) The patient lies on his back. The doctor stands in front of the patient, crosses the fingers and puts them on the lower abdomen, uses the side of the little fingers to exert force and slowly holds it upwards to the umbilicus along with the patient's breath, and then slowly puts the abdomen down. Repeat the operation for 5 - 10 minutes.

(5) Press-knead Zusanli (ST 36) on both sides for one minute respectively.

MODIFIED MANIPULATIONS WITH SYNDROME DIFFERENTIATION

(1) For patients with gastroptosis accompanied by subjective borborygmus or alternate appearance of constipation and stomachache, the following manipulations may be performed in addition.

i. The patient lies on his back with his legs flexed. The doctor stands by his side, kneads and grasps the abdominal muscles with both his hands 10 times. Then pushes and shakes transversely the stomach back and forth with his palms 5 - 10 times.

ii. Put one palm or two overlapped palms on the region below the umbilicus, press with slight force upward, in

10遍。

（2）患者俯卧，医者以指按揉法并配合弹拨法在脾俞、胃俞、三焦俞穴重点操作1～3分钟。

（3）患者坐或站位，医者立其后，以食、中、无名指三指掌背贴沿病人肩胛骨内下角，向肩胛骨内上插入，以能忍受为度，持续1～3分钟，再换手操作。

（4）患者仰卧，医者立其头前，以两手指交叉，合掌置于下腹部，以小指侧着力，随呼吸徐徐向上托起，托至脐部，慢慢放下。反复操作5～10分钟。

（5）按揉双侧足三里穴各1分钟。

【随症加减】

（1）胃下垂伴见自觉肠鸣辘辘有声，便秘与腹痛交替出现者，基本手法再加：① 患者仰卧，两腿屈曲，医者立其侧，用双手揉拿腹部肌肉10次。然后以掌横向来回推荡脘腹部5～10次。② 以单掌或双掌相叠置脐下，稍用力由下向上按压并施振颤法1～3分钟。

combination with vibrating manipulation for 1 – 3 minutes.

(2) For patients with gastroptosis accompanied by emaciation, vertigo, fatigue, palpitation and insomnia, the following manipulations can be applied additionally.

i. Circularly rub the abdomen clockwise for 5 – 10 minutes.

ii. Press-knead Neiguan (PC 6), Shenmen (HT 7) and Hegu (LI 4) for one minute respectively.

iii. Grasp-knead the four limbs for 1 – 3 minutes respectively.

iv. Scrub transversely the dorsal, lumbar, and sacral regions with a single palm till a hot sensation is gained.

v. Palm-twist and rub the two hypochondriac regions for 3 – 5 minutes.

Patients with gastroptosis are recommended to take little food at a time but more times a day, not to take cold, crude, pungent or indigestible foods, to develop a regular living habit, and to exercise their abdominal muscles properly. For those with severe gastroptosis, a gastric supporter may be used during treatment to strengthen the therapeutic effects.

4. 1. 9 Diarrhea

INTRODUCTION

Diarrhea, also termed Fuxie, is a symptom of many diseases. According to modern medical science, it is mainly caused by bacterial infection or dysfunction of the stomach and intestine. It is most commonly seen in acute or chronic enteritis. TCM holds that the main pathological changes of diarrhea lie in the spleen, the stomach and intestines, and the pathogenic factors can be classified as external and internal ones. Diarrhea can be induced by external factors, such as cold, dampness, summer-heat, heat and improper diet, which affect the digestive func-

（2）胃下垂伴见消瘦、眩晕、乏力、心悸、失眠等症，基本手法再加：① 顺时针摩腹5～10分钟。② 按揉内关、神门、合谷穴各1分钟。③ 抓揉四肢部各1～3分钟。④ 单掌横擦背、腰、骶部，以热为度。⑤ 搓擦双胁部3～5分钟。

胃下垂患者宜少食多餐，忌食生冷、辛辣及不易消化的食物。并注意起居规律，平时配合适当的腹肌锻炼。胃下垂严重者，治疗期间可用胃托帮助，以巩固疗效。

九、泄泻

【概述】

泄泻又称腹泻，是多种疾病的一种症状。现代医学认为本病多由细菌感染和胃肠功能障碍所致，最常见于急、慢性肠炎。中医认为泄泻的主要病变在脾胃与大小肠，其致病原因可分为外因和内因两大类。外因可由寒、湿、暑、热及饮食不节，影响脾的运化功能，造成水湿相夹并走大肠

tion of the spleen and leads to the co-existence of water and dampness in the large intestine. It can also result from internal factors. For example, weakness of the spleen and stomach plus injury by emotional factors leads to dysfunction of spleen-qi and stomach-qi. This long-term morbid condition will impair the spleen-yang and stomach-yang and finally cause chronic diarrhea.

MAIN POINTS FOR DIAGNOSIS

The common symptoms of diarrhea are abdominal pain, borborygmus, 3 - 5 times of defecation or more every day, poor appetite, general fatigue, soreness and weakness of the lumbus and knees.

1. Syndrome of Cold-damp Impairing the Spleen Abrupt onset, loose stools or mixed with mucus, abdominal pain with borborygmus, aching pain of the extremities, pale or yellowish and greasy tongue fur, soft and slippery pulse.

2. Syndrome of Food Retention Sudden onset, abdominal fullness and pain, diarrhea with stool fetid as rotten egg, which can be relieved after diarrhea, foul belching and acid regurgitation, greasy and thick tongue fur, slippery and rapid pulse.

3. Syndrome of Yang Deficiency of the Spleen and Kidney Intermittent diarrhea and loose stool with undigested food, abdominal pain at dawn, immediate diarrhea with borborygmus accompanied by abdominal aversion to cold, soreness and aching of the lumbus and knees, pale tongue fur, sunken and thready pulse.

BASIC MANIPULATIONS

The principle of tuina therapy: Reinforcing the spleen and regulating qi, warming yang and arresting diarrhea.

(1) The patient lies on his back. The doctor stands by his side, applies pushing manipulation with one finger

而发病;内因可由素体脾胃虚弱,复因情志所伤,致使脾胃气机失调而病久不愈,更伤及脾胃阳气而导致泄泻缠绵不止。

【诊断要点】

泄泻常见症状是:腹痛、肠鸣,每日排便3～5次以上,食欲减退,伴全身乏力、腰膝酸软等。

1. 寒湿伤脾型　症见发病急骤、大便稀薄或夹粘液,腹痛肠鸣,肢体酸痛,苔白或黄腻,脉濡滑。

2. 饮食积滞型　症见发病突然,脘腹胀痛,泻下粪便臭如败卵,泻后则痛减,嗳腐吞酸,舌苔腻垢,脉滑数。

3. 脾肾阳虚型　症见大便时溏时泻,完谷不化并多以黎明时腹痛,肠鸣即泻,伴有腹部畏寒,腰酸膝痛,舌苔淡白,脉沉细。

【基本治法】

推拿治疗泄泻的原则是健脾理气,温阳止泻。

(1) 患者仰卧位,医者位于其侧,以一指禅推法从中脘

slowly from Zhongwan (CV 12) to Qihai (CV 6) and Guanyuan (CV 4) to and fro for 3 – 5 minutes.

(2) Press the abdomen with the overlapped palms, combined with vibrating manipulation for one minute, and then lift palms suddenly. Repeat the first-pressing-then-loosening operation 5 – 10 times.

(3) The patient takes a prone position. The doctor rolls and pushes the muscles on his back and lumbar region, in combination with mainly pressing-kneading Pishu (BL 20), Dachangshu (BL 25), and Shenshu (BL 23) for 3 – 5 minute.

(4) Press-knead Zusanli (ST 36), Yinlingquan (SP 9) and Sanyinjiao (SP 6) for 1 minute respectively.

MODIFIED MANIPULATIONS WITH SYNDROME DIFFERENTIATION

1. Syndrome of Cold-damp Impairing the Spleen Besides the basic manipulations, the following can also be performed.

i. Press-knead the sacral coccygeal regions for 3 – 5 minutes.

ii. Push-scrub the sacral coccygeal region upward along the dorsal column with the hypothenar eminence until a hot sensation is gained.

iii. Press-knead Shangjuxu (ST 37) and Xiajuxu (ST 39) for one minute respectively.

iv. Press-knead Quchi (LI 11) and Hegu (LI 4) for one minute respectively.

2. Syndrome of Food Retention The following manipulations may be added to the basic ones.

i. Circularly rub the abdomen counterclockwise for 3 – 5 minutes.

ii. Scrub the lower abdomen with both palms separately and obliquely 5 – 10 times.

iii. The patient takes a prone position. The doctor

穴开始缓慢向下操作至气海、关元穴，往返3～5分钟。

（2）医者双掌相叠按压患者腹部，并施振颤法1分钟，然后双掌突然提起，如此一按一松，反复操作5～10次。

（3）患者俯卧位，医者擦、推其背、腰部肌肉，重点配合按揉脾俞、大肠俞、肾俞等穴，操作3～5分钟。

（4）按揉足三里、阴陵泉、三阴交等穴各1分钟。

【随症加减】

1. 寒湿伤脾型 基本治法再加：① 按揉尾骶部3～5分钟。② 以小鱼际从尾骶部沿脊椎向上推擦，以热为度。③ 按揉上巨虚、下巨虚各1分钟。④ 按揉曲池、合谷穴各1分钟。

2. 饮食积滞型 基本治法再加：① 逆时针摩腹3～5分钟。② 双掌分向斜擦少腹5～10次。③ 患者俯卧，医者以拇、食指捏紧其尾骶部肌肉，一松一捏渐向上移动直至大椎止，反复操作5～10次。

pinches tightly the muscles in the sacral coccygeal region with the index and the middle fingers, and then loosens them. Repeat the pinching-loosening operation upward to Dazhui (GV 14) 5 - 10 times.

ⅰ. Scrub the medial sides of the thigh and the shanks up and down until a hot sensation is felt.

3. Syndrome of Yang Deficiency of the Spleen and Kidney　The following manipulations may be added to the basic ones as the case requires.

ⅰ. Circularly rub the areas around the umbilicus and the lower abdomen with both palms for 3 - 5 minutes.

ⅱ. Scrub horizontally Dazhui (GV 14) and Mingmen (GV 4) until a hot sensation is achieved.

ⅲ. Press and knead Taixi (KI 3) for 1 minute respectively.

ⅳ. Scrub and palm-twist Yongquan (KI 1) for 3 - 5 minutes.

Attention should be paid to those with severe dehydration caused by diarrhea, to whom other treatments should be given promptly. In addition, the patient is recommended not to take cold, raw foods and not to overwork so as to reinforce the gained therapeutic effects.

4.1.10　Constipation

INTRODUCTION

Constipation refers to difficulty in defecation, prolonged intervals between defecations, or the condition of being difficult in defection since the stool is too dry and hard though there is a desire. Modern medical science believes that the problem is mainly caused by defecation adynamia (e. g. weakness of diaphragm and abdominal muscles), inadequate stimulation on the intestinal wall (that is mainly because of insufficient chemical or mechanical stimulation of food upon the large intestine and rectum),

④ 向上向下擦大腿、小腿内侧面,以热为度。

3. 脾肾阳虚型　基本治法再加:① 掌摩脐周及小腹部3～5 分钟。② 横擦大椎、命门穴,均以热为度。③ 按揉太溪穴各 1 分钟。④ 搓擦涌泉穴 3～5 分钟。

治疗中值得注意的是,泄泻严重脱水者,宜及时采取其他方法治疗。并嘱病人避免进食生冷、过分劳累,以配合巩固疗效。

十、便秘

【概述】

便秘是指大便秘结不通,排便间隔时间延长,或欲大便而粪便干燥艰涩难解的一种病症。现代医学认为致病原因多是由于排便动力缺乏(如膈肌、腹肌等衰弱),肠道所受刺激不足(主要由于食物对大肠、直肠的机械或化学的刺激不足),肠粘膜应激力减弱(各

and abirritation of the intestinal mucosa（which results from various pathological changes in intestinal mucosa，such as in dysentery）. TCM holds that the pathogenic factors include consumption of intestinal fluid due to febrile disease and excessive intake of pungent food，lung-dryness and lung-heat，which descend to the large intestine and impair body fluid，internal injury due to seven emotions，stagnation of qi activity，and deficiency of blood and qi of the aged and the asthenic. All those may lead to dysfunction of the stomach and intestine in transportation，transformation，descending and ascending，resulting in the occurrence of constipation.

MAIN POINTS FOR DIAGNOSIS

Besides difficult defecation，the common symptoms of constipation also include discomfort in the epigastrium，stuffiness in the chest，poor appetite，and irritability.

1. Syndrome of Gastriointestinal Dryness and Heat   Dry and hard stools，scanty and dark urine，reddened face，fever，dry mouth，restlessness，red tongue with yellowish or dry fur，and slippery and rapid pulse.

2. Syndrome of Stagnation of Qi   Difficult fecal discharge although there is an urge to defecate，full sensation in the costal and hypochondriac region，distending pain in the abdomen，poor appetite，thin and greasy tongue fur and floating pulse.

3. Syndrome of Deficiency of Blood and Qi   Retention of feces，difficult defecation for several days，dizziness with blurred vision，pale complexion，cold extremities，pale lips and tongue，thin tongue fur，and thready and weak pulse.

BASIC MANIPULATIONS

The principle of tuina therapy：Regulating the intestines and relieving constipation.

（1）The patient lies on his back. The doctor applies pushing manipulation with one finger to Zhongwan（CV

种肠粘膜的病变,如痢疾等）造成的。中医则认为,病因可由热性病后或过食辛辣燥伤肠液;肺燥肺热下移于大肠,耗伤津液;七情内伤;气机郁滞;年老体弱,气血亏虚等造成的胃肠运化、升降和传导功能的失常而致本病症的发生。

【诊断要点】

常见症状除大便难解外,还可见脘腹不适,胸憋气闷,饮食不馨,甚至脾气暴躁等。

1. 胃肠燥热型   症见大便干结,小便短赤,面红身热,口干心烦,舌红苔黄或燥,脉滑数。

2. 气机郁滞型   症见大便秘结不畅,临便努责,胁腹痞胀,食纳欠馨,舌苔薄腻,脉弦。

3. 气血亏虚型   症见大便秘结,多日难解,头晕目眩,面色无华,四肢欠温,唇舌淡,苔薄,脉细弱。

【基本治法】

推拿治疗便秘总的原则是和肠通便。

（1）患者仰卧,以一指禅推法在中脘、关元、天枢穴治

12), Guanyuan (CV 4) and Tianshu (ST 25) for 1 minute each, then circularly rubs the abdomen counterclockwise for about 5 minutes.

(2) The patient takes a prone position. The doctor applies pushing manipulation with one finger or rolling manipulation along both sides of the spinous column from Feishu (BL 13), via Pishu (BL 20), Weishu (BL 21), Sanjiaoshu (BL 22) and Shenshu (BL 23) to Shangliao (BL 31), Ciliao (BL 32), Zhongliao (BL 33) and Xialiao (BL 34) repeatedly for about 5 minutes. Meanwhile press-knead these points with a finger.

MODIFIED MANIPULATIONS WITH SYNDROME DIFFERENTIATION

1. Syndrome of Gastrointestinal Dryness and Heat　The following manipulations may be added to the basic ones.

i. Scrub the spinous and lumbar regions along two sides of the spinous column till a hot sensation is gained.

ii. Lift-grasp the medial muscles of the thighs with both hands for 3 – 5 minutes, combined with digitally-pressing Yanglingquan (GB 34) and Sanyinjiao (SP 6), until a sore, distending sensation is achieved.

iii. Digitally-press and pluck Hegu (LI 4), Quchi (LI 11) and Zhigou (TE 6) for 1 minute each.

2. Syndrome of Stagnation of Qi

Besides the basic therapy, the following methods may be used additionally.

i. Press-knead Zhongfu (LU 1), Yunmen (LU 2), Danzhong (CV 17), Zhangmen (LR 13) and Qimen (LR 14) on the chest or abdomen, and Feishu (BL 13) on the back for 1 minute respectively with slight stimulation. Then press Taichong (LR 3) and Xingjian (LR 2) with a finger for 1 minute respectively.

ii. Scrub horizontally the upper chest till a hot sensation is gained.

疗,每穴约 1 分钟。然后以逆时针摩腹约 5 分钟。

(2) 患者俯卧,一指禅推或㨰法沿脊柱两侧从肺俞开始向下,沿脾俞、胃俞、三焦俞、肾俞直到八髎穴,往返治疗,时间约 5 分钟,同时以指按揉上述穴位。

【随症加减】

1. 胃肠燥热型　基本手法再加: ① 沿背脊两旁直擦腰脊部,以热为度。② 双手提拿大腿内侧肌肉 3～5 分钟,配合点按阳陵泉、三阴交穴,以酸胀为度。③ 点按、弹拨合谷、曲池、支沟穴各 1 分钟。

2. 气机郁滞型　基本治法再加: ① 按揉胸腹部的中府、云门、膻中、章门、期门穴以及背部的肺俞穴各 1 分钟,按揉时刺激宜轻,再以指按太冲、行间穴各 1 分钟。②横擦胸上部,以热为度。③ 斜擦两胁,以热为度。

iii. Scrub obliquely the costal and hypochondriac regions till a hot sensation is gained.

3. Syndrome of Deficiency of Blood and Qi

The following may be added to the basic manipulations if necessary.

i. Scrub transversely the upper chest and scrub vertically the back to the lumbosacral region until a hot sensation is gained.

ii. Press-knead Shenshu（BL 23）for 3 minutes, combined with transversely scrubbing.

iii. Press-knead Zusanli（ST 36）and Sanyinjiao（SP 6）, palm-twist Yongquan（KI 1）, and press Quchi（LI 11）and Zhigou（TE 6）for one minute respectively.

Some preventing methods of constipation: drink a glass of salty boiled water on an empty stomach after getting up, eat more fresh vegetables and fruits, do more exercises, develop a regular life habit and defecate regularly.

4.1.11 Prostatitis

INTRODUCTION

As a common disease in the urinary system, prostatitis is often seen in young and middle-aged people. According to modern medical science, prostatitis is usually derived from invasion of the prostate by bacteria, viruses, mycoplasma, and chlamydia. It is also related to excess of sexual intercourse, over drinking of alcohol, perineum damage, and acute urethritis. TCM holds that prostatitis is mainly caused by failure of the kidney in controlling, urination due to kidney qi deficiency, or downward infusion of damp-heat.

MAIN POINTS FOR DIAGNOSIS

The common symptoms of prostatitis are frequent micturition, urgency of micturition, dribbling urination, white secretion at the meatus urinarius accompanied by

3．气血亏虚型　基本治法再加：① 横擦胸上部，直擦背部至腰骶部，均以热为度。② 按揉肾俞穴 3 分钟，并配合横擦法。③ 按揉足三里、三阴交穴，搓涌泉穴，按曲池、支沟穴各 1 分钟。

预防便秘方法：晨起可空腹喝一杯淡盐开水，平时多吃蔬菜、水果，增加运动，起居有节，养成按时大便的习惯。

十一、前列腺炎

【概述】

本病多见于青壮年。现代医学认为本病多因细菌、病毒、支原体、衣原体等侵入腺体所致，与房事不节、过度饮酒、会阴部损伤、急性尿道炎等有关。它是一种常见的泌尿系统疾病。中医认为本病由肾气亏虚、不能约束或湿热下注所致。

【诊断要点】

本病临床常见症状有尿频、尿急或小便淋漓不尽，尿道口常有白色分泌物及伴见

decreased sexual desire and emission. Usually, it can be differentiated as follows.

1. Syndrome of Downward Infusion of Damp-heat Frequent micturition, dark urine, urodynia, discomfort sensation in the lumbosacral region, perineum and the medial side of the thigh, yellowish and greasy tongue fur, floating and soft pulse.

2. Syndrome of Asthenic Kidney Qi Dribbling urination, aching pain in the lower back, bearing-down and distending sensation in the lower abdomen and perineum, thin and pale tongue fur, weak and thready pulse.

BASIC MANIPULATIONS

The principle of tuina therapy: removing dampness and strengthening the kidney.

(1) The patient takes a prone position. The doctor stands by his side, presses and kneads, and palm-twists and scrubs the caudal region with the two palms until a hot sensation is achieved.

(2) Digitally-press Baliao (BL 31 – BL 34) with the two thumbs for 3 – 5 minutes, and then strike the points with the metacarpal-phalangeal parts or a slightly-bent palm for one minute.

(3) The patient lies on his back. The doctor places one palm or two overlapped palms on Guanyuan (CV 4) to press-knead and circularly rub toward the pubic region repeatedly for 3 – 5 minutes.

(4) Place both palms beside the umbilicus, obliquely push-scrub toward the pubic region until a hot sensation is achieved.

(5) Press-knead Yinlingquan (SP 9) and Sanyinjiao (SP 6) with a finger for one minute respectively.

MODIFIED MANIPULATIONS WITH SYNDROME DIFFERENTIATION

1. Syndrome of Downward Infusion of Damp-heat

性欲减退,遗精等。分型可见:

1. 湿热下注型 症见尿频、色赤、尿痛,以及腰骶部会阴区和大腿内侧不适,苔黄腻,脉弦濡等。

2. 肾气亏虚型 症见小便淋漓不尽,下腰部酸痛,小腹及会阴坠胀,苔薄质淡,脉虚细等。

【基本治法】

推拿治疗前列腺炎的原则是利湿固肾。

(1) 患者俯卧,医者立其旁,以双掌按揉并搓擦尾骶部,以热为度。

(2) 以双手拇指点按八髎穴 3～5 分钟,然后以掌指或虚掌叩击该部 1 分钟。

(3) 患者仰卧,医者单掌或双掌相叠置关元穴上按揉、摩动至耻骨处,反复 3～5 分钟。

(4) 双掌置患者脐旁,同时斜向耻骨部推擦,以热为度。

(5) 以指按揉阴陵泉、三阴交穴各 1 分钟。

【随症加减】

1. 湿热下注型 基本治

The manipulations may include the following besides the basic ones.

i. Push-scrub the medial side of the thigh with one palm from top to below till a hot sensation is achieved.

ii. Press-knead Sanyinjiao (SP 6), Taichong (LR 3) and Yinlingquan (SP 9) for one minute respectively.

iii. Palm-rub and scrub the inguinal regions for one minute.

2. Syndrome of Asthenic Kidney Qi   The manipulations may include the following in addition to those basic ones.

i. Push-scrub the medial sides of the thighs with one palm from top to below until a hot sensation is felt.

ii. Scrub transversely Mingmen (GV 4) until a hot sensation is achieved.

iii. Press-knead Zusanli (ST 36) and Taixi (KI 3) for one minute respectively.

iv. Palm-twist and scrub Yongquan (KI 1) for 1 - 3 minutes.

v. Press-knead the perineum for one minute.

4.1.12   Uroschesis

INTRODUTION

Uroschesis refers to accumulation of profuse urine in the bladder and being unable or difficult to discharge. According to modern medical science, there are two reasons for uroschesis: mechanical obstruction and dynamic obstruction. The former is often seen in proliferation of prostate, urethra stenosis, lithous impaction, tumor in the bladder or bladder obstruction by blood clots. The latter is caused by dysfunction of urination due to anesthesia, operation, or injury and inflammation of the central or peripheral nerves. Tuina therapy is usually applicable to the latter. In TCM, the disease is called Longbi, and can be

法再加：① 单掌推擦大腿内侧，自上向下，以热为度。② 按揉三阴交、太冲、阴陵泉穴各 1 分钟。③ 搓擦腹股沟处 1 分钟。

2. 肾气亏虚型   基本治法再加：① 单掌推擦大腿内侧，自下向上，以热为度。② 横擦命门穴处，以热为度。③ 按揉足三里、太溪穴各 1 分钟。④ 搓擦涌泉穴 1～3 分钟。⑤ 按揉会阴部 1 分钟。

十二、尿潴留

【概述】

尿潴留是指大量尿液积蓄在膀胱中而不能排出或排出不畅的病症。现代医学认为发生尿潴留的原因有机械性梗阻和动力性梗阻两种，前者常见于前列腺增生、尿道狭窄、结石嵌顿、膀胱内肿瘤或血块堵塞膀胱等；后者由排尿功能障碍所引起，如麻醉、手术后或由于中枢神经或周围神经的损伤、炎症等。推拿治

caused by damp-heat, stagnation of qi, or deficiency of the kidney. It is also related to dysfunction of the spleen, the lung and the kidney.

MAIN POINTS FOR DIAGNOSIS

The commonly-seen clinical symptoms of uroschesis are distending eminence and pain in the lower abdomen, strong desire for urination with bearing-down sensation, difficult or dribbling urination. Clinically, the commonly seen syndromes are as follows:

1. Stagnation of Damp-heat Syndrome　Difficult urination, dark and hot urine or anuresis, distension of the lower abdomen, difficult defecation, bitter taste in the mouth or sticky mouth, thirst without desire for drinking, reddened tongue with yellowish and greasy tongue fur, sunken and rapid pulse.

2. Excess of Lung-heat Syndrome　Dribbling and difficult urination, dry throat, thirst with desire for drinking, shortness of breath, thin and yellowish tongue fur and rapid pulse.

3. Deficiency of Kidney-qi Syndrome　Blocked or dribbling urination, weakness in urination, pale complexion, listlessness, cold limbs, lassitude in the loin and knee, pale tongue, sunken and thready pulse.

BASIC MANIPULATIONS

The principle of tuina therapy is eliminating pathogenic factors and restoring vital qi, regulating flow of qi and relieving uroschesis.

(1) The patient lies on his back. The doctor uses one palm to push from the umbilicus to the pubic symphysis slightly and forcefully 20 times.

(2) Press-knead with the index and the middle fingers Qihai (CV 6), Guanyuan (CV 4) and Zhongji (CV 3)

疗多适用于后者。中医称此病为"癃闭",认为湿热、气郁、肾亏均可致病,且多与脾、肺、肾三脏功能失调有关。

【诊断要点】

临床常见症状有小腹部隆胀疼痛和高度尿意,并有下坠感,小便难以排出或点滴不畅。临床上常见证型如下:

1. 湿热蕴积型　症见小便不利,热赤或闭,小腹胀满,大便不畅,口苦口粘,或口渴不欲饮,舌质红,苔黄腻,脉沉数。

2. 肺热壅盛型　症见小便涓滴不通或点滴不爽,咽干,烦渴欲饮,呼吸急促,舌苔薄黄,脉数。

3. 肾气不充型　症见小便不通,或滴沥不畅,排出无力,面色㿠白,神气怯弱,四肢欠温,腰膝乏力,舌质淡,脉沉细。

【基本治法】

推拿治疗本病症的总的原则是,祛邪扶正,理气通尿。

(1) 患者仰卧,医者以单掌从脐部推向耻骨联合部,推时稍用力,操作20次。

(2) 以食、中指按揉气海、关元、中极穴各1分钟。

for one minute respectively.

(3) Use the palm to scrub obliquely both sides of the abdomen 10 – 20 times.

(4) Scrub horizontally the upper chest until a hot sensation is achieved.

(5) The patient takes a prone position, and the doctor rubs across the caudal region until a hot sensation is achieved.

(6) The patient sits. The doctor stands behind him, clamps his hypochondriac areas with both palms, and rubs back and forth and up and down to the lumbar region. Repeat the operation for 1 – 3 minutes.

(7) The patient lies on his back. The doctor puts one palm on the mid-point of the line between the umbilicus and the pubic symphysis, and then uses the palmar root to press toward the pubic symphysis region with increasing force. This manipulation can also be combined with vibrating manipulation. If it is appropriately manipulated, micturition will take place immediately and voluntarily.

MODIFIED MANIPULATIONS WITH SYNDROME DIFFERENTIATION

1. Stasis of Dampness-heat Syndrome   The following can be performed additionally besides the basic manipulations.

i. Circularly rub the abdomen clockwise and counter-clockwise for 3 – 5 minutes respectively.

ii. Press-knead Zusanli (ST 36), Sanyinjiao (SP 6) and Yinlingquan (SP 9) for one minute respectively.

2. Excess of Lung-heat Syndrome   The following can be added to the basic manipulations as the case requires.

i. Press-knead Zhongfu (LU 1) and Yunmen (LU 2) for one minute respectively.

ii. Push-scrub the anterior region of the medial sides of the upper limbs with one palm until a hot sensation is

（3）以掌斜擦两侧腹部10~20次。

（4）横擦胸上部，以热为度。

（5）患者俯卧，横擦尾骶部，以热为度。

（6）患者坐位，医者立其后，双手掌夹持两侧胸胁，同时搓动，并向下移至腰，反复操作1~3分钟。

（7）患者仰卧，医者以单掌按在脐与耻骨联合连线的中点处，用掌根向耻骨联合部按压，逐渐加大压力，且可配合振颤手法，如操作正确，小便即当自行排出。

【随症加减】

1. 湿热蕴积型   基本治法再加：① 顺逆时针摩腹各3~5分钟。② 按揉足三里、三阴交、阴陵泉穴各1分钟。

2. 肺热壅盛型   基本治法再加：① 按揉中府、云门穴各1分钟。② 单掌推擦上肢内侧前缘，以热为度。③ 按揉膻中穴1~3分钟。

achieved.

iii. Press-knead Danzhong（CV 17 ）for 1 – 3 minutes.

3. Deficiency of Kidney-qi Syndrome　Besides the basic manipulations, the following may be performed additionally.

i. Press-knead Shenshu（BL 23）and Mingmen（GV 4）for 3 minutes respectively.

ii. Rub-scrub Yongquan（KI 1）for 3 – 5 minutes.

In order to prevent recurrence of uroschosis and to strengthen therapeutic effects, the manipulations mentioned above can be conducted continuously 2 – 3 times every day.

4. 1. 13　Seminal Emission

INTRODUCTION

Emission refers to discharge of semen without sexual intercourse. It is originally a physiological phenomenon of male sexual function, but excessively frequent emission（several times a week or even several times one night）would be a morbid condition. According to modern medical science, seminal emission is one of male sexual dysfunctions, which is often caused by neurosis, excessive sexual activity（excessive masturbation and sexual intercourse）, and pathological changes in the reflex stimulating of the central nervous system. TCM holds that excessive intake of heavy or pungent foods can lead to accumulation of damp-heat in the spleen and the stomach, which infuses downward to disturb the seminal house and eventually causes emission. Or excessive sexual intercourse and exhaustion of the heart and the spleen lead to weakness of the kidney and declining of the vital fire, resulting in seminal emission.

MAIN POINTS FOR DIAGNOSIS

It is mainly manifested as spontaneous discharge of

3. 肾气不充型　基本治法再加：①按揉肾俞、命门穴各 3 分钟。②搓擦涌泉穴 3～5分钟。

为预防尿潴留再次发生和巩固疗效，以上方法可每日连续操作 2～3 次。

十三、遗精

【概述】

遗精是精液不因性交而遗出生殖器。它本是男子性功能生理现象，但如遗精过频，每周数次或一夜数次，则是一种病态。现代医学认为是男子性功能障碍之一，多因神经衰弱、恣情纵欲（如过度手淫、房事不节）、反射刺激中枢神经系统病变所致。中医认为本病发病的原因可因过食厚味或辛辣等，致使脾胃湿热内盛、下注扰动精室；或因劳欲过度，心脾亏虚致使肾虚不藏，命门火衰而发病。

【诊断要点】

主要症见精液每于寐中

semen in sleep accompanied by restlessness and soreness and flaccidity in the loin and the knee. It is clinically classified as deficiency syndrome and excess syndrome.

1. Excess Syndrome   Bitter taste in the mouth, thirst, dark and hot urine, easy erection, itching and pain in the penis, nocturnal emission, thick semen, reddened tongue with greasy tongue fur, wiry and strong pulse.

2. Deficiency Syndrome   Dizziness with blurred vision, listlessness, soreness and flaccidity of the loin and the knee, cold limbs, impotence, thin semen, pale tongue with thin tongue fur, thready and weak pulse.

BASIC MANIPULATIONS

The principle of tuina therapy: calming the mind and reinforcing the kidney, consolidating and astringing the seminal function.

(1) The patient lies on his back. The doctor stands or sits beside him. First press-knead Shenque (CV 8), also called Qizhong (the center of the umbilicus), with the palmar root until a warm, hot sensation is achieved below the umbilicus. The manipulation should be gentle, but able to reach the deep part, the duration is about three minutes. Next, use a finger to knead Qihai (CV 6), Guanyuan (CV 4) and Zhongji (CV 3) for one minute respectively. Finally, operate on Qihai (CV 6) and Guanyuan (CV 4) with circular palm-rubbing manipulation for 3 - 5 minutes.

(2) The patient takes a prone position. The doctor applies rolling manipulation to his lumbar and sacral regions for 3 - 5 minutes first. Next, press-knead Shenshu (BL 23) and Mingmen (GV 4) with a finger for one minute respectively until arrival of qi with a sore, distending sensation is achieved. Then digitally-press Baliao (BL 31 - BL 34), combined with kneading and rubbing maneuvers for 3 - 5 minutes.

自行遗出,伴见心烦意乱或腰膝酸软等,临床常分虚、实两证。

1. 实证   症状可见口苦口渴,小便赤热,阴茎易举,茎中痒痛,多梦而遗,精液粘稠,苔腻质红,脉弦而有力。

2. 虚证   症状可见头晕目眩,精神疲乏,腰膝酸软,四肢欠温,阴茎不举,精液稀薄,舌质淡,苔薄,脉细弱。

【基本治法】

推拿治疗遗精总的原则是宁心益肾,固摄精关。

(1) 病人仰卧,医者立或坐其侧。先用掌根按揉神阙穴部(脐中穴),以脐下有温热感为度,手法宜柔和深沉,时间约 3 分钟。再以指揉气海、关元、中极等穴,每穴各 1 分钟。然后在气海、关元穴处用掌摩法操作 3～5 分钟。

(2) 病人俯卧,医者先用擦法在其腰、骶部操作 3～5 分钟。再以指按揉肾俞、命门穴各 1 分钟,使其有酸胀得气感。然后点按八髎穴并加揉、摩 3～5 分钟。

MODIFIED MANIPAULATIONS WITH SYNDROME DIFFERENTIATION

1. Excess Syndrome　Besides the basic manipulations, the following may be performed additionally as the case requires.

i. Ask the patient to lie on his back, circularly rub the epigastrium counterclockwise for 3 - 5 minutes. Then push with one-finger manipulation, and pinch-grasp from the region below the umbilicus to the pubic region repeatedly 10 - 15 times.

ii. Apply the rolling and pinching manipulation to the medial side of the thigh and shank for 3 - 5 minutes, combined with digitally-pressing Sanyinjiao (SP 6), Yinlingquan (SP 9), etc.

iii. The patient takes a prone position. The doctor pushes and scrubs the muscles on both sides of the spinous column from the back to the lumbus and the sacral region until a hot sensation is felt.

iv. Press-knead Pangguangshu (BL 28), Dachangshu (BL 25) and Baliao (BL 31 - BL34), and press Huantiao (GB 30) forcefully for one minute respectively.

v. The patient sits, the doctor kneads and pushes Baihui (GV 20), and digitally-presses Neiguan (PC 6) and Waiguan (TE 5) for one minute respectively.

vi. Palm-rub both the hypochondriac areas until a hot sensation is achieved.

2. Deficiency Syndrome　The following manipulations can be added to the basic ones.

i. The patient lies on his back, the doctor circularly rubs the umbilicus and the lower abdomen clockwise until a hot sensation is achieved.

ii. Grasp-pinch the abdominal muscles, combined with digitally-pressing Guanyuan (CV 4) and Qihai (CV 6) for 5 - 10 minutes.

【随症加减】

1. 实证　基本治法再加：① 患者仰卧，逆时针摩脘腹部 3～5 分钟；一指禅推、捏拿自脐下至耻骨部，反复 10～15 遍。② 搓、捏拿大腿、小腿内侧 3～5 分钟，配合点按三阴交、阴陵泉等穴。③ 患者俯卧，推擦脊柱两旁肌肉，自背向腰至骶，以热为度。④ 揉按膀胱俞、大肠俞、八髎穴，重压环跳穴各 1 分钟。⑤ 患者坐位，揉推百会穴，点按神门、内关、外关穴各 1 分钟。⑥ 搓、擦两胁，以热为度。

2. 虚证　基本治法再加：① 患者仰卧，顺时针摩脐及下腹部，以热为度。② 拿捏腹部肌肉，配合点按关元、气海穴 5～10 分钟。③ 横擦腰骶部，以热透腹部为好。④ 点按足三里、三阴交穴，搓擦涌泉穴部各 1 分钟。⑤ 提拿合谷、内

iii. Scrub transversely the lumbosacral region until a hot sensation throughout the abdomen is felt.

iv. Digitally-press Zusanli (ST 36) and Sanyinjiao (SP 6), and palm-twist and rub Yongquan (KI 1), for one minute respectively.

v. Lift-grasp Hegu (LI 4), Neiguan (PC 6), Quchi (LI 11) and Jianjing (GB 21) 3 - 5 times respectively.

During the treatment of seminal emission with tuina therapy, the patient is recommended to relax himself mentally and take a correct attitude towards the disease. He is also supposed to stress his spiritual regulation, to be free from avarice and wild fancy and to get rid of the bad habit of masturbation.

4. 1. 14 Hemiplegia

INTRODUCTION

Hemiplegia is also called Banshen Busui, which is a sequela of stroke in TCM. According to modern medical science, hemiplegia is mainly caused by pathological changes in cerebral blood vessels such as rupture, embolism and spasm of cerebral blood vessels, which lead to the injury of central nervous system resulting in paralysis of limbs and face on one side. TCM holds that the problem is because of endogenous excess of damp-phlegm, deficiency of qi and excessive fire, which lead to hyperactivity of liver yang, and endogenous movement of liver wind, resulting in disharmony of qi, blood, yin, and yang.

MAIN POINTS FOR DIAGNOSIS

The common clinical symptoms are palsy on one side, deviated mouth and eyes, disturbance of speech, drooling from mouth angle, and difficulty in swallowing (dysphagia) accompanied by numbness in the face, hand and foot, heavy sensation in the body and tremor of the fingers.

关、曲池、肩井穴部各 3 ～ 5 次。

在治疗遗精过程中,还应鼓励病人放松思想,正确对待疾病,且嘱以加强精神调养,排除杂念,清心寡欲,克服手淫等不良习惯。

十四、偏瘫

【概述】

偏瘫又称半身不遂,是中风后遗症状,现代医学认为偏瘫多因脑血管病变引起,如脑血管破裂、栓塞、痉挛等,造成中枢神经系统损害则发生一侧的肢体瘫痪。中医认为偏瘫的原因是由于湿痰内盛,气虚火旺,以致肝阳上亢,肝风内动而导致气血阴阳失调致病。

【诊断要点】

临床表现为半身肢体不遂,口眼歪斜,语言障碍,口角流涎,吞咽困难,并可伴有颜面、手足麻木,肢体沉重或手指震颤等。

BASIC MANIPULATIONS

The principle of tuina therapy: Dispelling wind and relieving the exterior, activating circulation of blood and regulating the meridians.

(1) The patient sits or lies, and the doctor presses and kneads with a finger Fengchi (GB 20) on both sides for 3 - 5 minutes, and then applies sweeping manipulation to both sides of the head for 1 - 3 minutes respectively.

(2) Lift-grasp Jianjing (GB 21) on both sides with both hands for 5 - 10 times.

(3) Press-knead Zusanli (ST 36), Fenglong (ST 40), Hegu (LI 4) and Quchi (LI 11) for one minute respectively.

(4) Use the fingers or palm to strike the back, the lumbus and the sacral muscles on both sides of the spinous column with a relatively strong stimulation 5 - 10 times.

MODIFIED MANIPULATIONS WITH SYNDROME DIFFERENTIATION

1. Limb Paralysis Besides the basic manipulations, the following may be performed additionally.

i. The patient takes a prone position, and the doctor stands by his side. Press both sides of his spinal column, especially those Back-Shu acupoints on the back such as Feishu (BL 13), Pishu (BL 20), Weishu (BL 21), Shenshu (BL 23), Sanjiaoshu (BL 22), and Dachangshu (BL 25) from top to below 2 - 3 times.

ii. Apply the rolling or pushing manipulation with one finger along both sides of the spinal column downward to the buttocks, the posterior side of the thighs and the posterior sides of the shanks. More manipulations should be given to the Back-Shu acupoints on both sides of the lumbar vertebrae, popliteal fossa , and tendo calcaneus regions, in combination with the passive movements of retroversion of the lumbar and the hip joints. Repeat the

【基本治法】

推拿治疗偏瘫的原则是疏风解表,活血通络。

(1)患者坐或卧位,医者以指按揉双侧风池穴 3～5分钟。然后再以扫散法在两侧头部各操作 1～3 分钟。

(2)双手提拿两侧肩井穴5～10 次。

(3)按揉足三里、丰隆、合谷、曲池穴各 1 分钟。

(4)指掌叩击脊柱两侧背、腰及骶部肌肉 5～10 遍,手法刺激应强强。

【随症加减】

1. 半身不遂 基本治法再加:① 患者取俯卧位,医者站于一侧,先用按法施于患者脊柱两侧,并着重在肺、脾、胃、肾、三焦、大肠俞等背俞穴上,自上而下操作 2～3 遍。② 再以㨰法或一指禅推法沿脊柱两侧并向下至臀部、股后侧、小腿后部,以腰椎两侧各背俞穴位、腘窝、跟腱部为重点治疗,同时配合腰部后伸和髋关节后伸的被动活动,反复操作 3～5 分钟。③ 患者侧卧,患肢在上,医者用㨰法或拿揉法从患侧肩关节起,沿上臂外侧,经肘部至腕部进行治

operation for 3 - 5 minutes.

iii. The patient takes a latericumbent position with the paralyzed limbs on the top. The doctor performs the rolling manipulation or the grasping-kneading manipulation first from the shoulder joint on the affected side, along the lateral side of the upper limb, via the elbow to the wrist repeatedly 3 - 5 times. The stress of manipulation should be put on the shoulder, elbow and wrist joints.

iv. Scrub and palm-twist the shoulder, upper limb and wrist 3 - 5 times.

v. Apply the rolling or grasping-kneading manipulations to the anterior aspect of the thigh and the lateral aspect of the shank on the affected side downward, combined with pressing-kneading the knee joint with a palm and plucking Yanglingquan (GB 34), Zusanli (ST 36), Juegu (GB 39) and Sanyinjiao (SP 6) repeatedly for 3 - 5 minutes.

vi. Press-pinch the ends of the affected fingers and toes with greater force 3 - 5 times respectively.

vii. Twist and rotate the affected lower limb 5 - 10 times.

2. Facial Paralysis   The following manipulations may be used in addition to the basic ones.

i. The patient takes a supine position. The doctor sits beside him, and pushes with one-finger manipulation to and fro from Yintang (EX-HN 3), Yangbai (GB 14), Sibai (ST 2), Yingxiang (LI 20), Xiaguan (ST 7), Jiache (ST 6) to Dicang (ST 4) for 3 - 5 minutes.

ii. Knead with the major thenar eminence or press-knead with a finger along the previous route, repeatedly, first the affected side, then the healthy side for 3 - 5 minutes.

iii. Rub or wipe the facial area 3 - 5 times with even and gentle force to avoid abrasion.

疗,以肩、肘、腕关节为治疗重点,反复操作 3～5 分钟。④ 再以擦、搓手法在肩部、上肢部、手腕部操作 3～5 遍。⑤ 以㨰法或拿揉法沿患侧大腿正面、小腿外侧面向下,并配合手掌按揉膝关节,弹拨阳陵泉、足三里、绝骨、三阴交等穴,反复操作 3～5 分钟。⑥ 以较重力量按捏患者指、趾末节端各 3～5 次。⑦ 扳摇患侧下肢 5～10 次。

2. 口眼歪斜 基本手法再加:① 患者取仰卧位,医者坐其侧,以一指禅推法从印堂、阳白、四白、迎香,下关、颊车、地仓等穴位往返操作 3～5 分钟。② 用大鱼际揉法或指按揉法沿以上路线,先患侧后健侧,往返操作 3～5 分钟。③ 擦法或抹法在颜面部操作 3～5 遍,操作时用力应均匀,手法柔和,防止损伤皮肤。

4.1.15　Stiff Neck

INTRODUCTION

Stiff neck is also called Shizhen In TCM. According to modern medical science, it is mainly caused by myospasm of the muscle groups in one side of the neck in those with a weak physique, overstrain, improper height of the pillow or posture during sleep, which results in long-time over extension of the muscle. TCM holds that when the neck is attacked by wind-cold in sleep at night, stagnation of blood and qi, and blockage of the meridians will occur, and stiff neck will follow.

MAIN POINTS FOR DIAGNOSIS

Common symptoms: tension, spasm, and rigidity of the muscles in one side of the neck after sleep, limitation to neck movements, pain in the neck aggravated by moving especially to the diseased side. In severe cases, the pain can involve the shoulder and the upper back, and the head of the patient inclines towards the diseased side.

BASIC MANIPULATIONS

The principle of tuina therapy is to relax the tendon and activate blood circulation and to warm and remove obstruction from the meridians.

(1) The patient takes a sitting position. And the doctor first applies the rolling or one-finger pushing manipulations to the affected neck and shoulder, combined with the patient's anteflexing, retroflexing and rotating his head to promote circulation of the local qi and blood. Then lift-grasp with the grasping manipulation the neck and the shoulder or pluck the tense muscles to make them relaxed. Repeat the operation 5 - 10 times.

(2) Press-grasp Fengchi (GB 20), Fengfu (GV 16), Fengmen (BL 12), Tianzong (SI 11) and Jianjing (GB

十五、落枕

【概述】

落枕又称失枕。现代医学认为这种病症的发生多由于体质虚弱,劳累过度,睡眠时枕头高低不适、躺卧姿势不良等因素,使一侧颈部肌肉在较长时间内处于过度伸展的紧张状态,以致发生痉挛而起病。中医认为夜卧颈部当风受寒,气血凝滞,经络痹阻而发病。

【诊断要点】

常见症状是:多于起床后发现颈项部一侧肌肉紧张、痉挛、僵硬,头部转动不利,动则疼痛加剧,尤以向患侧旋转更为明显,严重者疼痛可牵引至肩背部,病人头向患侧偏斜。

【基本治法】

推拿治疗落枕的原则是舒筋活血,温经通络。

(1) 患者坐位,医者先用㨰法或一指禅推法在患侧颈项及肩部治疗,配合头部前屈、后伸及左右旋转活动,以加强局部气血循行,再用拿法提拿颈项和肩背或弹拨紧张的肌肉,使之放松,反复操作5~10分钟。

(2) 按拿风池、风府、风门、天宗、肩井等穴,反复3~

21) repeatedly 3 - 5 times.

(3) The patient takes a sitting position with his cervical muscles relaxed. The doctor stands behind him, inserts both his hands from the back of the patient's neck with the two thumbs pressing on Fengchi (GB 20), and with the slightly separated index and middle fingers holding the mandible, lifts it with steady force and turns it left and right 3 - 5 times to extend the cervical muscles and alleviate the spasm.

(4) The patient takes a prone position. The doctor digitally-presses with the tips of both thumbs Chengshan (BL 57) on the shanks with a gradually-increased force. Meanwhile ask the patient to move his head and neck.

(5) Use the palms to press-knead and push-rub the cervical area on the affected side until a hot sensation is achieved.

MODIFIED MANIPULATIONS WITH SYNDROME DIFFERENTIATION

(1) For patients with stiff neck accompanied by facial tension and numbness, in addition to the basic manipulations, the following may also be used.

i. Apply the kneading manipulation with the major thenar eminence to the facial region for 3 - 5 minutes. Then press-knead Taiyang (EX-HN 5), Yintang (EX-HN 3), Xiaguan (ST 7) and Jiache (ST 6) for one minute respectively.

ii. Grasp-knead Hegu (LI 4) on both sides with relatively strong stimulation.

(2) For those with serious stiff neck, which can't be relieved by basic manipulations, the following manipulations may be performed additionally.

i. Manipulation of pulling the cervical vertebrae

After applying the above-mentioned manipulations to the cervical muscles, the patient takes a sitting position,

5 次。

（3）在颈部肌肉放松情况下,患者取坐位,医者立其后,两手从颈后侧分别插入,双手拇指抵风池穴,食、中指略分开,托住下颌骨,稳力向上端提,并作左右旋转 3～5 次,使颈部肌肉舒展,痉挛缓解。

（4）患者俯卧位,医者双手拇指点按小腿承山穴,用力由轻到重,边点按边让患者活动头颈部。

（5）以掌按揉并推擦患侧颈部,以热为度。

【随症加减】

（1）落枕伴见同侧颜面紧张、麻木者,基本治法再加:① 大鱼际揉法,在颜面部操作 3～5 分钟,并按揉太阳、印堂、下关、颊车穴各 1 分钟。② 较强刺激力量拿揉双侧合谷穴各 1 分钟。

（2）落枕严重,经基本治法不能缓解者,再加:① 扳颈椎法,即在颈部肌肉实施以上手法后,患者取坐位,医者立其后,以一掌平托其下颌,另一掌按扶其后头部,使颈项作

and the doctor stands behind him, holds his submaxillary horizontally with one palm, with the other palm pressing-supporting the posterior part of his head to make his neck turn slowly. Ask the patient to coordinate actively by relaxing his neck. After the cervical muscles have been relaxed thoroughly (namely, there is no resistance when rotating), quickly increase the turning amplitude to the affected side, and sounds like "ka da" can often be heard. This manipulation should be applied with properly-coordinated force, and violent turnings beyond the physiological limit should be avoided. Twisting left and right once each is enough.

ii. The patient sits upright, and the doctor is in front of him, places the fingers separately on the muscles around the knees with the thumbs pressing on Xuehai (SP 10). Then suddenly press-knead them with strong force 3 -5 times until the patient feels his body vibrating all of sudden with the manipulation.

After receiving tuina therapy, hot compress may be applied in combination to the neck and the shoulders. During treatment, manipulations with different size of force should be applied to different patients with different conditions. The sound produced while twisting the head shouldn't be achieved intentionally. And great care must be given to the aged.

4. 1. 16 Omalgia

INTRODUCTION

Omalgia is also called Dongjiejian (frozen shoulder), Jianningzheng (congealed shoulder), or Wushijian (omalgia in one's fifties) since it usually occurs in people at the age of fifties. It is called scapulohumeral periarthritis in modern medicine.

In TCM, omalgia is mainly due to invasion of the

徐缓的旋转,并嘱患者主动放松项部配合,待颈项肌肉确已放松(摇动时没有阻力),可迅速向患侧加大旋转幅度,此时常可听到"喀嗒"声。操作此手法时,应刚柔相济,切忌旋转扳动的幅度超过生理限度。左右各扳动 1 次即可。② 患者正坐位,医者居其前,双手手指散置膝周肌肉,拇指按在血海穴上,猛然用力按揉 3～5 次,以患者感到身体随手法突然振动为好。

落枕经手法治疗后,可在颈项和肩部配合热敷法。治疗中要注意手法轻重因人而异,摇动头部不可强求响声,对老年患者尤要仔细。

十六、漏肩风

【概述】

漏肩风,又称"冻结肩"、"肩凝症"。因为发病年龄多在 50 岁左右,故又称"五十肩"。现代医学称之为肩关节周围炎,简称肩周炎。

中医认为本病的起因主

body by wind, cold and dampness when a person is under the conditions of insufficiency of vital qi and over consumption and deficiency of blood and qi, and just at that time his shoulder is uncovered during sleep or exposed to wind in sweating, which cause blockage of the meridians and stagnation of blood and qi, inducing the problem. In modern medical science, omalgia is often related to functional disorders of the endocrine system, trauma, overstrain and chronic degeneration of the tissues around the shoulder, which cause aseptic inflammation in the tendon sheath or synovial bursa around the shoulder, eventually giving rise to omalgia.

MAIN POINTS FOR DIAGNOSIS

(1) In the early stage, omalgia mostly occurs in one side, and only in fewer cases seen in both sides. It is manifested by shoulder pain, difficulty in movement sometimes involving the upper limb, nomadic pain aggravated at night to the extent that the patient can not fall asleep, or is woken by it.

(2) In the advanced stage, its symptoms are manifested by adhesion of the shoulder joints, marked limitation to their movement, inability for the patient to place his hands behind himself, comb his hair, fasten the waist belt and dress himself. There are also rigid, tense sensation or atrophy in the muscles of the shoulder and marked tenderness around the shoulder joints. The abduction test is proved to be positive.

BASIC MANIPULATIONS

The principle of tuina therapy for this disease is dredging the meridians, activating blood circulation and relieving pain. The manipulations applied is to enhance local metabolism, strengthen function of the muscles and tendons, relieve adhesion and lubricate the joints.

要是在正气不足、气血亏虚的情况下,睡卧露肩,汗出当风,感受风寒湿导致经络不畅、气血痹阻而发病。现代医学认为本病的发生多与身体内分泌功能紊乱、外伤、劳损以及肩周组织的慢性退行性变等因素有关,进而造成肩部的一些腱鞘、滑囊的无菌性炎症而引起疾病。

【诊断要点】

(1) 初期多为单侧发病。也有极少数病人两侧同时发病。早期多表现为肩部疼痛、活动不便,有的牵涉到上肢部,疼痛的部位多不固定,尤其是夜间疼痛突出,病人常因疼痛而不能入睡或痛醒。

(2) 后期则表现为肩关节粘连,活动功能明显受限。病人常不能做背手、梳头、系腰带、穿衣等动作。肩部肌肉有僵硬、紧张感觉或肌肉萎缩现象,同时肩关节周围有明显压痛,肩关节外展试验为阳性。

【基本治法】

推拿治疗这种疾病的原则是疏通经络,活血止痛,采取的手法可以促进局部代谢,加强肌腱、肌肉功能以及松解粘连,滑利关节。

(1) The patient takes a sitting or supine position, and the doctor stands beside him. Apply the rolling or one-finger pushing manipulations to his anterior part of the shoulder and the medial side of the upper limb to and fro 5 -10 times, combined with passive abduction and extorsion of the patient's affected limb. The manipulation is mainly performed on the anterior region of the shoulder.

(2) The patient takes a supine or sitting position with the affected limb on the top. The doctor holds the wrist of his affected limb with one hand, and applies with the other hand the rolling manipulation to the lateral side of his shoulder and the posterior part of his axilla, combined with pressing and grasping Jianyu (LI 15) and Jianzhen (SI 9), superducting and adducting the affected limb repeatedly 5 - 10 times.

(3) The patient sits, and the doctor stands behind him. Apply the rolling or one-finger pushing manipulation to the cervical and the scapular regions, in combination with passive bending backward and superduction of the affected limb repeatedly 5 - 10 times.

(4) Grasp Jianjing (GB 21) 5 - 10 times.

MODIFIED MANIPULATIONS WITH SYNDROME DIFFERENTIATION

(1) For patients with cold pain in the shoulder radiating to the fingers, the following manipulations may be used additionally.

i. The patient sits upright, and the doctor stands by his side, holds the wrist of the patient's affected limb with his left hand, kneads slightly the acromion with his right hand, and increases the kneading range gradually from the pain point outward. Then, pinches and kneads Jianjing (GB 21) and Tianzong (SI 11) repeatedly 5 - 10 times.

ii. Hold the patient's shoulder with the palmar bases, and perform holding-kneading manipulation for 3 - 5 mi-

（1）患者仰卧或坐位，医者立于患侧、用㨰法或一指禅推法施于肩前部及上臂内侧，往返 5～10 次，配合患肢的外展、外旋被动活动，重点在肩前部使用本手法。

（2）患者仰卧或坐位，患肢在上，医者一手握住患肢的腕部，另一手在肩外侧和腋后部施㨰法，配合按、拿肩髃、肩贞穴及患肢上举、内收等活动，往返操作 5～10 遍。

（3）患者坐位，医者立其后，在颈项部及肩胛部施㨰法或一指禅推法配合患肢后弯、上抬的被动运动，反复操作 5～10遍。

（4）拿肩井穴 5～10 次。

【随症加减】

（1）肩部冷痛延及手指，基本手法再加：① 患者正坐位，医者立其患侧，左手握住患肢腕部，右手轻揉肩峰部，从痛点向周围扩大，并捏揉肩井、天宗穴，反复 5～10 次。② 医者用双掌根夹起患者肩部并施抱揉法，操作 3～5 分钟，使之有轻松、微热感。③ 掌擦患肩部，以热为度。

nutes until a relaxing and slight hot sensation is achieved.

iii. Rub the affected shoulder with the palm until a hot sensation is achieved.

(2) For patients with stiff shoulder and severe limit to movements, the following manipulations are also used besides the basic ones.

i. Hold the affected shoulder with one hand, clamp the wrist with the other hand, and perform the rotating manipulation to the shoulder and arm to its greatest amplitude for 3 - 5 minutes.

ii. Hold the patient's wrist and evenly shake it up and down for 1 - 3 minutes.

Besides timely treatment, patients with omalgia should do self-exercises of the shoulders. The following methods may be practised.

i. Climbing the Wall: Face the wall, climb it with one or two hands upward gradually, raise the upper limbs as high as possible, and then return slowly to the starting position. Repeat the exercise many times.

ii. Pulling the Hands Behind the Body: Place two hands behind the body, and use the healthy hand to pull the wrist of the affected limb gradually upward. Repeat the exercise.

iii. Rotating the Shoulder: Take a bow-step position, clamp the waist with one hand, place the hollow-fist of the other hand close to the waist, rotate the shoulder forward and backward in a gradually increasing amplitude and frequency.

iv. Exercising with a Stick: Prepare a stick, hold its two ends with both hands, and make forward-and-backward, left-and-right, and raising movements.

4.1.17   Cervical Spondylopathy

INTRODUCTION

Cervical spondylopathy is a commonly and frequently

（2）肩部僵硬，活动受限严重，基本手法再加：① 医者一手扶住患者肩部，一手握住其腕部，作摇动法，并使肩臂旋转至最大允许范围，操作3～5分钟。② 双手握住患者手腕部作均匀的上下抖动1～3分钟。

肩周炎除要及时治疗外，还要适当地进行肩部自我锻炼。可采取下列方法进行 ① 爬墙锻炼 面对墙壁，双手或单手沿墙壁缓缓向上爬动，使上肢尽量高举，然后缓缓向下回到原处，反复进行。② 体后拉手 双手向后，由健手拉住患肢腕部，渐渐向上拉动，反复进行。③ 环摇膀子 弓箭步，一手叉腰，另一手握空拳靠近腰部，肩膀作前后环转摇动，幅度由小到大，动作由慢到快。④ 木棍运动 备木棍一根，两手把握其两端，作前后、左右或上举活动。

十七、颈椎病

【概述】

颈椎病是中、老年人的常

encountered disease in the middle-aged and the aged people. According to modern medical science, the problem is
mostly caused by the senile degeneration of the cervical
vertebrae, e. g. hyperplastic bony substance crushes the
nerves and blood vessels or stimulates the local muscles
inducing aseptic inflammation and causing a series of clinical symptoms, so it is also called cervical spondylotic syndrome. TCM holds that the occurrence of cervical spondylopathy results from advanced age, deficiency of kidney qi
and insufficiency of nourishment; another reason is disorders of qi and blood in the human body, or stagnation of
pathological products such as dampness, phlegm, blood
stasis, etc., which cause obstruction of the meridians and
dysfunction of tendons and bones, resulting in the problem.

MAIN POINTS FOR DIAGNOSIS

Common symptoms of cervical spondylopathy in mild
cases are numbness and pain in the head, neck, shoulder,
and arm. Those in severe cases are soreness and weakness in the body and limbs, even dizziness, palpitation,
incontinence of feces and urine, and paralysis. The results of special functional tests such as compressing vertex
test and pressing intervertebral foramina test are both
positive.

BASIC MANIPULATIONS

The principle of tuina therapy is dredging the meridians, activating blood circulation and removing blood stasis.

(1) Ask the patient to sit with his head bending
slightly forward to expose the neck thoroughly (patients
with poor physique may takes a prone position with a pillow under his chest). Apply the one-finger pushing and
pressing-kneading manipulations to the midline of the neck
from Fengfu (GV 16), Yamen (GV 15) to Dazhui (GV

见病、多发病。现代医学认为
本病的发生多是因颈椎组织
的老年退行性变化,即增生的
骨质压迫神经、血管或刺激局
部肌肉发生无菌性炎症而产
生的一系列临床症状,故又称
为颈椎综合征。中医认为本
病多是由于年老体虚,肾气不
足,濡养欠乏,另则是人体气
血紊乱,湿、痰、瘀等病理产物
积聚而导致经络不通,筋骨不
利而发病。

【诊断要点】

临床常见症状是:轻者
头、颈、肩、臂麻木疼痛;重者
可见肢体酸软无力,甚至头
晕、心慌、大小便失禁、瘫软
等。特殊功能检查可见叩顶
试验、椎间孔挤压试验等
阳性。

【基本治法】

推拿治疗颈椎病的原则
是疏通经络,活血化瘀。

(1) 患者坐位,头稍向前
俯使项部充分暴露(体弱者可
取俯卧位,胸前垫枕),先以一
指禅推、按揉法在颈项部中线
自风府、哑门到大椎穴;两侧
自风池而下到大杼穴,反复操

14). On both sides of the neck, apply the same manipulation repeatedly from Fengchi (GB 20) down to Dazhu (BL 11) for 5 - 10 minutes.

(2) Digitally-press Tianzhu (BL 10), Jianzhongshu (SI 15), Jianwaishu (SI 14) and Tianzong (SI 11) 5 - 10 times respectively.

(3) Perform rolling manipulation on the neck, shoulders and arms, combined with passive movements, repeatedly for 3 - 5 minutes to relax the muscles completely.

(4) The patient sits with the head bending slightly forward. The doctor stands behind him, presses the tenderness point of the vertebrae on the affected side with one thumb, supports the patient's mandible with the elbow of the other arm, and pulls anteriosuperiorly. Meanwhile rotates gently the patient's head toward the affected side, and springy sounds of reduction can often be heard. If the patient lies on his back, his shoulder and back can be supported high with a pillow, and the doctor can stand at the head of his bed, hold the occipital part tightly with the right hand while the left hand supporting the mandible, pulls the patient's head up from the pillow to form an angle of 45° with the horizontal level. After doing slight traction, rotate the head left and right and swing it forward and backward, and springy sounds can often be heard, too. However, the left and right rotation shouldn't be beyond its physiological limitation.

MODIFIED MANIPULATIONS WITH SYNDROME DIFFERENTIATION

(1) For patients with numbness, distension, trembling or flaccidity of the upper extremities, the basic manipulations should be added with the following.

i. The patient sits upright, and the doctor stands behind him, holds the lower jaw of the patient with both hands, and pulls upward slightly for 1 - 3 minutes.

作 5～10 分钟。

（2）点按天柱、肩中俞、肩外俞、天宗等穴各 5～10 次。

（3）以㨰法于颈项、肩臂部，配合被动运动，反复操作 3～5 分钟，使肌肉充分放松。

（4）患者坐位，头部稍向前屈，医者立其身后，一手拇指按住患侧椎体压痛处，一手用肘部托住患者下颏，向前上方牵引，同时向患侧轻柔转动头部，往往可以听到整复的弹响声。如仰卧位时，肩后用枕稍垫高，医者立于床头，右手紧托患者枕部，左手托住颏部，将其头自枕上拉起，使颈与水平呈 45°角，略作牵引后，轻轻将头作左右旋转和前后摆动，亦常可听到弹响声，但左右转动不要超过生理限度。

【随症加减】

（1）如出现上肢麻木、发胀、发抖或无力症状者，基本治法外再加：① 患者正坐位，医者立其后，两手分别端住患者的下颌，轻轻向上端提 1～3 分钟。② 经上法后，患者病症

ii. After performing the above manipulations, the patient's conditions may be improved, and he will feel somewhat relaxed. Then hold the patient's forehead with one hand, pinch-knead downward both lateral sides of his neck with the other hand from Fengchi (GB 20) to Jian-jing (GB 21) repeatedly 10 - 15 times.

（2）For patients who has a long pathological duration and muscular atrophy in the forearms and hands, accom-panied by headache, dizziness, and pains in the scalp, the following should be performed additionally besides the basic manipulations.

i. Grasp-knead the affected shoulder, the arm and the hand 5 - 10 times, in combination with doing rubbing manipulation until a hot sensation is achieved.

ii. Press and knead Neiguan （PC 6） and Waiguan （TE 5） on the affected side for 1 - 3 minutes respective-ly. Meanwhile apply arc-sweeping manipulation to the af-fected side of the head for 1 - 3 minutes.

Although cervical spondylopathy is a retrograde affec-tion, some health care methods can postpone its occur-rence and development, and can relieve symptoms after the pathological changes take place. The work can be done from the following respects：

i. Protect the neck from repeated sprain and contu-sion, overwork or exposure to cold.

ii. The height of the pillow should be proper. That is, it should be low when the patient lies on his back, and relatively high when he lies on his side in order to avoid occurrence or aggravation of the case due to improper sleeping posture.

iii. Constantly do physical exercises, especially do shaking and rotating the neck movements frequently, Specifically as follows：

Qianshen Tanhaishi （Bending the Head Forward to

改善,感到轻松,再以一手扶患者前额,一手捏揉其两侧颈部,从风池到肩井穴,顺序向下捏揉,反复10～15次。

（2）如发病已久,前臂及手出现肌肉萎缩,并伴见头痛、头晕或头皮痛等症状者,基本手法再加：① 医者单手抓揉患肩及手臂5～10次,并做擦法,以热为度。② 按、揉患肢内关、外关穴各1～3分钟,并在患侧头侧部作扫散法1～3分钟。

颈椎病虽然多是一种退行性病变,但可以通过一些保健方法延缓其发生,发展及改善病变后的症状,主要可以从以下几个方面着手① 避免颈项部反复扭挫伤、过度劳累和局部受寒。② 枕头高度要适宜,一般仰卧时枕头要低,侧卧时可略高,防止因不正确的睡眠姿势引起病情发生或加重。③ 锻炼身体,尤其是常做颈项的摇头转颈活动,具体可做：

前伸探海势：下颌尽量上

See the Sea): Lift the lower jaw as high as possible, and rotate the neck left and right slowly while keeping the high-jaw position.

Huitou Wangyueshi (Turning the Head Back to Watch the Moon): Make the lower jaw as close as possible to the chest, and rotate the neck left and right slowly while keeping the above position.

4. 1. 18 Lumbago

INTRODUCTION

Lumbago is one of the commonly seen clinical symptoms, and a syndrome caused by various kinds of diseases. According to modern medical science, the occurrence of lumbago is mostly due to injury of the lumbar muscles, ligaments, fasciae, and joints, or congenital deformity of the lumbosacral vertebrae, protrusion of the lumbar intervertebral disc, or pathological changes of some internal organs such as the kidney and bladder.

In the theory of TCM, in addition to the fact that lumbago is closely related to functional changes of the kidney, invasion of exogenous pathogenic wind, cold, dampness, etc. and injury of fall and sprain may all lead to blood stasis and qi stagnation of the meridians in the lower back, which will cause obstruction resulting in the disorder.

MAIN POINTS FOR DIAGNOSIS

According to the diagnostic methods mentioned in the previous chapter, combined with experimental tests, tuina therapy has significant effects on lumbago excluding those caused by visceral diseases. Lumbago may clinically be divided into the acute and the chronic types.

(1) Acute Lumbago, also called Shanyao (lumbar sprain): Lumbago usually occurs when people bend their waist to work with improper posture or strength, or when they overload their waists, which cause intensive contraction

抬,保持这个姿势,作徐缓的左右转颈。

回头望月势：下颌尽量贴向胸部,保持这个姿势,作徐缓的左右转颈。

十八、腰痛

【概述】

腰痛是临床常见病症之一,是一种可由多种疾病引起的证候群。现代医学认为腰痛的发生大多是腰部肌肉、韧带、筋膜和关节的损伤或先天性腰骶椎骨畸形、腰椎间盘突出以及肾、膀胱等内在脏器的病变所致。

中医认为,腰痛除与肾脏的功能改变密切相关外,风、寒、湿等外邪的侵袭,跌仆闪挫的伤损,都可导致腰部经脉气滞血瘀,产生不通则痛的病变。

【诊断要点】

根据前述诊断方法结合实验室的检查,排除内脏疾病所致的腰痛,推拿治疗有着良好的疗效。临床上常以急、慢性腰痛来概括。

（1）急性腰痛,俗称闪腰。可因弯腰劳动时姿势不正确或用力不当,腰部负重过大引起肌肉的强烈收缩,使肌纤

of the muscles leading to rupture of soft tissues such as the muscle fibers and fascia and other injuries. Or it may also result from sprain of the waist, which brings on impaction and malposition of the lumbar vertebral joints as well as rupture of the ligaments and joint capsules around the joints, or even protrusion of the lumbar intervertebral disc. This type of acute pain may have a sudden attack after trauma, injury of soft tissue is signed by marked tenderness, and tension of the muscles increases because of their protective contraction. When small joints are impaction or mallocated, local swelling is not evident, but there is severe pain. While in patients with protrusion of lumbar intervertebral disc, the pain may radiate to the lower limb. In the special lumbar functional tests of ordinary cases, positive results can be seen in flexing test (Nrudzinski's sign) and straightening the abdomen test. In the patient with protrusion of lumbar intervertebral disc, tests of lifting a straightening leg and increasing pressure on it and tests of dorsiflexion and plantar flexion of the great toe are both positive.

(2) Chronic Lumbago: It refers to the intermittent, sore and distending pain in the lumbus caused by delayed or uncured acute lumbago and chronic strain of the soft tissues, which is characteristic of extensive, but not sharp pain aggravated by fatigue and relieved by rest and also related to changes of weather. There is no marked disturbance, but a pulling sensation in waist movements. The diseased part is of preference for warmth and aversion to cold. Of special functional tests, the calcaneus-hip test and the lifting straightened leg test prove positive.

BASIC MANIPULATIONS

The principle of tuina therapy: activating flow of qi

维、筋膜等软组织发生撕裂等损伤；或因腰部闪挫等因素引起腰部脊柱骨关节嵌顿、错位，关节周围韧带、关节囊撕裂，甚至腰椎间盘突出。这种腰部的急性疼痛，多在受伤后突然发作，软组织损伤多有明显压痛，肌肉因保护收缩而张力增高。小关节嵌顿、错位时，局部肿胀常不明显，但疼痛较剧。而腰椎间盘突出者更可兼见疼痛向下肢放射。一般急性腰痛腰部特殊功能检查，可见屈颈试验和挺腹试验等阳性体征。而腰椎间盘突出者则可查见直腿抬高加压试验和跗趾背伸或蹠屈等试验阳性体征。

（2）慢性腰痛，多指急性腰痛迁延未愈或治疗不及时，以及软组织的慢性劳损造成的时作时止的酸胀疼痛。这种疼痛可有广泛的压痛，但不明显，劳累后加剧，休息后减轻，并与气候的变化有关。腰部活动无明显障碍，但活动时可有牵制感。患部喜热怕冷。腰部特殊功能检查，有时亦可见跟臀试验、直腿抬高试验等阳性体征。

【基本治法】
　　推拿治疗腰痛的原则是

and promoting blood circulation, restoring and reducing injured soft tissues.

(1) The patient takes a supine position. The doctor applies one-finger pushing or rolling manipulations to the painful area and its surroundings in the lumbar region (for those with redness, swelling and severe pain, pressing-kneading manipulation may be performed first), combined with pressing Shenshu (BL 23), Dachangshu (BL 25), Juliao (GB 29) and pressure pain points. According to different dysfunction, passive movements can be made properly and co-operatively for 3 - 5 minutes.

(2) Press-knead Weizhong (BL 40), Zusanli (ST 36) and Juegu (GB 39) with strong stimulation for one minute respectively to relieve pain in the lumbus.

(3) The patient takes a supine position. The doctor scrubs the lumbosacral region along the direction of the fibers of sacrospinalis until a hot sensation is achieved.

(4) The patient lies on his side, and the doctor applies twisting manipulation to the lumbar region.

MODIFIED MANIPULATIONS WITH SYNDROME DIFFERENTIATION

(1) For acute lumbago, the following manipulations may be performed additionally.

i. Apply the back-carrying manipulation for 1 - 3 minutes to pull and extend the patient's lumbar vertebrae and correct dislocation and other anatomical disorders, which can relieve or even remove the symptoms quickly.

ii. For patients with protrusion of the lumbar intervertebral disc, apply first the rolling or palm-pushing manipulation to the lumbar muscles to relax them, and then press forcefully with the thumb pressure pain points in the lumbus, and acupoints Juliao (GB 29) and Huantiao (GB 30) repeatedly. Next, perform manipulation of backward extension of the waist —— press the lumbar vertebral

行气活血,理筋整复。

(1) 患者俯卧位,医者先在其腰部疼痛处及其周围以㨰法或一指禅推(如红肿痛剧者可先用按揉法)医治,配合按肾俞、大肠俞、居髎等穴位及压痛点,根据功能障碍的具体情况,适当配合被动运动,操作 3~5 分钟。

(2) 按揉委中、足三里、绝骨穴各 1 分钟,刺激量要大,以缓解腰部疼痛。

(3) 患者俯卧位,医者沿骶棘肌纤维方向直擦腰骶部,以热为度。

(4) 患者侧卧位,医者行腰部斜扳法。

【随症加减】

(1) 急性腰痛,除基本治法外再加: ① 用背法操作 1~3 分钟,达到牵伸患者腰部脊柱,纠正错位等解剖位置的异常。这种方法常能很快使症状减轻或消失。② 如系腰椎间盘突出症,先用㨰法或掌按法使腰部肌肉放松,再用拇指重按腰部压痛点及居髎、环跳穴,反复操作。接着可用腰部后伸扳法,即医者一手掌按压在腰椎部,另一手用力托起患者双大腿膝关节部位作向后

part with one palm, and support the patient's knee both joints with the other hand to lift upward, or pull the affected limb first, then the healthy one. This manipulation can also be operated by two massagists cooperatively. That is, they stand face to face at either side of the patient. Each has his one hand overlapped together with the others and places them on the patient's pain area in the lumbar region and presses. Each supports with his one hand the patient's lower limb on the side close to oneself and lift backward coordinately at the same time. Palm-pressing is operated 3 - 5 times. If radiating pain appears in the lower limb, force of pressing and kneading can increase.

(2) For chronic lumbago, the followings are added to the basic manipulations.

i. Apply rubbing and horizontally-pushing manipulations to the affected area until heat is generated.

ii. Combine manipulations with hot compress.

iii. Pat the affected area with a hollow palm 5 - 10 times.

Patients with acute or chronic lumbago should attach importance to prevention of the disease and self-protection after its attack. The usual methods are as follows: to change one's working position as much as possible at work, especially, to take a correct posture while exerting force, to increase exercises of the lumbar muscles daily, to fasten the waist with a wider belt, to sleep on a hard bed, and for patients with protrusion of the intervertebral disc, place a pillow under the waist while lying on his back.

4.1.19　Irregular Menstruation

INTRODUCTION

Irregular menstruation is a common disease in

伸扳动（或先扳患肢,后扳健肢）。此法亦可由两人配合操作,即两人相对站立患者两侧,各以一掌相叠按压患者腰部痛点部位,各以一手单独托起本侧患者下肢,同时协调用力向后伸扳,掌部按压 3～5 次。若症见下肢有放射疼痛,加重按揉。

（2）慢性腰痛,除基本治法外再加：① 施以擦、平推法,以患部发热为度。② 配合热敷。③ 虚掌拍打患部 5～10 次。

急、慢性腰痛患者,应重在预防,病后要注意加强保护。一般的方法是在劳动中尽可能地变换作业姿势,特别是用力时要采取正确的体位;平时要加强腰肌锻炼;病后以宽皮带束腰,宜睡硬板床。腰椎间盘突出者,仰卧时腰部宜垫枕头。

十九、月经失调

【概述】

月经失调是妇女的一种

women. It is manifested by abnormality in period, amount, color and property of menstruation, which includes disorder of menstrual period, prolonged or shortened menstrual duration, increased or decreased menstrual volume, or even ceased menstruation. Modern medical science holds that disorder in secretion of estrogen, functional disorder of vegetative nerves, mental irritation, cold, fatigue, and some general diseases may all lead to menoxenia.

In TCM, disorders of menstruation mainly result from abnormality in transformation of qi, blood, and body fluid of thoroughfare and conception vessels due to pathological changes of the heart, spleen, liver, kidney and other visceral organs. Preceded menstruation is mostly caused by fire generated by stagnation of liver qi, failure of blood to flow in the vessel due to heat, exhaustion of kidney yin, heat due to deficiency of blood, or failure of spleen in controlling blood. Delayed menstruation often results from cold obstruction causing qi stagnation and deficiency of qi and blood. Irregular menstruation is mainly due to stagnation of liver qi or hepatorenal asthenia. Excess or deficiency of menstrual blood is mainly caused by failure of qi in controlling blood, hemopyrexia, deficiency of the heart and spleen, asthenia of thoroughfare vessel or cold obstruction.

MAIN POINTS FOR DIAGNOSIS

Irregular menstruation, abnormality in amount, color, and property of menstrual blood are often seen, accompanied by various general symptoms such as listlessness or restlessness. In clinic, it may be divided into the following syndromes.

1. Blood-heat Syndrome　Preceded menstruation, profuse and thick menstrual blood with dark red or purple color, restlessness, reddened tongue with yellowish fur

常见疾病,表现为月经在期、量、色、质上的异常,包括月经周期紊乱,出血期延长或缩短,出血量增多或减少,甚至月经闭止。现代医学认为体内雌激素分泌失调、植物神经功能紊乱、精神刺激、寒冷疲劳和某些全身性疾病等,都可以导致此病的发生。

中医则认为月经失调,主要是由于心脾或肝肾等脏腑的病变引起冲任二脉气血津液生化的失常。月经先期,多因肝郁化火,血热妄行或肾阴亏耗,血虚而热及脾不统血所致。月经后期,多为寒凝气滞,气血不足所致。先后无定期,多为肝郁气滞或肝肾亏损所致。经量过多过少,多因气不摄血或血热及心脾亏损、血海空虚或寒凝瘀阻所致。

【诊断要点】

月经失调,经期不定或有量、色、质的异常,并伴有精神疲乏或烦躁不安等各种全身症状,临床可见以下分型。

1. 血热型　症见月经先期、量多、色深红或紫、质浓,烦躁不安,舌红苔黄,脉滑数

and slippery, rapid and strong pulse.

2. Qi Deficiency Syndrome　Preceded or irregular menstruation, profuse and thin menstrual blood with light red color, lassitude, pale complexion and pale tongue and weak, forceless pulse.

3. Cold Stagnation Syndrome　Delayed menstruation, scanty menstrual blood with dark red color, pain in the lower abdomen which can be relieved by warmth, aversion to cold, cold limbs, pale complexion, pale tongue with thin and whitish fur, and deep and tense pulse.

4. Qi Stagnation Syndrome　Delayed menstruation, scanty menstrual blood with normal or dark red color, pain and distending sensation in the lower abdomen, chest distress with discomfort, distending sensation in the breast and pain in the hypochondrium, dark purple tongue and floating or unsmooth pulse.

BASIC MANIPULATIONS

The principle of tuina therapy: regulating zang and fu organs, replenishing qi and promoting blood circulation.

(1) The patient takes a supine position. The doctor stands by his side, presses and kneads Baliao (BL 31 - BL 34) area with the overlapped palms for 3 - 5 minutes, and gradually increases force within the patient's endurance.

(2) Apply the rolling manipulation to the muscles on both sides of the spinal column repeatedly for 3 - 5 minutes, especially to Ganshu (BL 18), Pishu (BL 20) and Shenshu (BL 23).

(3) Digitally-press Mingmen (GV 4) with both thumbs for one minute to make it produce a sinking and distending sensation in the patient and radiate toward the lower abdomen.

(4) The patient lies on his back. The doctor puts the thumb on the superior and lateral part of the patient's knee, the other fingers on its medial side, grasps and

有力。

2. 气虚型　症见月经先期或先后不定,量多、色淡红、质稀薄,肢体倦怠,面色㿠白,舌质淡,脉弱无力。

3. 寒凝型　症见月经后期、量少、色暗红,小腹疼痛,得热则减,畏寒肢冷,面色苍白,舌淡苔薄白,脉沉紧。

4. 气滞型　症见月经后期、量少、色正常或暗红,小腹胀痛,胸闷不舒,乳胀胁痛,舌质紫暗,脉弦或涩。

【基本治法】

推拿治疗月经失调总的原则是调和脏腑,益气活血。

(1) 患者俯卧,医者立其侧,以双掌相叠按揉八髎穴部位3～5分钟。在患者能耐受情况下加重手法。

(2) 以㨰法在脊柱两旁肌肉往返操作3～5分钟,重点在肝俞、脾俞、肾俞穴上。

(3) 双手拇指点按命门穴1分钟,使之有沉胀感,并向小腹传导。

(4) 患者仰卧,医者以拇指置膝上部外侧,其余四指置膝内侧,自膝内上方阴廉、足

kneads from Yinlian (LR 11) and Zuwuli (LR 10) on the medial and superior sides of the knee via Yinbao (LR 9) and Xuehai (SP 10), down to Yinlingquan (SP 9) for 3 - 5 minutes.

(5) Push-rub the medial side of the thigh back and forth until a hot sensation is gained.

(6) Digitally-press and pluck Sanyinjiao (SP 6) for one minute.

(7) Rub annularly with one palm around Qihai (CV 6) for 5 - 10 minutes.

MODIFIED MANIPULATIONS WITH SYNDROME DIFFERENTIATION

1. Blood-heat Syndrome   Besides the basic manipulations, the following can be done additionally in this case.

i. Press-knead Dazhui (GV 14) for one minute and push-scrub the area until a hot sensation is gained.

ii. Digitally-press Quchi (LI 11) and Shenmen (HT 7) for one minute respectively.

iii. Twist-scrub Yongquan (KI 1) for 3 - 5 minutes.

iv. Scrub-knead the medial side of the thigh up and down for 3 - 5 minutes.

2. Qi Deficiency Syndrome   The following methods may be used in addition to the basic treatment.

i. Press-knead Xuehai (SP 10) on the medial aspect of the thigh above the knee, and then move downward to Yinlingquan (SP 9) and Sanyinjiao (SP 6) and operate repeatedly for 1 - 3 minutes.

ii. Digitally-press Taixi (KI 3) for one minute.

iii. Rub the whole abdomen clockwise for 3 minutes first, and then apply vibrating manipulation to Guanyuan (CV 4) with the palm for 1 - 3 minutes.

3. Cold Stagnation Syndrome   Besides the basic manipulations, the following is performed additionally.

i. Push-scrub both sides of the lower abdomen and

五里穴向下拿揉经阴包、血海穴至阴陵泉穴止,操作3～5分钟。

(5) 往返推擦大腿内侧,以热为度。

(6) 点按、弹拨三阴交穴1分钟。

(7) 以气海穴为圆心,做单掌环形摩法5～10分钟。

【随症加减】

1. 血热型   基本治法再加:① 按揉大椎穴1分钟,并推擦该部,以热为度。② 点按曲池、神门穴各1分钟。③ 搓擦涌泉穴3～5分钟。④ 搓揉大腿内侧,自上而下3～5分钟。

2. 气虚型   基本治法再加:① 按揉膝上股内侧血海穴并渐次向下移动至阴陵泉、三阴交穴处止,重复操作1～3分钟。② 点按太溪穴1分钟。③ 作全腹顺时针摩法3分钟后,再以掌置关元穴处施振颤法1～3分钟。

3. 寒凝型   基本治法再加:① 推擦小腹两侧及腹股沟处,以热为度。② 双掌指

the inguinal region until a hot sensation is gained.

ii. Pinch and grasp forcefully the muscles around Jianjing (GB 21) with the palms and fingers of both hands 5 - 10 times.

iii. Push separately from the umbilicus with both palms around the abdomen and the waist circularly until a hot sensation is gained.

4. Qi Stagnation Syndrome　In this case, the following manipulations may be performed additionally.

i. Digitally-press Danzhong (CV 17) for one minute.

ii. Push-scrub with both palms from the infra-axillary region down to the lumboiliac region 15 - 20 times.

iii. Push-scrub the thoracic and the abdominal regions alternately with two palms 10 - 15 times.

4. 1. 20　Dysmenorrhea

INTRODUCTION

Dysmenorrhea refers to pain in the lower abdomen appearing during, prior to, or after menstruation possibly accompanied by such general symptoms as abdominal distension, discomfort sensation in the breast, etc. In modern medical science it is sorted as primary and secondary types. Primary dysmenorrhea usually occurs in unmarried women, and is mainly caused by congenital factors, such as excessive anteversion or retroflexion or hypoplasia of the uterus. Secondary dysmenorrhea often occurs in married women, and is mostly caused by some acquired factors, such as inflammation of the uterus and polypus.

According to the theory of TCM, dysmenorrhea is mainly caused by unsmooth circulation of blood and qi. Since menses are transformed from blood, and blood moves following qi; if qi is sufficient, its circulation is smooth, blood will be flourishing and regular, and menses will flow unhindered, so no pain appears in movement of

捏、拿肩井穴处肌肉 5～10 次,力量稍重。③ 沿脐以掌分推腹、腰一周,以热为度。

4. 气滞型　基本治法再加: ① 点按膻中穴 1 分钟。② 双掌从腋下向下推擦至腰髂部 15～20 次。③ 双掌前后交替推擦胸、腹部 10～15 次。

二十、痛经

【概述】

痛经是指月经来潮及行经前后出现的下腹部疼痛或伴有腹胀、乳房不适等全身症状。现代医学分痛经为原发性和继发性两种。原发性痛经以未婚女青年多见,为先天因素如子宫过度前倾、后屈,子宫发育不良等造成。继发性痛经以已婚妇女为多见,多因子宫炎症、息肉等后天因素所致。

中医学认为本病症是因气血运行不畅所致。因月经为血所化,血随气行,气充血沛,气顺血和,则经行通畅,自无疼痛之患。若气滞血瘀或气虚血少,则有经行不畅,不

menstrual blood. However, if qi and blood are stagnated or qi is insufficient and blood is scanty, flow of menses will be unsmooth, and pain will follow. Qi-stagnancy and blood stasis, accumulation of cold and dampness, deficiency of qi and blood, etc. can all cause obstructed circulation of qi and blood.

MAIN POINTS FOR DIAGNOSIS

Clinical manifestations of dysmenorrhea are characterized by periodic pain in the lower abdomen during menstruation. The cold, heat, asthenia and sthenia properties of dysmenorrhea can be determined by the time and nature of menstrual pain. Generally, pain before or during menstruation shows sthenic property, while pain after menstruation belongs to asthenic property. Pain and aversion to pressure is a sthenia syndrome, while pain with preference for pressure is an asthenia one. Pain relieved by warmth is a cold syndrome, and pain aggravated by warmth is a heat syndrome. If pain is more severe and distension is less, and there is a relief of pain after discharge of blood clots, it is caused by blood stasis. If distension is more severe and pain is less, it results from qi stagnancy. Colicky and cold pain belongs to cold property, stabbing pain belongs to heat property, and persistent, mild and dull pain belongs to deficiency property.

1. Syndrome of Qi Stagnancy and Blood Stasis Distending pain in the lower abdomen before or during menstruation, scanty and dark-purple menstrual blood mixed with clots, dribbling of menstrual blood, pain relieved after discharge of blood clots, distension in the chest, hypochondrium and breast, deep purple tongue with petechia on the edges, deep and wiry pulse.

2. Syndrome of Stagnation of Cold and Dampness Cold pain in the lower abdomen before or during menstruation, even involving the lumbus and back, which can be

通则痛。而造成气血不畅的原因,有气滞血瘀、寒湿凝滞、气血虚损等等。

【诊断要点】

痛经临床表现的特点是行经时少腹疼痛,随月经周期而发作。根据疼痛发生的时间、疼痛性质可辨别其寒、热、虚、实的属性。即一般以经前、经期痛者属实,经后痛者为虚。痛时拒按属实,喜按属虚。得热痛减为寒,得热痛剧为热。痛甚于胀,血块排出疼痛减轻者为血瘀,胀甚于痛为气滞。绞痛、冷痛属寒,刺痛属热。绵绵作痛或隐痛为虚。

1. 气滞血瘀型 症见经期或经前少腹胀痛,行经量少,淋漓不畅,血色紫暗有瘀块,块下则疼痛减轻,胸胁乳房作胀,舌质紫暗,舌边有瘀点,脉沉弦。

2. 寒湿凝滞型 症见经前或经期少腹冷痛,甚则牵连腰背疼痛,得热则舒,经行量

relieved by warmth, scanty and dark menstrual blood mixed with blood clots, aversion to cold, loose stools, whitish and greasy tongue fur, deep and tense pulse.

3. Syndrome of Deficiency of Qi and Blood   Mild pain in the lower abdomen during or after menstruation, relieved by pressing, light colored and thin menstrual blood, pale complexion, listlessness, pale tongue with thin fur, weak and thready pulse.

BASIC MANIPULATIONS

The principle of tuina therapy: invigorating qi and promoting blood circulation, regulating and governing thoroughfare and conception vessels.

(1) The patient takes a supine position, and the doctor sits or stands by the patient's side. First rub with one palm the lower abdomen around Guanyuan (CV 4) clockwise and counterclockwise 36 times respectively. Next apply one-finger pushing or palm-pushing manipulation from below the umbilicus via Guanyuan (CV 4) and Qihai (CV 6) to the pubic bone for 3 - 5 minutes. Then place the two hands on both sides of the umbilicus and do arc-shaped pushing along both sides of the lower abdomen. Repeat the whole procedure until a hot sensation is achieved.

(2) The patient takes a supine position with a pillow under the patient's waist. Insert the four fingers of both hands from the sides of the chest to the back with the middle fingers pointing to each other and put beside the spinous process of the seventh thoracic vertebra and at the same level of the inferior angle of the scapulae. Support the chest and ribs with the thumbs, while the other three fingers placing at random, and then exert force to push-wipe from the back to the front to Qimen (LR 14) on the thoracic-costal region. Repeat this procedure 10 - 15 times.

少,色暗有血块,畏寒便溏,苔白腻,脉沉紧。

3. 气血虚弱型　症见经期或经净后,小腹绵绵作痛,按之痛减,经色淡,质清稀,面色苍白,精神倦怠,舌淡苔薄,脉虚细。

【基本治法】

推拿治疗痛经总的原则是行气活血,调摄冲任。

(1) 患者仰卧,医者坐或立其侧,先以关元穴为中心,顺、逆时针单掌摩少腹部各36次;继从脐向下经关元、气海穴直至耻骨施以一指禅推或掌推3~5分钟;再将双掌分放脐旁沿少腹两侧向下作弧形擦法,反复操作,以热为度。

(2) 患者仰卧,腰部垫枕,医者以两手四指由胸两旁伸至背部,中指相对置于第七胸椎棘突旁肩胛下角相平处,两手拇指扶定胸胁,其余三指自然散开,用力从后向前推抹至胸肋部期门穴止,反复操作10~15遍。

(3) The patient takes a supine position. The doctor kneads and grasps from the medial sides of the thighs down to the medial malleolus 5 - 10 times, and mainly dig-itally-presses Sanyinjiao (SP 6). In doing so, the three yin meridians will be dredged, while qi and blood will be regulated and nourished.

(4) The patient takes a prone position with a pillow under the patient's abdomen. The doctor applies the one-finger pushing or the rolling manipulations along the two sides of the spinal column to the lumbo-sacral region up and down, and presses and kneads Ganshu (BL 18), Pishu (BL 20), Weishu (BL 21), Shenshu (BL 23), Qihaishu (BL 24) and Dachangshu (BL 25) for one minute respec-tively. Then scrub across the lumbo-sacral region with the minor thenar eminence, especially Shenshu (BL 23), Zhi shi (BL 52) and Baliao (BL 31 - BL 34), until a hot sen-sation throughout the lower abdomen is achieved.

MODIFIED MANIPULATONS WITH SYNDROME DIFFERENTIATION

1. Syndrome of Qi Stagnancy and Blood Stasis The following methods may be used additionally in this case.

i. Press-knead Zhangmen (LR 13), Ganshu (BL 18) and Geshu (BL 17) with a finger or a palm for one minute respectively.

ii. Grasp-knead Xuehai (SP 10) and Yinlingquan (SP 9) for one minute respectively.

iii. Place the overlapped palms on the patient's Qihai (CV 6) and Guanyuan (CV 4) and apply the vibrating ma-nipulation for 1 - 3 minutes.

2. Syndrome of Stagnation of Cold and Dampness The following methods may be used additionally in this case.

i. Rectilinearly rub the muscles on both sides of the spinal column with a palm from the back down to the lum-

（3）患者仰卧,医者自其大腿内侧,自上向下到内踝部揉拿5～10遍,着重点按三阴交穴,以通畅三条阴经,调益气血。

（4）患者俯卧,腹下垫枕,医者以滚法、一指禅推法自背沿脊柱两旁向下至腰骶部操作,往返数遍,同时按揉肝俞、脾俞、胃俞、肾俞、气海俞、大肠俞等穴各1分钟。再以掌侧小鱼际横擦腰骶,着重于肾俞、志室、八髎穴,以热透小腹为度。

【随症加减】

1. 气滞血瘀型 基本治法再加:① 指、掌按揉章门、肝俞、隔俞穴各1分钟。② 拿揉血海、阴陵泉穴各1分钟。③ 双掌相叠置于患者气海、关元穴处,以振法操作 1～3分钟。

2. 寒湿凝滞型 基本治法再加:① 以掌从背部向下至腰骶,直擦脊柱两旁肌肉,以热为度。② 点按关元穴1分钟。③ 按揉命门穴 1～3

bo-sacral region until a hot sensation is gained.

ⅱ. Digitally-press Guanyuan (CV 4) for one minute.

ⅲ. Press-knead Mingmen (GV 4) for 1 – 3 minutes.

3. Syndrome of Deficiency of Qi and Blood: The following methods can be included in addition.

ⅰ. Digitally-press Quchi (LI 11) and Zusanli (ST 36) for one minute each.

ⅱ. Pinch-grasp the muscles on both sides of the back and lumbus from top to below 10 – 15 times.

Since dysmenorrhea occurs periodically, the manipulation is supposed to be performed one week before menstruation, once every day or every other day to reinforce the therapeutic effects.

4.1.21 Hysteroptosis

INTRODUCTION

Hysteroptosis refers to the descending of the uterus along the vagina through the outer orifice of cervix uteri to the level below the sciatic spine, even virtually out of the vaginal orifice. Modern medical science believes that the problem is mainly caused by weak constitution and emaciation, excessive childbearing, insufficient rest and malnutrition after giving birth, long periods of squatting and standing and cough, which cause too high abdominal pressure and decreased elasticity and relaxation of the ligaments and muscles which support the uterus. In TCM, hysteroptosis is also called yinting (vaginal hernia) or yintuo (hysterotosia), which results from asthenic spleen qi, which leads to sinking of qi in the middle energizer and exhaustion of kidney qi, resulting in weakness of the supporting tissues.

MAIN POINTS FOR DIAGNOSIS

Common symptoms include subjective sensation of a thing out of the vagina, accompanied by soreness and pain

分钟。

3. 气血虚弱型   基本手法再加：① 点按曲池、足三里穴各 1 分钟。② 捏拿两侧腰背肌，从下向上 10～15 遍。

痛经因有周期性发作的规律，治疗可在月经来潮前 1 周进行，每日或隔日 1 次，以巩固和加强疗效。

二十一、子宫下垂

【概述】

子宫下垂是指子宫从正常位置沿阴道下降至子宫颈外口、达坐骨棘水平以下，甚至子宫全部脱出于阴道口外者。现代医学认为因体弱消瘦、生育过多或产后休息和调养不当，且蹲站过多以及咳嗽等造成腹压过大，支持子宫的韧带、肌肉组织弹力下降和松弛而致。

中医称本病症为"阴挺"、"阴脱"等，认为是由于脾气不足、中气下陷及肾气亏损、维系无力造成。

【诊断要点】

常见症状是：阴道自觉有物脱出，伴见腰酸背痛，小腹

in the lumbus and back, bearing-down sensation in the lower abdomen, constant desire for urination, frequent urination or constipation with difficult urination.

BASIC MANIPULATIONS

The principle of tuina therapy is regulating the spleen and kidney, invigorating qi and strengthening its lifting function.

(1) The patient sits or lies. The doctor stands beside the patient, presses and kneads Baihui (GV 20) on the head with the overlapped index and middle fingers clockwise first and then counterclockwise 72 times respectively.

(2) The patient takes a supine position and the doctor lifts and grasps the muscles on Zhongji (CV 3) with the fingers of one hand 10 times.

(3) Push-press gently with the palmar base from the pubic bone upward 10 times to make the lower abdomen achieve a sensation of contracting upward.

(4) Press the palmar base against the pubic bone, and vibrate forcefully upward for one minute. Then digitally-press with the finger acupoint Tituo [4 cun lateral to Guanyuna(CV 4)], and Zigong [3 cun lateral to Zhongji (CV 3)], for 1 - 3 minutes respectively.

(5) Press-knead with the fingers Sanyinjiao (SP 6), Yinlingquan (SP 9) and Zusanli (ST 36) for one minute respectively. Then digitally-press Huiyin (CV 1) with the index and the middle fingers, combined with performing vibrating manipulation for one minute.

(6) Press-knead with the fingers Pishu (BL 20) and Shenshu (BL 23) for one minute each, and scrub transversely Baliao (BL 31 - BL 34) until a hot sensation is achieved.

(7) For patients with less severe hysteroptosis, self-tuina is recommended every day. That is, knead Baihui (GV 20) 100 times, scrub-knead Dazhui (GV 14) 50

坠胀,屡有便意,小便频数,或见大便秘结,小便困难等。

【基本治法】

推拿治疗子宫下垂的原则是调理脾肾,补气升提。

(1)患者坐或卧位,医者立其侧,以食、中指相叠按揉头部的百会穴,先顺时针,后逆时针方向各72次。

(2)患者仰卧,医者以单手掌、指提拿中极穴处肌肉10遍。

(3)以掌根自耻骨向上行按推法10次,力量要柔和,可使下腹有向上收缩的感觉。

(4)以掌根按于耻骨,向上用力施振颤法1分钟。再以指点按提托穴(关元穴旁开4寸处)、子宫穴(中极穴旁开3寸处)各1~3分钟。

(5)以指按揉三阴交、阴陵泉、足三里穴各1分钟。再以食、中指点按会阴穴且做振颤法1分钟。

(6)以指按揉脾俞、肾俞穴各1分钟。横擦八髎穴处,以热为度。

(7)轻度子宫脱垂者,每日可做自我推拿,每次揉百会穴100次,擦揉大椎穴50次,

times, push-grasp Jianjing (GB 21) 50 times, knead Guanyuan (CV 4) 100 times and press Sanyinjiao (SP 6) 50 times, each time.

MODIFIED MANIPULATIONS WITH SYNDROME DIFFERENTIATION

（1）For patients with hysteroptosis accompanied by poor appetite, general lassitude, flaccidity and weakness in the limbs, to the basic manipulations the spine-pinching manipulation can be added. The patient takes a prone position, and the doctor stands by patient, pinches and grasps with the thumb and the index finger, from Changqiang (GV 1), along the middle of the spinal column, upward to Dazhui (GV 14) progressively 10 - 15 times.

（2）For those having hysteroptosis with dizziness, discomfort and restlessness, pressing-kneading Hegu (LI 4), Shenmen (HT 7) and Taichong (LR 3) respectively for one minute are added.

（3）During the treatment of above discussed symptoms with tuina therapy, a sitting-bath method can also be recommended to the patient. That is, have the Chinese medicinal herbs Zhike (*Fructus Aurantii*) 50 g, Shechuangzi (*Fructus Cnidii*) 50 g, Wumei (*Fructus Mume*) 50 g, and Huangbai (*Cortex Phellodendri*) 30 g boiled, and then fumigate and wash with the boiled medicated water twice a day.

In addition, patients can do self-tuina exercises. One is the method of contracting the anus and urethra: sitting naturally, contracting the abdominal muscles and doing the movements of restraining the bowels when inhaling, and relaxing when exhaling; repeating alternately the relaxing and contracting movements for 5 - 10 minutes. The other is the method of strengthening the uterus: the patient takes a prone position with the upper limbs placed horizontally before the head and the knees and the trunk

推拿肩井穴 50 次,揉关元穴 100 次,按压三阴交穴 50 次。

【随症加减】

（1）子宫下垂伴见食少体倦,肢软无力者,基本治法再加捏脊法:患者俯卧,医者立其侧,自长强穴起,沿脊柱正中以拇、食指捏拿肌肉,边捏拿边渐行向上至大椎穴止,操作 10～15 遍。

（2）子宫下垂伴见头晕不适,心绪不宁者,基本治法再加按揉合谷、神门、太冲穴各 1 分钟。

（3）以上诸症治疗过程中,均可嘱患者增加坐浴法,即以中药枳壳 50 克,蛇床子 50 克,乌梅 20 克,黄柏 30 克,煎水薰洗,每日 2 次。然后再做自我推拿锻炼:① 缩二阴法:患者持自然坐位,随吸气收缩腹肌并做忍住大便及小便的动作,随呼气放松,如此一紧一松,交替进行 5～10 分钟。② 固脱法:患者俯卧,上肢平放头前,屈膝躬身,臀部上抬、下降,重复 10～15 次后,保持抬臀姿势 5～10 分钟。

flexed, raises and lowers the buttocks repeatedly 10 - 15 times, then keeps the buttocks raised for 5 - 10 minutes.

4.1.22 Acute Mastitis

INTRODUCTION

Acute mastitis usually occurs in the feeding period of women, and most commonly in primiparaes. Acute mastitis, according to modern medical science, is mainly caused by infection of aureus staphylococci. In TCM, it results from retention of milk, stagnation of the milk duct, invasion of exogenous wind and heat, and accumulation of pathogenic factors.

MAIN POINTS FOR DIAGNOSIS

In the early stage, heat, redness, swelling and pain in the breast are often seen, accompanied by some general symptoms, such as fever, aversion to cold, and headache. Then, suppuration and ulceration in the breast will occur after a long duration.

BASIC MANIPULATIONS

The principle of tuina therapy: regulating qi activity, eliminating pathogenic factors and removing toxic materials.

(1) The patient sits upright, First press-knead Ganshu (BL 18), Shaoze (SI 1) and Hegu (LI 4) for one minute each. Next, apply the rubbing and kneading manipulations to the affected mammary region for 1 - 3 minutes. Then, support the breast with one hand, press and wipe closely to the skin with the palmar surface of the four fingers of the other hand orderly from below the armpits, the clavicles, beside the sternum and then above the ends of ribs to the mammary areola. The manipulation is supposed to be performed with gradually increased force, and repeated in the same direction 5 - 7 times, in the mean-

二十二、乳痈

【概述】

乳痈一般发生在妇女哺乳期,其中尤以初产妇女最为多见。现代医学称本病为急性乳腺炎,认为大多由金黄色葡萄球菌感染引起。中医则认为本病乃因乳汁积滞,乳络不畅,外感风热或肝胃蕴热,邪毒壅积而成。

【诊断要点】

乳痈初起可见乳部焮红肿痛,同时是可伴有发热、恶寒、头痛等全身症状,日久作脓溃烂。

【基本治法】

推拿治疗乳痈总的原则是调畅气机,祛邪解毒。

(1)患者正坐,先按揉肝俞、少泽、合谷穴各1分钟。然后施摩、揉法于患乳部1~3分钟;继以一手托乳房,另一手以四指掌面先后从患者腋下、锁骨下、胸骨旁和肋缘上紧贴皮肤顺抹至乳晕部,顺抹手法先轻后重,每一方向重复5~7次,顺抹时可见乳汁流出。

time milk is seen flowing out.

(2) Support the breast with one hand to get the nipple slightly sticking up, assemble the five fingers of the other hand to hold the nipple and the mammary areola with the whirled surface loosely and do pushing inwards and pulling outwards repeatedly 8 - 10 times. At this time, some coagulated and granular obstructing substances can be discharged along with outflow of milk. Another method is to nip the papilla with one hand, move the other hand from the breast to the mass and then to the papilla. Meanwhile squeeze while kneading alternately with both hands cooperated. The operation is performed repeatedly many times first gently and superficially, and then strongly and deeply until all the milk and pus drain off.

(3) Pinch-grasp the greater pectoral muscles and the broadest muscle of the back with the thumb, the index and the middle fingers, and pluck forcefully the tendons 3 times respectively. In addition, palm-twist the streak parts in the axillary fossa until numbness is sensed in the finger and palm.

(4) Press-knead Danzhong (CV 17) for one minute, and palm-twist and rub the hypochondriac areas of the patient with both palms for 3 - 5 minutes.

MODIFIED MANIPUALTIONS WITH SYNDROME DIFFERENTIATION

(1) If aversion to cold, fever, dry mouth and restlessness are also manifested in this case, the following manipulations are added.

i. Digitally-press Fengchi (GB 20) on both sides for one minute each.

ii. Press-knead Dazhui (GV 14) for one minute, and perform regional rubbing manipulation until a hot sensation is gained.

iii. Grasp the muscles around Jianjing (GB 21)

（2）医者仍一手托住乳房，使乳头稍翘起，另一手以五指指尖作聚拢状，用指螺纹面松弛地抓住乳晕乳头部，反复推进拿出 8～10 次，此时随乳汁可排出凝结的粒样堵塞物。另一方法是一手捏住乳头，另一手由乳房逐渐向肿块继至乳头，两手配合边揉边挤，由轻到重，由浅入深，反复多次直到乳汁和脓液排出排净。

（3）医者以拇、食、中指捏拿胸大肌和背阔肌，且用力弹拨肌腱各 3 次。并在腋窝搓动条索状物，以患者指掌感觉麻木为度。

（4）按揉膻中穴 1 分钟；双掌搓擦患者两胁肋部 3～5 分钟。

【随症加减】

（1）症见恶寒、发热、口干、烦躁者，基本治法再加：① 点按双侧风池穴各 1 分钟。② 按揉大椎穴 1 分钟，并施局部擦法，以热为度。③ 拿肩井穴部位肌肉 10～15 次。④ 从上向下推脊背至尾骶，以热为度。⑤ 搓擦双侧涌泉穴各 1～3分钟。泡洗双足后操作，

10 – 15 times.

iv. Push the spinal column from the back down to the caudal region until a hot sensation is gained.

v. Palm-twist and rub Yongquan (KI 1) on both sides for 1 – 3 minutes respectively. The therapeutic effect will be more satisfactory if the feet are first soaked and washed with hot water.

（2）If mastitis is accompanied by continuous fever, growth of mammary mass, and softness in the center of the hard lump and a waving sensation present when pressed, the following manipulations may be used in addition to the basic ones.

i. Gently comb-scrub the breast from the outer parts to the inner parts with a cutin comb, better with an ox horn comb, for 3 – 5 minutes.

ii. Digitally-press Quchi (LI 11) on both sides for one minute each.

iii. Press-knead and pluck Zusanli (ST 36) for 1 – 3 minutes each.

iv. Digitally-press Taichong (LR 3) and Xingjian (LR 2) for one minute each.

v. Push-rub with a palm from the chest region (above the breast) along the medial side of the upper limb to the fingers 10 – 15 times respectively.

Before applying tuina therapy, the doctor should wash his own hands and clean the mammary region of the patient, and the manipulation should be gentle and quick. Violent kneading and rubbing must be avoided in the indurate mass. Meanwhile other anti-infective therapies can be used in combination for severe cases.

4.1.23   Climacteric Syndrome

INTRODUCTION

Climacteric syndrome refers to a series of symptoms

效果尤佳。

（2）症见发热持续、乳肿增大、硬结中央渐软、按之有波动感者，基本治法可加：① 以角质梳（牛角为好）轻梳擦乳部，自外向内操作 3～5 分钟。② 点按双侧曲池穴各 1 分钟。③ 按揉、弹拨足三里穴 1～3 分钟。④ 点按太冲、行间穴各 1 分钟。⑤ 以掌从胸膺部（乳上方）沿上臂内侧向手指方向推擦各 10～15 次。

治疗乳痈时，医者先要清洗双手及患者乳房部，手法宜轻快柔和，切忌在硬结部位暴力揉、搓。病情严重时，还当配合抗感染等其他疗法。

二十三、更年期综合征

【概述】

更年期综合征是指更年

caused by disorders of the endocrine system and vegetative nervous system due to hypofunction of ovary in climacteric women. In TCM, it is called syndrome of before and after menopause or zangzao (hysteria). The disease often occurs in the women at the age of 45 - 55 and relieved after 3 - 5 years or more. It is believed in TCM that the syndrome results from abnormal flow of qi and blood due to declination of kidney qi and exhausation of kidney essence as well as imbalance between yin and yang.

MAIN POINTS FOR DIAGNOSIS

Common symptoms of climacteric syndrome are restlessness, irritability, dizziness, insomnia, palpitation, perspiration, gradual corpulence, and abnormal sensation in the skin, etc.

BASIC MANIPULATIONS

The principle of tuina therapy is regulating qi, activating blood and regulating yin and yang.

(1) The patient sits. And the doctor stands behind the patient, supports the patient's shoulder with one hand, and pushes and scrubs with the palm of the other hand obliquely from the superior part of the chest along the middle part of the two breasts downward for 1 - 3 minutes.

(2) Digitally-press Danzhong (CV 17) for one minute.

(3) Palm-twist and rub the hypochondriac regions with both hands for 3 - 5 minutes.

(4) Press-knead Shenshu (BL 23) and Mingmen (GV 4) first with a finger for one minute each, and then scrub this area horizontally with a palm until a hot sensation is attained.

(5) Press-knead Ganshu (BL 18) and Sanjiaoshu (BL 22) for one minute each.

(6) The patient lies in supine position, and the doctor pinches and grasps the medial muscles of the thigh 5 - 10

期妇女因卵巢功能衰退导致内分泌失调、植物神经功能紊乱而引发的一系列症状。中医学称为"经断前后证候"或"脏躁证"。一般发生在 45～55 岁之间，持续 3～5 年或更长时间可缓解。中医认为更年期综合征是因为肾气渐衰，天癸将竭，阴阳平衡失调而引起气血逆乱的结果。

【诊断要点】

更年期综合征常见症状是：烦躁、易怒、头晕、失眠、心悸、出汗、体渐肥胖或皮肤感觉异常等。

【基本治法】

推拿治疗的原则是理气和血，调整阴阳。

(1) 患者坐位，医者立其后，一手扶其肩头，另一手以掌斜向从其胸上方沿两乳正中，向下推擦 1～3 分钟。

(2) 点按膻中穴 1 分钟。

(3) 双手搓擦两胁肋部 3～5 分钟。

(4) 先以指按揉肾俞、命门穴各 1 分钟，继以掌横擦该部，以热为度。

(5) 按揉肝俞、三焦俞穴各 1 分钟。

(6) 患者仰卧，医者捏拿其下肢内侧肌肉 5～10 遍，再

times, and then pushes and scrubs the medial and the lateral aspects of the four limbs until a hot sensation is attained.

(7) Digitally-press Waiguan (TE 5), Quchi (LI 11), Zusanli (ST 36) and Sanyinjiao (SP 6) for one minute respectively.

MODIFIED MANIPULATIONS WITH SYNDROME DIFFERENTIATION

(1) For patients with restlessness and insomnia in this case, besides the basic manipulations, digitally-press Shenmen (HT 7) and Xinshu (BL 15) for 1 - 3 minutes respectively, and palm-twist and scrub Yongquan (KI 1) for 3 - 5 minutes.

(2) For patients with skin itching in this case, in addition to the basic manipulations, digitally-press Xuehai (SP 10) and Baichongwo (EX-LE 9) (1 cun above Xuehai) for 1 - 3 minutes respectively.

(3) Besides the manipulations mentioned above, patients with menopausal syndrome may practice self-tuina to prevent and treat it according to symptoms, by referring to the Self-Tuina Manipulations in Chapter V, such as regulating acupoint Danzhong (CV 17), relaxing the scalp skins, soothing the chest oppression, dispersing intercostal stagnation, regulating the triple energizer, nourishing the heart.

4. 1. 24   Simple Obesity

INTRODUCTION

Simple obesity refers to accumulation of fat inside the body due to excessive intake of calorie. According to modern medical science, dysfunction of the nervous and endocrine systems can cause decrease in the ability of regulating human activity and metabolism of food. Besides, some inherited factors can also cause incidence of simple obesity. According to the theory of TCM, crapulence,

推擦四肢内外侧面,均以热为度。

(7) 点按外关、曲池、足三里、三阴交穴各 1 分钟。

【随症加减】

(1) 症见心烦失眠者,基本治法加点按神门、心俞穴各1～3分钟;并搓擦涌泉穴 3～5分钟。

(2) 症见皮肤瘙痒者,基本治法加点按血海、百虫窝穴(血海穴上 1 寸)各 1～3 分钟。

(3) 除以上治疗方法外,更年期综合征尚可对症参照第五章自我推拿方法中之舒气会、疏头皮、宽胸法、疏肋间、理三焦、养心法等自行操作防治。

二十四、单纯性肥胖症

【概述】

单纯性肥胖症多是由于摄食热量超过消耗量而造成体内脂肪堆积的病症。现代医学认为神经系统、内分泌系统功能失常,对人体活动、摄食代谢等过程的调节能力降低,以及遗传等因素均可引起

excessive intake of rich or sweet food, improper balance between activity and rest may all cause disorders in the digestive functions of the spleen and the stomach. After a long period of time, dampness and phlegm will accumulate inside the body, and simple obesity will develop.

MAIN POINTS FOR DIAGNOSIS

Common symptoms in clinic are the weight of the patient 20% more than that of the normal weight (the normal weight of male(cm) = height - 105, the female one (cm) = height - 110), overstaffed body, marked accumulation of fat in the abdomen and haunch, accompanied by lassitude, dyspnea, dizziness, and constipation.

BASIC MANIPULATIONS

The principle of tuina therapy is reinforcing function of the spleen and the stomach, removing phlegm and dampness.

(1) The patient lies on his back. The doctor stands by his side, places one palm or the overlapped palms on the patient's umbilicus, and rubs his abdomen slightly forcefully clockwise and counterclockwise with the circle from small to large, then from large to small for 5 minutes respectively.

(2) Lift-grasp the muscles around Zhongwan (CV 12) with the fingers of one hand and the muscles around Qihai (CV 6) with those of the other hand. The lifted and grasped area should be properly large enough and the force used should be penetrating. Finger-twisting and pressing actions can be added while lifting up, but the putting-down action should be slow. Repeat the procedure 20 -30 times.

(3) The patient sits. And the doctor stands behind him, grasps his abdominal muscles from under both hypochondria with both hands, and then relaxes them. Grasping

单纯性肥胖症的发生。中医认为暴饮暴食,过食肥甘,劳逸不当,使脾胃运化功能失常,日久湿、痰积聚体内而导致发病。

【诊断要点】

临床常见症状,体重超过正常标准20%者(正常标准:男性身高(cm)－105＝正常体重,女性身高(cm)－110＝正常体重),体态臃肿,腹部、臀部脂肪明显堆积,常伴见乏力、喘息、头晕、便秘等。

【基本治法】

推拿治疗单纯性肥胖症的原则是健运脾胃,祛化痰湿。

(1) 患者仰卧,医者立其侧,单掌或叠掌置脐上,顺、逆时针,从小到大、从大到小,稍用力各摩腹5分钟。

(2) 以一手掌指提拿中脘穴处肌肉组织,另一手提拿气海穴处肌肉组织,提拿时宜面积大,力量深沉。拿起时可加捻压动作,放下时,动作应缓慢,反复操作20～30次。

(3) 患者坐位,医者立其后,双掌从其双胁下抄拿腹部肌肉,一拿一放,拿起时亦应

and relaxing are alternately done. While grasping up, finger-twisting and pressing actions should be added with a little more force, in the meantime, the doctor's hands are gradually moving upwards and downwards respectively. Repeat the operation 20 times.

(4) Push-rub forcefully from the hypochondria toward the abdomen with the two palms until a hot sensation is achieved.

(5) Scrub the shoulders, the back and the lumbosacral region with a palm until a hot sensation is attained, and pat from top to below with a hollow palm for 1 - 3 minutes.

(6) The patient takes a prone position. The doctor applies grasping manipulation to the muscles of the four limbs, or pinches and grasps or presses and kneads them properly.

(7) Press-knead and pluck Hegu (LI 4), Zusanli (ST 36) and Fenglong (ST 40) for one minute respectively.

MODIFIED MANIPULATIONS WITH SYNDROME DIFFERENTIATION

(1) For patients with obesity accompanied by asthma and palpitation, the following may also be used besides the basic manipulations.

i. Press-knead Danzhong (CV 17) and point Feimen (Ex) for one minute each.

ii. Press-knead Waiguan (TE 5) and Shenmen (HT 7) for one minute each.

iii. Press-knead Pishu (BL 20), Weishu (BL 21) and Sanjiaoshu (BL 22) for one minute each.

iv. Scrub transversely the superior part of the chest until a hot sensation is attained.

(2) For patients with obesity accompanied by dizziness, insomnia and constipation, the following methods can be used additionally.

i. Press-knead Yintang (EX-HN 3), Taiyang (EX-

加力捻压,并渐次向上向下操作,反复进行 20 次。

(4) 双掌自胁下向腹部用力推擦,以热为度。

(5) 掌擦肩、背、腰骶部,以热为度,并以虚掌从上向下拍击 1～3 分钟。

(6) 患者卧位,医者以抓法或捏拿、按揉四肢部肌肉,各以适量为宜。

(7) 按揉并弹拨合谷、足三里、丰隆穴各 1 分钟。

【随症加减】

(1) 肥胖伴见气喘,心慌者,基本治法再加:① 按揉膻中、肺门穴各 1 分钟。② 按揉外关、神门穴各 1 分钟。③ 按揉脾俞、胃俞、三焦俞穴各 1 分钟。④ 横擦胸上方,以热为度。

(2) 肥胖伴见头晕、失眠、便秘者,基本治法再加:① 按揉印堂、太阳、百会穴各 1 分钟。② 按揉合谷、曲池穴并配

HN 5) and Baihui (BL 9) for one minute each.

ii. Press-knead Hegu (LI 4) and Quchi (LI 11) cooperated with plucking for 1 - 3 minutes respectively.

iii. Palm-twist and rub the two hypochondria for 3 - 5 minutes.

iv. Press-knead with the hand and press with the elbow the buttocks and Huantiao (GB 30) for 1 - 3 minutes.

Prevention is very important in avoiding incidence of simple obesity. On one hand, one can start from his diet, and avoids taking excessive calorie from foods. On the other hand, one can do proper exercises in daily life. For those who has the problem of obesity, besides tuina therapy, they are suggested to do some self-tuina exercises actively, such as rubbing the stomach and abdomen, scrubbing the lumbosacral region, pushing the upper limbs, grasping the lower limbs, grasping the lumbar muscles, rubbing the lower abdomen, pinching the three lines, grasping Hegu (LI 4), pressing Zusanli (ST 36) as well as practicing some Shaolinneigong.

4. 1. 25　Toothache

INTRODUCTION

There are many kinds of causative factors of toothache. Besides saprodontia, according to modern medical science, acute periapicalitis, peridentitis, pericorona dentitis of opsigenes, hypersensitivity of dentin and so on may all cause toothache. In the theory of TCM, splenogastric heat, which is stagnant and transformed into fire, and exhaustion of renal qi, which leads to hyperactivity of asthenia fire, can cause toothache. In clinic, pain in the affected tooth can be aggravated by stimuli like cold, heat, acid, and sweetness.

MAIN POINTS FOR DIAGNOSIS

1. Gastric Heat Syndrome Symptoms are paroxys-

合弹拨各 1～3 分钟。③ 搓擦两胁 3～5 分钟。④ 按揉、肘压臀部和环跳穴 1～3 分钟。

单纯性肥胖的发生，重在预防，一方面应注意饮食结构的调整，避免摄入多余的热量；另一方面在日常生活中，要保持适当的运动量。对已出现的肥胖，除推拿防治外，还应积极进行自我推拿练功锻炼，如摩脘腹、擦腰骶、推上肢、拿下肢、拿腰肌、擦小腹、捏三线、拿合谷、按足三里，以及练习少林内功功法。

二十五、牙痛

【概述】

牙痛的病因很多，现代医学认为除龋齿之外，急性根尖周围炎、牙周围炎、智齿冠周炎、牙本质过敏等，均可导致牙痛发作。中医认为脾胃有热，郁而化火，以及肾元亏虚，虚火上炎等均可引起发病。临床常见患齿疼痛且遇冷、热、酸、甜等刺激则加剧。

【诊断要点】

1. 胃火型　症见牙痛阵

mal severe toothache accompanied by halitosis, constipation, yellowish and greasy tongue fur and floating and rapid pulse.

2. Renal Asthenia Syndrome   Symptoms are dull pain in the tooth accompanied by odontoseisis, listlessness and lassitude, pale tongue with thin fur and floating and thready pulse.

BASIC MANIPULATIONS

The principle of tuina therapy: Dredging the meridians, reinforcing for asthenia and reducing for sthenia.

(1) Ask the patient to sit or lie. Push with one-finger manipulation or press-knead Fengchi (GB 20) and Fengfu (GV 16) on the neck for one minute each, with the purpose of expelling wind and depriving exogenous pathogenic heat, cold, etc. of existing sites.

(2) Press-knead Hegu (LI 4) on both sides for one minute respectively, which is in accordance with the clinical principle of "treating diseases of the face and other facial organs by stimulating Hegu (LI 4)".

(3) Perform rolling manipulation on the shoulders and the back for 3 - 5 minutes, especially on Dazhui (GV 14) because the point has dual-directional therapeutic effects of expelling wind and clearing away heat as well as activating yang and warming the meridians.

(4) Lift-grasp Jianjing (GB 21) 5 - 10 times with light manipulations for those having asthenia syndrome and weak constitution, and strong stimulations for those with sthenic syndrome.

MODIFIED MANIPULATIONS WITH SYNDROME DIFFERENTIATION

1. Gastric Heat Syndrome   The following can be performed in addition.

i. Press-knead Waiguan (TE 5) for one minute.

ii. Pinch-press Neiting (ST 44) with the nail of a

剧伴口臭、便秘、苔黄腻、脉弦数。

2. 肾虚型　症见牙痛隐隐,伴见齿浮、神疲乏力,苔薄质淡,脉细弦。

【基本治法】

推拿治疗牙痛的原则是疏经通络,补虚泻实。

(1) 患者坐位或卧位,一指禅推或按揉颈项部风池、风府穴各 1 分钟,先以祛散风邪,使寒热等外邪无所依附。

(2) 按揉双侧合谷穴各 1~3分钟。取"面口合谷收"的临床治疗经验,以对症治疗五官疾患。

(3) 以㨰法在肩背部操作3~5 分钟,着重于大椎穴部,取其祛风清热、通阳温经的双向治疗作用。

(4) 提拿肩井穴 5~10遍,虚证体弱者手法宜轻,实证者手法刺激要强。

【随症加减】

1. 胃火型　基本治法再加:① 按揉外关穴 1 分钟。② 以拇指甲掐按内庭穴 1 分钟。③ 逆时针摩腹 3~5 分

thumb for one minute.

iii. Rub the abdomen counterclockwise for 3 - 5 minutes.

iv. Rub longitudinally from the lumbar region to the sacral region back and forth 5 - 10 times.

2. Renal Asthenia Syndrome　The following can be performed additionally.

i. Press-knead Taixi (KI 3) and Xingjian (LR 2) for one minute each.

ii. Palm-twist and rub Yongquan (KI 1) for 3 - 5 minutes.

iii. Rub transversely the lumbosacral region until a hot sensation is attained.

If toothache is present in the maxillofacial teeth, press and knead Xiaguan (ST 7), Quanliao (SI 18), Yingxiang (LI 20) and Renzhong (GV 26) for one minute each.

If toothache is present in the mandibular teeth, press and knead Jiache (ST 6), Yifeng (TE 17) and Chengjiang (CV 24) for one minute each.

4.2　Infantile Diseases

Physiologically, the infantile viscera are delicate and under fast development and growth. Pathologically, infants are more susceptible to injury by six exogenous pathogenic factors, yet less liable to be internally harmed by seven emotions. Infantile diseases are often characterized by abrupt onset and fast conversion and transmission. Therefore, tuina therapy for infants should be distinctly different from that of adults. Infantile manipulations lay stress on their reinforcing and reducing effects, especially on slight, quick and moderate exertion of force and steady and penetrating property. The selection of manipulations,

钟。④ 直擦腰背至骶部,往返 5～10 次。

2. 肾虚型　基本治法再加:① 按揉太溪、行间穴各 1 分钟。② 搓擦涌泉穴 3～5 分钟。③ 横擦腰骶部,以热为度。

如见症为上牙痛,加按揉下关、颧髎、迎香、人中穴各 1 分钟。

如见症为下牙痛,加按揉颊车、翳风、承浆穴各 1 分钟。

第二节　小儿疾病

小儿在生理上脏腑娇嫩,发育迅速;病理上易于外感六淫邪气,较少七情内伤,但发病急迫,传变迅速。所以,运用推拿治疗就应与成人有所不同。其手法讲究补泻,特别强调轻快柔和,平稳着实,应根据患儿病情的轻重、体质的强弱和年龄的大小等,注意采用适当的手法、力量和操作时间。为减轻摩擦,避免损伤皮

force and duration of treatment should be based on the
infant's pathological condition, physique, and age. In order to decrease friction, avoid skin injury, and enhance
therapeutic effects, media are mostly recommended during operation. Manipulations are usually applied on the
head and face first, next on the upper limbs, then on the
chest, the abdomen, the lumbus and the back, and finally
on the lower limbs. They can also be handled flexibly according to the seriousness of the case, the principal or
compatible order of point selection, or the position of the
infant. As to the reinforcing and reducing effects of manipulations, generally, reinforcement is produced by
clockwise, upward, gentle and slow manipulations, while
reduction is induced by counterclockwise, downward,
strong and quick ones. Usually, circular pushing means
reinforcement while direct pushing toward the base of a
finger is reduction. The duration of infantile tuina is long
and the times are numerous in pushing, kneading, and
rubbing manipulations, but short and fewer in pressing,
grasping, nipping and pinching. In addition, strong manipulations like pressing, grasping, nipping and pinching
are normally executed at the end of treatment, for these
strong manipulations might cause infants to cry and inter-
fere with the later treatment.

4.2.1　Fever

INTRODUCTION

Fever is actually the abnormal increase of body temperature, and is one of the most common symptoms in pediatrics department. It is often seen in many acute and
chronic infantile diseases. According to modern medicine,
infection of viruses and bacteria may induce fever in infants. Or even some foreign factors like hot weather, too
much wearing or covering may cause irregular changes of

肤,增强疗效,操作时多采用介质。操作的次序一般是先头面,次上肢,再胸腹腰背,最后是下肢。也可根据病情轻重,取穴主次,或患儿体位而定,灵活掌握。至于手法的补泻,一般是以顺、上、轻、缓为补,逆、下、重、急为泻;旋推为补,向指根方向直推为泻。小儿推拿手法操作的时间,一般推、揉、摩等手法操作时间长而次数多,按、拿、掐、捏等手法操作时间短而次数少。按、拿、掐、捏等刺激强的手法应放在最后操作,以免刺激过重引起患儿哭闹而影响后面的操作。

一、发热

【概述】

发热即体温异常升高,是儿科最常见的症状之一,可见于多种急、慢性小儿疾病。现代医学认为细菌、病毒等感染可导致小儿发热,也可由于小儿体温调节中枢还未完全发育成熟,易受外界影响,诸如

infantile temperature due to their underdeveloped temperature controlling center that is likely to be affected by external changes. TCM holds that infants are of innate deficiency and their healthy qi is not sufficient enough, therefore, they are more susceptible to attacks by the six exogenous pathogens of wind, cold, summer-heat, dampness, dryness and fire, suffering from diseases than adults.

In clinic, types of wind-cold fever and wind-heat fever invaded by exogenous pathogenic factors, internal injury fever due to accumulated heat caused by retention of food, and internal heat due to deficiency of yin after long-time fever are commonly seen.

MAIN POINTS FOR DIAGNOSIS

1. Syndrome of Exogenous Wind-cold Symptoms are manifested as fever, headache, aversion to cold, stuffy nose, running nose, thin and whitish tongue fur and bright red finger veins.

2. Syndrome of Exogenous Wind-heat Common symptoms are fever, slight perspiration, dry mouth, sore throat, yellow nasal discharge, thin and yellowish tongue fur, red and purple finger veins.

3. Syndrome of Sthenia Pulmonary and Gastric Heat Symptoms are manifested as high fever, flushed face, shortness of breath, poor appetite, constipation, irritability and restlessness, thirst with a desire for drink, red tongue with dry fur and dark, purple finger veins.

4. Syndrome of Internal Heat Due to Deficiency of Yin Common symptoms are afternoon fever, feverish sensation in the palm and sole, emaciation, night sweating, decreased appetite, thready and rapid pulse, red tongue with exfoliated fur and light purple finger veins.

BASIC MANIPULATIONS

The principle of tuina therapy is dispersing wind and clearing away heat.

天气炎热、衣被过多等,都会导致体温异常波动。中医认为小儿禀赋不强,正气未充,较成人更易受风、寒、暑、湿、燥、火等六淫之邪损伤而致病。

临床分型可见有感受外邪所致的风寒发热、风热发热,食积蕴热的内伤发热以及发热日久导致的阴虚内热。

【诊断要点】

1. 外感风寒型 症见发热,头痛,恶寒,鼻塞,流涕,苔薄白,指纹鲜红。

2. 外感风热型 症见发热,微汗出,口干,咽痛,鼻流黄涕,苔薄黄,指纹红紫。

3. 肺胃实热型 症见高热,面红,气促,不思饮食,便秘,烦躁,渴而引饮,舌红苔燥,指纹深紫。

4. 阴虚内热型 症见午后发热,手足心热,形瘦,盗汗,食欲减退,脉细数,舌红苔剥,指纹淡紫。

【基本治法】

推拿治疗多以疏散、清热为原则。

Manipulation of Qingtianheshui is performed 300 – 500 times; manipulation of reducing Liufu, 300 times; manipulation of pushing Sanguan, 100 times; manipulation of separating yinyang, 100 times; manipulation of Longruhukou, 100 times. Clear Feijing, 300 times; knead Wailaogong, 300 – 500 times and push the spinal column, 100 times.

清天河水 300～500 次，退六腑 300 次，推三关 100 次，分阴阳 100 次，龙入虎口 100 次，清肺经 300 次，揉外劳宫 300～500 次，推脊 100 次。

MODIFIED MANIPULATIONS WITH SYNDROME DIFFERENTIATION

【随症加减】

(1) Syndrome of Exogenous Wind-cold: Besides the basic manipulations, the following are also performed.

Manipulation of opening Tianmen is performed 100 times; pushing Kangong 100 times; arc-pushing Taiyang (EX-HN 5) 100 times; nipping-kneading Ershanmen 100 times; manipulation of Huangfeng Rudong 100 times; grasping Fengchi (GB 20) and Hegu (LI 4) 10 times each; pushing Sanguan 300 times. And reducing Liufu is reduced to 100 times.

(1) 外感风寒型，基本治法加开天门 100 次，推坎宫 100 次，运太阳 100 次，掐揉二扇门 100 次，黄蜂入洞 100 次，拿风池、合谷各 10 次，推三关至 300 次，退六腑减至 100 次。

(2) Syndrome of Exogenous Wind-heat: Manipulation of opening Tianmen is performed 100 times; pushing Kangong 100 times; arc-pushing Taiyang (EX-HN 5) 100 times; nipping Zongjin 100 times; pushing Tianzhugu 100 times and grasping Jianjing (GB 21) and Quchi (LI 11) 10 times each.

(2) 外感风热型，开天门 100 次，推坎宫 100 次，运太阳 100 次，掐总筋 100 次，推天柱骨 100 次，拿肩井、曲池各 10 次。

(3) Syndrome of Sthenia Pulmonary and Gastric Heat: The following are used in addition.

Manipulation of Damaguotianhe is performed 100 times; manipulation of Shuidilaomingyue 100 times; clearing Feijing 200 times; clearing Weijing 200 times; clearing Dachang 100 times; manipulation of Longruhukou 300 times; kneading Tianshu (ST 25) 300 times and pushing Xiaqijiegu 100 times.

(3) 肺胃实热型，基本治法加打马过天河 100 次，水底捞明月 100 次，清肺经 200 次，清胃经 200 次，清大肠 100 次，龙入虎口至 300 次，揉天枢 300 次，推下七节骨 100 次。

(4) Syndrome of Internal Heat due to Deficiency of Yin: The following maneuvers are added.

(4) 阴虚内热，加补脾经 100 次，补肺经 100 次，补肾经

Manipulation of reinforcing Pijing is performed 100 times; Feijing 100 times; Shenjing 100 times; kneading Erren Shangma 100 times; arc-pushing Laogong (PC 8) 100 times; clearing Ganjing 100 times; kneading Shending 50 times; pushing Yongquan (KI 1) 100 times; and pressing-kneading Zusanli (ST 36) 30 times. In addition, clearing Xinjing 100 times and pressing-kneading Baihui (GV 20) 50 times are used for insomnia due to restlessness. Reinforcing Shenjing 300 times, kneading Shending 100 times and nipping-kneading Shenwen 100 times are applied to patients with night sweating or spontaneous perspiration.

As for patients with food retention, clear and reinforce Pijing 100 times respectively, arc-push Bagua 100 times and rub the abdomen for 3 minutes. For those with vomiting, push the lower Danzhong (CV 17) 50 times, and push from Hengwen to Banmen 100 times. For those who have convulsion, clear Ganjing 100 times, nip-knead Xiaotianxin and Wuzhijie 50 times respectively.

The treatment of fever with Tuina is given once a day, but 2 or 3 times a day to severe cases. And three days form a therapeutic course. During treatment, the infant patients are recommended to have good rest, drink plenty of water, eat light food, and stay in well-aired rooms. Moreover, physical hypothermia (cold compress, alcoholic bath) may be combined with for patients of two or three months old.

4.2.2　Cough

INTRODUCTION

Cough is one of the most common symptoms of the respiratory diseases caused by many diseases. It may occur in any season, but mostly in winter and spring. Modern medicine holds that the infantile respiratory tracts are

100 次，揉二人上马 100 次，运内劳宫 100 次，清肝经 100 次，揉肾顶 50 次，推涌泉 100 次，按揉足三里 30 次。烦躁不眠，加清心经 100 次，按揉百会 50 次；自汗盗汗，补肾经至 300 次，揉肾顶至 100 次，加掐揉肾纹 100 次。

夹食滞者加清补脾经各 100 次，运八卦 100 次，摩腹 3 分钟；呕吐者加推下膻中 50 次，横纹推向板门 100 次；夹惊者加清肝经 100 次，掐揉小天心、五指节各 50 次。

推拿每日 1 次。重者每日 2～3 次，3 日为 1 个疗程。治疗期间，患儿应注意休息，多饮水，吃易消化食物，并保持室内空气流通。2～3 月龄的患儿最好配合物理降温法（冷敷法、酒精浴）。

二、咳嗽

【概述】

咳嗽是呼吸系统疾病最常见的一个症状，可由多种疾病而引起。一年四季都可发生，但以冬春季最为多见。现

distributed with profuse blood vessels and the mucous membranes of the trachea and bronchi are delicate, so they are liable to be infected and develop inflammation. TCM believes that the lung qi in infants is insufficient, so their lung is susceptible to being attacked by exogenous pathogenic factors, leading to disturbances in its dispersing and descending functions and eventually resulting in cough. Clinically, cough is divided into two types: exogenous cough and endogenous cough. And infantile cough mostly belongs to the former.

MAIN POINTS FOR DIAGNOSIS

1. Exogenous Cough   In cough caused by exopathogenic wind-cold, its common symptoms are cough, clear and thin sputum, stuffy nose, thin nasal discharge, headache and general pain, aversion to cold with no or slight fever, no perspiration, no thirst, thin and whitish tongue fur, floating and tight or floating and slow pulse and superficial red dactylogram. In cough due to exopathogenic wind-heat, symptoms are manifested as cough, yellow and thick sputum difficult to expectorate, fever and aversion to wind, perspiration, turbid nasal discharge, sore and dry or itching throat, thirst, constipation, yellow urine, reddened tongue with thin and yellowish fur, floating and rapid pulse and red or purple finger veins.

2. Endogenous Cough   Long-time cough with profuse sputum, or dry cough or with scanty or thick sputum which is hard to expectorate, pallor complexion, cold limbs, short breath, perspiration, chest stuffiness, physical leanness, listlessness, whitish and greasy tongue fur, weak or weak and rapid pulse and purple, sticky finger veins.

BASIC MANIPULATIONS

The principle of tuina therapy is mainly dispersing pulmonary qi to stop cough.

代医学认为小儿呼吸道血管丰富,气管、支气管粘膜较嫩,极易受感染而发生炎症。中医学认为小儿肺气未充,易为外邪侵袭,导致肺脏的宣肃功能失常而发生咳嗽。临床上一般将咳嗽分为外感咳嗽和内伤咳嗽两大类,小儿以外感咳嗽为多见。

【诊断要点】

1. 外感咳嗽　属风寒者,症见咳嗽,咯痰清稀,鼻塞涕清,头身疼痛,恶寒不发热或有微热,无汗,口不渴,苔薄白,脉浮紧或浮缓,指纹浮红;属风热者,症见咳嗽,痰黄稠,咯吐不爽,发热恶风,汗出,流浊涕,咽喉干痛或痒,口渴,便秘尿黄,舌质红,苔薄黄,脉浮数,指纹鲜红或紫红。

2. 内伤咳嗽　久咳痰多或干咳无痰、少痰或痰稠难以咳出,面色苍白,四肢欠温,气短汗出,胸闷纳呆,形体消瘦,神疲乏力,苔白腻,脉细或细数,指纹紫滞。

【基本治法】

推拿治疗咳嗽以宣肺止咳为主。

Press-knead Tiantu (CV 22) 20 times, parting-push Danzhong (CV 17) 100 times; knead Rugen (ST 18) 20 times; knead Rupang 20 times; clear Feijing 300 times; reinforce Feijing 500 times and arc-push Bagua 200 times; nip Wuzhijie on each finger 10–20 times; nip Jingning 10 times; press-knead Tianshu (ST 25) 100 times, Fenglong (ST 40) and Zusanli (ST 36) 50 times each, Fengmen (BL 12), Dingchuan (EX-B 1) and Feishu (BL 13) 100–200 times each; parting-push the scapulae 100 times and palm-rub the back of the infant until a hot sensation is attained.

MODIFIED MANIPULATIONS WITH SYNDROME DIFFERENTIATION

(1) Syndrome of Exopathogenic Wind-cold: Additionally open Tianmen 30 times, push Kangong 30 times, push Taiyang (EX-HN 5) 30 times, knead Wailaogong (EX-UE 8) 30 times, push Sanguan 300 times, reduce Liufu 100 times, grasp Hegu (LI 4) 10 times, and Fengchi (GB 20) 10 times.

(2) Syndrome of Exopathogenic Wind-heat: Additionally clear Feijing 200 times, reduce Liufu 300 times, push Sanguan 100 times, and push Tianzhu (BL 10) 100 times as well.

(3) Internal Injury Syndrome: Additionally reinforce Pitu 300 times, Shenjing 800 times, knead Zhongwan (CV 12) 200 times, Dantian 200 times, and Banmen 30 times, press-knead Pishu (BL 20) and Weishu (BL 21) 20 times each, and knead Shenshu (BL 23) 30 times.

The manipulations are performed once a day, but twice for severe cases, and three days form one treatment course. In the course of treating cough with Tuina, the cause of cough should also be looked for so as to conduct a comprehensive treatment. Meanwhile proper rest and light food should also be given to infantile patients in the

按揉天突 20 次，分推膻中 100 次，揉乳根 20 次，揉乳旁 20 次，清肺经 300 次，补肺经 500 次，运八卦 200 次，掐五指节每指各掐 10～20 次，掐精宁穴 10 次，按揉天枢 100 次，按揉双侧丰隆、足三里各 50 次，按揉风门、定喘、肺俞各 100～200 次，分推肩胛骨 100 次，掌擦患儿背部，以温热为度。

【随症加减】

（1）外感风寒者，加开天门 30 次，推坎宫 30 次，推太阳 30 次，揉外劳宫 30 次，推三关 300 次，退六腑 100 次，拿合谷 10 次，然后拿风池 10 次。

（2）外感风热者，加清肺经 200 次，退六腑 300 次，推三关 100 次，推天柱 100 次。

（3）内伤咳嗽者，加补脾土 300 次，补肾经 800 次，揉中脘 200 次，揉丹田 200 次，揉板门穴 300 次，然后按揉脾、胃俞各 20 次，揉肾俞 30 次。

推拿每日 1 次，重者每日 2 次，3 日为 1 个疗程。在推拿治疗咳嗽的同时，应认真查找引起咳嗽的原因，以便综合治疗。小儿在咳嗽发作期间应适当注意休息，吃易于消化

presence of cough. In seasons with changeable weather, infantile thoracoabdominal areas should be kept warm in case of catching cold.

4. 2. 3   Anorexia

INTRODUCTION

Anorexia, namely aversion to food, refers to the symptom of long-term lack of appetite or even refusal of food-taking in infants. According to modern medicine, it is caused by improper feeding of infants whose digestive system is under full development. While TCM holds that infants are of delicate physique with asthenic yin and yang, and their spleen qi is often in insufficient condition. Therefore, many factors may lead to disharmony of the stomach and the spleen, and their dysfunction in reception, transportation and transformation, giving rise to anorexia. Generally, infants with anorexia are in a normal spiritual state, but if the condition is lingering, they will become spiritless, lose weight, and have poor resistance to diseases. For infants with longer duration of anorexia, their growth will be hindered to some degree, so the problem should be treated timely. Anorexia is often seen in 1 - 6 years old children. Anorexia caused by exopathic diseases or some other chronic diseases is not included in the range of this problem.

According to clinical symptoms, anorexia is classified as three syndromes: dysfunction of the spleen in transportation and transformation, insufficient gastric yin, and asthenia of splenogastric qi.

MAIN POINTS FOR DIAGNOSIS

(1) Syndrome of Dysfunction of the Spleen in Transportation and Transformation: Symptoms are pale complexion, no desire for food, tastelessness in the mouth, refusal of taking food, physical leanness, whitish or thin

的食物。在气候变化季节,尤其应注意胸腹部保暖,防止受凉。

三、厌食

【概述】

厌食又称恶食,是指小儿较长时期食欲不振,甚至拒食的一种病症。现代医学认为小儿消化系统功能尚未健全,加之喂养不当而导致本病的发生。中医学则认为小儿为稚阴稚阳之体,脾常不足,多种原因都可导致其脾胃不和,受纳运化失职而出现厌食的症状。厌食患儿一般精神状态均较正常,但日久精神疲惫,体重减轻,抗病力弱。病程长者对小儿的生长发育有一定的影响,故应及时治疗。本病以1～6岁小儿为多见。若因外感或某些慢性病而出现的食欲不振者,则不属本病范围。

根据临床症状,小儿厌食可分为脾失健运、胃阴不足和脾胃气虚三个证型。

【诊断要点】

(1)脾失健运者,症见面色少华,不思纳食,或食物无味,拒进饮食,形体偏瘦,舌苔白或薄腻,脉尚有力,指纹

and greasy tongue fur, normal pulse and colorless, sticky dactylogram.

(2) Syndrome of Insufficient Gastric Yin: Symptoms are dry mouth, frequent drinking of water, dislike of food, dry and lusterless skin, dry stools, uncoated and smooth tongue, or red and glossy tongue with less fluid, reddish tongue proper, thin pulse and deep and red finger veins.

(3) Syndrome of Asthenia of Splenogastric Qi: Symptoms are listlessness, sallow complexion, dislike of food, refusal of taking food, stools mixed with undigested food or shapeless stools after slight eating, aptness to perspiration, thin and whitish tongue fur, weak pulse and deep and sticky finger veins.

BASIC MANIPULATIONS

The principle of tuina therapy: strengthening the spleen and regulating the stomach. The effects of this therapy is very remarkable.

Reinforce Pijing 400 times, Weijing 200 times, and Dachang 200 times. Nip-knead Sihengwen 30 - 50 times each, rub the abdomen for 5 - 10 minutes, and press-knead Zusanli (ST 36), Pishu (BL 20) and Weishu (BL 21) 30 times respectively.

MODIFIED MANIPULATIONS WITH SYNDROME DIFFERENTIATION

(1) For patients with dysfunction of the spleen in transportation and transformation, reinforce Pijing up to 600 times, arc-push Neibagua 400 times, and perform Longruhukou manipulation 100 times.

(2) For patients with insufficient gastric yin, additionally separate yinyang 100 times, knead Banmen 300 times, arc-push Neibagua 200 times, press-knead Zhongwan (CV 12), Guanyuan (CV 4), Sanjiaoshu (BL 22), and Shenshu (BL 23) 30 - 50 times respectively.

淡滞。

（2）胃阴不足者，症见口干多饮而不喜进食，皮肤干燥，缺乏润泽，大便干结，舌苔多见光剥，亦有光红少津者，舌质偏红，脉细，指纹沉红。

（3）脾胃气虚者，症见精神较差，面色萎黄，厌食、拒食，若稍进食，大便中即夹有不消化残渣，或大便不成形，容易出汗，舌苔薄白，脉无力，指纹沉滞。

【基本治法】

推拿治疗以健脾和胃为原则，疗效显著。

补脾经 400 次，补胃经 200 次，补大肠 200 次，掐揉四横纹各 30～50 次，摩腹 5～10 分钟，按揉足三里、脾俞、胃俞各 30 次。

【随症加减】

（1）脾失健运者，补脾经加至 600 次，加运内八卦 400 次，龙入虎口 100 次。

（2）胃阴不足者，加分阴阳 100 次，揉板门 300 次，运内八卦 200 次，按揉中脘、关元、三焦俞、肾俞各 30～50 次。

（3）For patients with asthenia of splenogastric qi, reinforce Pijing 600 times, and Shenjing 300 times additionally, push Shangqijiegu 300 times, and pinch the spine 3 – 5 times.

The treatment is given once a day, and one course takes ten days.

Regulating diet is an important measure for preventing and treating infantile anorexia. The habit of monophagia should be corrected timely, and children are restricted to taking any snacks, candy and chocolate before meals. They also need to develop a good habit of regular eating and living. If poor appetite is manifested in infants after catching some diseases, the causes should be examined promptly and treated timely.

4. 2. 4   Vomiting

INTRODUCTION

Vomiting is one of the common symptoms in infantile diseases, and is caused mostly by the retroperistalsis of the stomach and the intestine, which, according to modern medicine, can result from many diseases, such as diseases of the gastrointestinal tract, fever, intracranial infection, drugs, food poisoning, and other metabolic disturbances. TCM holds that vomiting is mainly caused by improper feeding, leading to retention of food in the stomach, or accumulation of heat, stagnation of cold in the spleen and stomach, etc. , which result in failure of gastric qi to descend, inducing vomiting. The common symptoms are productive vomiting with sounds after foodtaking, sour and offensive or stinking vomitus, accompanied by pale complexion or flushed face and ears, sweating, and pain in the stomach. Clinically, vomiting is classified as cold vomiting, heat vomiting and indigestive vomiting, etc.

（3）脾胃气虚者，补脾经加至 600 次，加补肾经 300 次，推上七节骨 300 次，捏脊 3～5 遍。

推拿每日 1 次，10 日为 1 个疗程。

调节饮食，是预防治疗小儿厌食的重要措施。纠正不良的偏食习惯，禁止饭前吃零食和糖果、巧克力，定时进食，生活要有规律性。患病后发现食欲不振，应及时检查原因和治疗。

四、呕吐

【概述】

呕吐是小儿疾病中常见的一种症状，多为胃肠的逆行蠕动所致。现代医学认为这种胃肠的逆行蠕动可由于许多疾病如胃肠道疾患、发热、颅内感染、药物及食物中毒，或其他代谢性疾病等引起。中医学认为呕吐多由于喂养不当，食滞中脘或脾胃蕴热、寒滞等原因导致胃失和降，上逆作吐。常见症状是食后呕吐，有声有物，吐物酸臭或臭秽，并伴有面色苍白或面红耳赤，以及汗出、脘痛等。临床常见证型有寒吐、热吐和伤食吐等。

MAIN POINTS FOR DIAGNOSIS

1. Cold Vomiting Syndrome　Symptoms are vomiting after overeating, intermittent vomiting, vomitus with slight sour smell, pale complexion, cold limbs, abdominal pain which can be relieved by warmth, loose stools, pale tongue, thin and whitish tongue fur and red, sticky finger veins.

2. Heat Vomiting Syndrome　Symptoms are vomiting right after food-taking, sour and stinking vomitus, feverish sensation in the body, thirst, restlessness, stinking or dry stools, dark yellow urine, dry and red lips, yellowish and greasy tongue fur, rapid pulse and light purple finger veins.

3. Indigestive Vomiting Syndrome　Symptoms are frequent vomiting, foul breath, chest distress, anorexia, abdominal distension and pain, sour and stinking stools, loose or dry stools, thick and greasy tongue fur, slippery pulse, and deep, sticky dactylogram.

BASIC MANIPULATIONS

The principle of tuina therapy: regulating the stomach and relieving adverse rising of gastric qi.

Digitally-press Neiguan (PC 6), Zhongwan (CV 12) and Zusanli (ST 36) for one minute respectively. Pinch-grasp the muscles around acupoint Weishu (BL 21) on the back 15 - 20 times. Rub the abdomen clockwise and counterclockwise for 3 minutes respectively.

MODIFIED MANIPULATIONS WITH SYNDROME DIFFERENTIATION

（1）Cold Vomiting Syndrome: Additionally push Tianzhugu 100 times, reinforce Pijing 100 times, push from Banmen to Hengwen 100 times, knead Wailaogong 100 times, and push Sanguan 100 times.

（2）Heat Vomiting Syndrome: Additionally clear Pijing, Weijing and Dachang 100 times each. Reduce Liufu

【诊断要点】

1. 寒吐型　症见食多即吐,时作时止,呕吐物稍酸臭,面色苍白,四肢欠温,腹痛喜暖,大便溏薄,舌淡苔薄白,指纹红滞。

2. 热吐型　症见食入即吐,吐物酸臭,身热自渴,烦躁不安,大便臭秽或秘结,小便黄赤,唇色红而干,苔黄腻,脉数,指纹紫淡。

3. 伤食吐型　症见呕吐频繁,口气臭秽,胸闷厌食,肚腹胀痛,大便酸臭,或溏或秘,苔厚腻,脉滑,指纹沉滞。

【基本治法】

推拿治疗呕吐的原则是和胃降逆。

点按内关、中脘、足三里各1分钟,捏拿背部胃俞穴处肌肉15～20次,顺、逆时针摩腹各3分钟。

【随症加减】

（1）寒吐型,加推天柱骨100次,补脾经100次,板门推向横纹100次,揉外劳宫、推三关各100次。

（2）热吐型,加清脾经、清胃经、清大肠,退六腑各100次,

100 times, nip Shiwang 3 - 5 times each, and push down Tianzhugu and Qijiegu 100 times each.

（3）Indigestive Vomiting Syndrome: Additionally clear Pijing 100 times, arc-push Neibagua (clockwise) 300 times, push from Banmen to Hengwen 100 times, separating-push Danzhong (CV 17) 300 times, perform manipulation of Anxuan Zhoucuomo (Twist and Rub like Plucking the String) for one minute, and push down Qijiegu 100 times.

The tuina treatment is given once or twice a day, and three days' treatment forms a course.

Infants with vomiting must be controlled on diet, and for those with frequent vomiting, fasting should be practised till their conditions are improved, then food-taking gradually increases. Infant's head should be turned to one side while vomiting in case vomitus is inhaled into the trachea. In addition, fluid infusion should be given to patients with severe vomiting to avoid occurrence of disorder of water or electrolyte. In the course of tuina therapy, causes of vomiting should be ascertained further. For example, if the vomiting is jet-shaped and massive, accompanied by fever, convulsion, listlessness or eclampsia, some acute infectious diseases like epidemic encephalitis B or epidemic cerebrospinal meningitis should be under consideration. Infants should usually be kept in a proper temperature condition and fed reasonably.

4.2.5 Diarrhea

INTRODUCTION

Infantile diarrhea refers to the sudden increased frequency of defecation, usually more than three times a day with thin, or watery stools. It is one of the most common digestive diseases in infants under three years old, and mostly occurs in hot, damp autumn and summer. According to modern medicine, infants' digestive system is still

掐十王各 3～5 次,推下天柱骨 100 次,推下七节骨 100 次。

（3）伤食吐型,加清脾经 100 次,运内八卦（顺时针方向）300 次,板门推向横纹 100 次,分推膻中 300 次,按弦走搓摩 1 分钟,推下七节骨 100 次。

推拿每天 1～2 次,3 天为 1 个疗程。

小儿呕吐时要适当控制饮食,呕吐频繁者,应予禁食,待病情缓解后,再酌增饮食量。呕吐时应将患儿头置于侧位,避免呕吐物吸入气管。呕吐严重者应给予静脉补液,防止水、电解质紊乱。在小儿呕吐的推拿治疗过程中,必须进一步查明病因,如见患儿呕吐呈喷射状,量多,伴见发热、抽搐、神萎或惊厥等情况,当考虑流行性乙型脑炎、流行性脑脊髓膜炎等急性传染病的发生。小儿平时应冷热适度,并注意合理喂养。

五、腹泻

【概述】

小儿腹泻是指便次比正常时突然增多,每天 3 次以上,粪便性质呈稀便或水样便。它是 3 岁以下婴幼儿最常见的一种消化道疾病,尤以夏秋暑湿当令,最易发病。现

undeveloped, and the regulating function of their nervous system is relatively weak. If their diet is improper, or too hot or too cold, or infected by bacteria or virus, diarrhea will occur, and dysfunction of the stomach and the spleen and indigestion will follow.

TCM holds that the occurrence of diarrhea is mainly due to invasion of exogenous pathogenic factors, especially of wind, cold, summer-heat, dampness, etc., which cause disturbance of transporting and transforming functions of the stomach and spleen, and indigestion, as a result, the clear and the turbid are mixed up in the large intestine, and followed by abdominal pain or diarrhea. Another reason for infantile diarrhea is irregular or unclean diet or food retention, which impairs the spleen and the stomach. Infants are under development, of immatureness and yin in nature. Diarrhea with excessive water and fluids, or hot diarrhea injuring the fluid yin may lead to exhaustion of yin fluid and occurrence of injury of yin in patients with symptoms like dry skin, thirst, red lips, and difficult urination, etc.

MAIN POINTS FOR DIAGNOSIS

1. Diarrhea Due to Pathogenic Cold-damp　Symptoms are manifested as thin and foamy stools with light color and smell, borborygmus, pain in the stomach, pale complexion, no thirst, thin and prolonged urine, whitish and greasy tongue fur and soft pulse.

2. Diarrhea Due to Pathogenic Damp-heat　Symptoms are diarrhea right after abdominal pain, urgent defecation, hot and stinking stools with yellow color, slight fever, thirst, scanty and yellow urine, yellowish and greasy tongue fur, and slippery and rapid pulse.

3. Diarrhea Due to Indigestion　Symptoms are manifested as pain, distension and fullness in the abdomen,

代医学认为婴幼儿消化系统发育不成熟，神经调节作用较差，加之饮食失调、冷暖不匀或细菌、病毒感染等因素即可导致腹泻，以致胃肠功能紊乱，消化不良。

中医认为本病发生可由于感受外邪，尤其是风、寒、暑、湿等，致使脾胃运化失常，饮食难于消化，清、浊混走大肠而腹痛、腹泻；另外，由于饮食不节或不洁，宿食积滞，伤及脾胃，腹泻不止。小儿为稚阴之体，因泄泻大量水液，或热泻者火热伤阴，则阴津枯竭，出现皮肤干枯，口渴唇红，小便不利等阴伤证。

【诊断要点】

1. 寒湿泻　症见大便清稀多沫，色淡不臭，肠鸣腹痛，面色苍白，口不渴，小便清长，苔白腻，脉濡。

2. 湿热泻　症见腹痛即泻，大便急迫，色黄热臭，身有微热，口渴，尿少色黄，苔黄腻，脉滑数。

3. 伤食泻　症见腹痛胀满，泻前哭闹，泻后痛减，大便

crying before diarrhea, pain relieved after defecation, massive and sour stools, halitosis, poor appetite, or accompanied by sour regurgitation, thick and greasy tongue fur and slippery pulse.

4. Diarrhea Due to Deficiency of the Spleen Symptoms are lingering diarrhea or repeated attacks of diarrhea, pale complexion, poor appetite, loose stools mixed with milk masses or food residues or diarrhea after food-taking, pale tongue with thin fur and floating pulse.

5. Diarrhea Due to Yang-deficiency of the Spleen and Kidney Symptoms are watery, frequent stools with undigested food, incessant diarrhea, pale complexion, cold limbs, listlessness, pale tongue with thin fur and soft and weak pulse.

BASIC MANIPULATIONS

The principle of tuina therapy is strengthening the spleen, eliminating dampness and arresting diarrhea.

Reinforce Pijing 100 times, clear and reinforce Dachang 200 times each, clear Xiaochang 200 times, circularly rub the abdomen for 5 - 10 minutes, knead the umbilicus 500 times, knead Guiwei 300 times, push up Qijiegu 300 times, press-knead Pishu (BL 20), Weishu (BL 21), Dachangshu (BL 25) and Zusanli (ST 36) for 1 minute respectively.

MODIFIED MANIPULATIONS WITH SYNDROME DIFFERENTIATION

(1) Diarrhea Due to Pathogenic Cold-damp: Rub the abdomen counterclockwise. Additionally push Sanguan 100 times, knead Wailaogong 100 times, and knead Tianshu (ST 25) 100 times.

(2) Diarrhea Due to Pathogenic Damp-heat: Rub the abdomen clockwise, and push down Qijiegu. Instead of reinforcing Pijing, do clearing Pijing 100 times, reduce Liufu 100 times, clear Tianheshui 100 times, knead Tianshu

量多酸臭,口臭纳呆,或伴呕吐酸馊,苔厚腻,脉滑。

4. 脾虚泻 症见久泻不愈,或经常反复发作,面色苍白,食欲不振,便稀夹有奶块及食物残渣,或每于食后即泻,舌淡苔薄,脉濡。

5. 脾肾阳虚泻 症见大便水样,次数频多,或完谷不化,泻下不止,面色㿠白,四肢厥冷,精神委靡,舌淡苔薄,脉软无力。

【基本方法】

推拿治疗小儿腹泻的原则是健脾燥湿止泻。

补脾经 400 次,清补大肠各 200 次,清小肠 200 次,摩腹 5～10 分钟,揉脐 500 次,揉龟尾 300 次,推上七节骨 300 次,按揉脾俞、胃俞、大肠俞、足三里各 1 分钟。

【随症加减】

(1) 寒湿泻,逆时针摩腹,加推三关 100 次,揉外劳宫 100 次,揉天枢 100 次。

(2) 湿热泻,顺时针摩腹,推下七节骨,去补脾经,加清脾经 100 次,退六腑 100 次,清天河水 100 次,揉天枢 300 次,

(ST 25) 300 times, and push the spine 100 times.

(3) Diarrhea Due to Indigestion: Rub the abdomen clockwise, push down Qijiegu, add clearing Dachang 100 times, perform Longruhukou manipulation 200 times, arc-push Neibagua 200 times, knead Zhongwan (CV 12) 200 times and grasp Dujiao 10 - 20 times.

(4) Diarrhea due to Deficiency of the Spleen: Rub the abdomen counterclockwise, add kneading Banmen 300 times, arc-push Neibagua 200 times, and pinch the spine 10 - 15 times.

(5) Diarrhea Due to Yang-deficiency of the Spleen and Kidney: Rub the abdomen counterclockwise, add reinforcing Shenjing 300 times, knead Shending 50 times, press-knead Shenshu (BL 23) and Mingmen (GV 4) 100 times each, and rub Baliao (BL 31 - BL 34) points until heat penetrates the acupoints.

The treatment is generally given once a day, but twice for severe cases, and five days form a course. Chronic diarrhea needs 3 - 4 therapeutic courses. If many times of tuina therapy are not effective or the infant's conditions get even worse, accompanied by oliguresis, anuresis, frequent vomiting, sunken eyes or listlessness, combined Chinese and western medicine should be given, including timely venous transfusion, adopting measures of anti-infection and correcting the balance of electrolyte, etc.

For infants suffering from diarrhea, their diet should be controlled, including not taking rich foods. Washing the anus with warm water after each defecation, frequently changing their napkins and keeping their skin clean are recommended. At ordinary times, attention should be paid to proper feeding of infants, including feeding and lactating on regular time and with a certain amount, not too soon adding of non-staple food and not too

推脊 100 次。

（3）伤食泻，顺时针摩腹，推下七节骨，加清大肠 100 次，龙入虎口 200 次，运内八卦 200 次，揉中脘 200 次，拿肚角 10～20 次。

（4）脾虚泻，逆时针摩腹，加揉板门 300 次，运内八卦 200 次，捏脊 10～15 遍。

（5）脾肾阳虚泻，逆时针摩腹，加补肾经 300 次，揉肾顶 50 次，按揉肾俞、命门各 100 次，擦八髎透热为度。

推拿每日 1 次，重者 2 次，5 天为 1 个疗程。慢性腹泻需 3～4 个疗程。推拿治疗多次疗效不显著或发现患儿病情转重，出现少尿、无尿，呕吐频繁，眼窝凹馅，精神委靡等症时，宜配合中、西药物治疗，包括及时静脉输液、纠正电解质平衡和抗感染等措施。

对腹泻期间的小儿，应控制饮食，不食油腻之品，患儿每次便后须用温水洗净肛门，勤换尿布，保持皮肤清洁干燥。小儿平时应注意合理喂养，喂食哺乳尽量做到定时定量，添加副食品不宜太快，品种不宜太多，并注意气候变

many varieties. Attention should also be paid to changes of weather, timely increasing or decreasing clothes for infants and alimentary hygiene to avoid intestinal infections.

4.2.6   Infantile Malnutrition（Ganji）

INTRODUCTION

Ganji（malnutrition and food stagnation in infants）is the general term of malnutrition（Ganzheng）and food stagnation（Jizhi）. Malnutrition and food stagnation differ from each other in severity.

Food stagnation refers to infantile milk and food stagnation, which injures the spleen and the stomach, and further causes distension and fullness in the stomach and indigestion, emaciation, disturbed sleep, persistent crying, sour and stinky stools, and other symptoms. Malnutrition is the advanced phase of food stagnation. In other words, long-term functional disturbance of the stomach and the spleen in transportation and transformation, and failure of generation of blood and qi lead to emaciation, pallor complexion, cold limbs, sparse and withered hairs, listlessness, weak and lower cry, abdominal distension with visible superficial veins, and loose stools in infants. Generally, Ganji is similar to infantile malnutrition in modern medicine.

TCM holds that milk and food stagnation and splenogastric asthenia mutually have the cause and effect relationship. Namely, milk stagnation may injure the spleen and the stomach, on the other hand, weakness of the spleen and stomach may induce food stagnation. Clinically, Ganji（malnutrition and food stagnation）can be classified as type of injury of the spleen due to food stagnation, and type of deficiency of both qi and blood.

MAIN POINTS FOR DIAGNOSIS

1. Syndrome of Injury of the Spleen Due to Food

化,及时增减衣服,注意饮食卫生,预防肠道疾病。

六、疳积

【概述】

疳积是疳证和积滞的总称。积滞与疳证有轻重程度的不同。

积滞是指小儿伤于乳食,损伤脾胃,而导致脘腹胀满、食而不化、形体消瘦、夜卧不安、啼哭不宁、大便恶臭等症状;疳证则是积滞的进一步发展,即由于脾胃运化功能不健,气血无以生化,日久可见患儿形体羸瘦、面色㿠白、四肢不温、毛发稀枯、精神委靡、啼声低微、腹大筋暴、大便溏泄等症状。本病大致相当于现代医学之"小儿营养不良"。

中医认为乳食积滞与脾胃虚弱互为因果,即积滞可伤及脾胃,脾胃虚弱又能产生积滞。据临床症状可将疳积分为积滞伤脾和气血两亏两型。

【诊断要点】

1. 积滞伤脾型   症见形

Stagnation　It is manifested by emaciation, non-increased body weight, distension and fullness in the stomach and the abdomen, poor appetite, listlessness, restlessness in sleep, irregular bowel movements with fetid odor, thick and greasy tongue fur, purple and unsmooth finger veins.

2. Syndrome of Deficiency of Both Qi and Blood The manifested symptoms are sallow or pallor complexion, sparse and withered hairs, skinny physique, listlessness or irritability, restless sleep, weak and low cry, cold limbs, retarded development, depressed abdomen, loose stools, light tongue with thin fur, light finger veins.

BASIC MANIPULATIONS

The principle of tuina therapy is removing stagnation, promoting digestion, and regulating the spleen and the stomach.

Reinforce Pijing 400 – 600 times, arc-push Neibagua 400 times, perform Longruhukou manipulation 200 times, circularly rub the abdomen clockwise and counterclockwise for 5 minutes respectively. Separating-push Fuyinyang 200 times, pinch the spine 10 - 15 times, and press-knead Zusanli (ST 36), Pishu (BL 20) and Weishu (BL 21) 30 - 50 times respectively.

MODIFIED MANIPULATIONS WITH SYNDROME DIFFERENTIATION

(1) Syndrome of Injury of the Spleen Due to Food Stagnation: Additionally, knead Banmen 100 – 300 times, push Sihengwen and arc-push Neibagua 100 times respectively.

(2) Syndrome of Deficiency of Both Qi and Blood: Additionally, reinforce Shenjing 100 times, push Sanguan 100 times, knead Wailaogong (EX-UE 8) 100 times, and nip-knead Sihengwen 100 times.

(3) In the above two syndromes, if constipation is seen, cancel kneading Wailaogong (EX-UE 8) and pushing Sanguan, add clearing Dachang 200 times and pushing

体消瘦,体重不增,腹部胀满,饮食不香,精神不振,夜眠不安,大便不调常有恶臭,舌苔厚腻,指纹紫滞。

2. 气血两亏型　症见面色萎黄或㿠白,毛发枯黄稀疏,骨瘦如柴,精神委靡或烦躁,睡卧不宁,啼声低小,四肢不温,发育迟缓,腹部凹陷,大便溏薄,舌淡苔薄,指纹色淡。

【基本治法】

推拿治疗常采用消积导滞、调整脾胃的原则。

补脾经 400～600 次,运内八卦 400 次,龙入虎口 200 次,顺、逆时针摩腹各 5 分钟,分腹阴阳 200 次,捏脊 10～15 遍,按揉足三里、脾俞、胃俞各 30～50 次。

【随症加减】

(1) 积滞伤脾型,加揉板门 100～300 次,推四横纹、运内八卦各 100 次。

(2) 气血两亏型,加补肾经 100 次,推三关 100 次,揉外劳宫 100 次,掐揉四横纹 100 次。

(3) 以上两型,若大便秘结,去揉外劳宫、推三关,加清大肠 200 次,推下七节骨 100

down Qijiegu 100 times; if diarrhea and loose stools are present, add reinforcing Dachang 200 times and pushing up Qijiegu 200 times. For patients with hyperhidrosis, kneading Shending 100 times can be added. For patients with feverish sensation in the chest, palms and soles, and night sweating, cancel pushing Sanguan and kneading Wailaogong (EX-UE 8), add clearing Ganjing 100 times, nipping-kneading Xiaotianxin 100 times and Wuzhijie 50 times each. And for those with aphtha, add nipping, kneading Xiaohengwen 50 times each, and kneading Zongjing 100 times.

This tuina therapy is performed once a day. One treatment course takes ten days. Generally, food stagnation needs one treatment course, while malnutrition demands 1 - 3 courses. The interval between two courses is usually one or two days.

Ganji (malnutrition and food stagnation) in infants should be prevented and treated as soon as possible, in case the problem lasts for a long time and involves other organs with the result of being lingering and difficult to cure. Infants should be fed properly, especially fed with breast milk. Others like timely-adding auxiliary food, replenishing nutrients, feeding regularly with fixed quantity, avoiding some bad habits such as monophagia, addephagia should all be paid attention to. In addition, sufficient sleeping should be ensured, outdoors activities and physical exercises should be arranged properly to improve infants' appetite and their digestive abilities. Dietary hygiene should also be paid attention to so as to protect infants from infectious diseases and parasitosis.

4.2.7   Rectal Prolapse

INTRODUCTION

Rectal prolapse refers to the pathological eversion of

次;便溏者,加补大肠 200 次,推上七节骨 200 次;汗多者,加揉肾顶 100 次;症见五心烦热、盗汗等症者,去推三关、揉外劳宫,加清肝经 100 次,掐揉小天心 100 次,掐揉五指节各 50 次;口舌生疮者,加掐揉小横纹各 50 次,揉总筋 100 次。

推拿每日 1 次,10 日为 1 个疗程。一般积滞治疗 1 个疗程,疳证需要 1～3 个疗程即可治愈。每个疗程之间可间隔 1～2 天。

疳积之症宜早防早治,以免迁延日久累及他脏而缠绵难愈。要合理喂养小儿,尽可能给予母乳喂养,及时添加辅食,注意营养补充,进食要定时定量,防止偏食、嗜食异常等不良习惯。要保证小儿充足的睡眠;适当安排小儿户外活动和锻炼身体,以增进食欲,提高消化能力;注意饮食卫生,预防各种传染病和寄生虫病。

七、脱肛

【概述】

脱肛是指肛管、直肠各层

every layer of the anal canal and the rectum or that of the rectal mucous membrane, and their prolapse out of the anus. Its characteristic of clinical signs is a prolapsed coniform or oblong lump, or the prolapsed rectum, which often occurs in infants under three years old. In mild cases, the rectum is prolapsed outside during defecation, and returns to its original position voluntarily after defecation. In severe cases, the rectum can be prolapsed while crying or coughing, and it needs help to return to its original position. Infantile rectal prolapse is often seen in clinic, mainly because the vertebral curvatures of the infants are not well-developed yet, the rectum is in a vertical position, and the tissues that support the rectum are soft and weak. Therefore, when the pressure inside the abdominal cavity increases, the rectum, without the effective support from the vertebrae and the tissues, is prone to slip downwards and prolapse. Moreover, this disease may be caused by persistent high abdominal pressure like crying, coughing, diarrhea, and constipation.

TCM holds that rectal prolapse is due to infantile congenital deficiency, poor constitution after illness, or long-term diarrhea which consumes the vital qi, leading to asthenia and collapse of qi, and failure of supporting the rectum. Or it may be because of accumulated heat in the large intestine, or damp-heat flowing downward, or dry stools which force the rectum to prolapse outward and cause the disease. According to syndrome differentiation in TCM, rectal prolapse can be divided into two syndromes: asthenia syndrome and sthenia syndrome.

MAIN POINTS FOR DIAGNOSIS

1. Asthenia Syndrome Symptoms are light red prolapsed rectum with a little mucus, no pain sensation, pallor or sallow complexion, emaciated physique, cold limbs, lassitude and fatigue, spontaneous perspiration, pale

或直肠黏膜向外翻出,脱垂于肛门外的一种症状。肛门外可见脱出的圆锥形或长形肿块,即脱垂出的直肠为其临床特征。多见于 3 岁以下的小儿,轻者在大便时脱出,便后可自行还纳;重者因啼哭或咳嗽即能脱出,必须帮助才可回纳。小儿脱肛在临床上较为多见,这主要是由于小儿骶骨弯尚未长成,直肠呈垂直位,支持直肠的组织软弱,故当腹腔内的压力增高时,直肠没有骶骨和周围组织的有效支持,易于向下滑动,发生脱肛。另外,长期腹内压增高(如哭闹、咳嗽、腹泻、便秘等)也可导致本病。

中医认为本病的发生是由于小儿先天不足,病后体弱或因泻痢日久,耗伤正气,气虚下陷,托举无力,导致直肠脱垂。亦可因大肠积热,湿热下注,大便干结,迫肛外脱而发病。依据中医辨证,把脱肛分为虚证和实证两型。

【诊断要点】

1. 虚证 症见脱出的直肠色淡红,伴少量黏液,无痛感,面色苍白或萎黄,形体消瘦,肢体欠温,神疲乏力,自

tongue proper with thin and whitish fur, and weak and thin pulse.

2. Sthenia Syndrome   Symptoms are bright red prolapsed rectum with a little red exudation, redness and swelling and hot pain around the rectum, dry or hard stools, short and dark urine, constant crying, reddened tongue and yellow, greasy tongue fur and hollow pulse.

BASIC MANIPULATIONS

The principle of tuina therapy: nourishing qi, clearing away pathogenic heat, and ascending sunken qi to stop prolapse.

Press-knead Baihui (BL 9) for 2 minutes, knead Dantian for 5 minutes, knead Guiwei 600 times, grasp Jianjing (GB 21) 20 - 30 times, and press-knead Zusanli (ST 36) 30 times.

MODIFIED MANIPULATIONS WITH SYNDROME DIFFERENTIATION

(1) Asthenia Syndrome: Additionally, push the upper Sanguan 300 times, reinforce Pijing 300 times, reinforce Dachang 200 times, reinforce Shenjing 300 times, push up Qijiegu 300 times, and pinch the spine 3 - 6 times.

(2) Sthenia Syndrome: Additionally, reduce the lower Liufu 100 times, clear Dachang 300 times, clear Xiaochang 300 times, knead Quchi (LI 11) 60 times, knead Tianshu (ST 25) 100 times, and push the lower Qijiegu 300 times.

The therapy is given once a day, and five times form one treatment course. During the treatment, infant patients should not defecate in a squat position. A lying posture on the side or on the back can be adopted, for the rectum is not likely to prolapse out in this position.

Careful nursing should be given to infant patients after each occurrence of rectal prolapse. Wash the anus

汗,舌质淡,苔薄白,脉濡细。

2. 实证   症见脱出的直肠色鲜红,伴少量鲜红色渗出液,肛周红肿热痛,大便干燥或干结,小便短赤,且患儿哭闹不安,舌质红,苔黄腻,脉弦。

【基本治法】

推拿治疗脱肛的原则是益气清热,升提固脱。

按揉百会2分钟,揉丹田5分钟,揉龟尾600次,拿肩井20～30次,按揉足三里30次。

【随症加减】

(1) 虚证脱肛者,加推上三关300次,补脾经300次,补大肠200次,补肾经300次,推上七节骨300次,捏脊3～6遍。

(2) 实证脱肛者,加退下六腑100次,清大肠300次,清小肠300次,揉曲池60次,揉天枢100次,推下七节骨300次。

推拿每天1次,5次为1个疗程。在推拿治疗期间,小儿应避免蹲位排便,可采用侧卧或仰卧位排便,这样直肠不易脱出。

小儿脱肛后应注意护理,每次大便后应用温开水将肛

with warm water after each defecation. Keep clean while pushing the prolapsed rectum back to its original position and prevent abrasion from causing infection. Usually the defecating time of patients should not be too long. And ask them to stand up right after defecation. Moreover, attention should also be paid to their nutrients regulation and dietary hygiene. If rectal prolapse is following some diseases like diarrhea or constipation, these diseases should be treated at the same time.

4. 2. 8　Enuresis

INTRODUCTION

Enuresis refers to involuntary urination during sleep in children over three years old. It is more common in boys. In modern medicine, urination is mainly related to the reflex of the central nervous system. As the cerebral cortex gradually develops, urination of the bladder is controlled by the cerebral cortex and becomes a voluntary action. However, involuntary urination may be developed from dysfunction of the voluntary urination of the bladder, which results from functional disorders of the cerebral cortex caused by various causes. As to infants less than three years old who are mentally under development and growth, and have not developed a habit of regular urination, or children who play excessively in the daytime, or pre-school children who pass water occasionally at night, they are excluded in patients with enuresis.

In TCM, enuresis is mainly due to deficiency of kidney qi and asthenia-cold of the bladder, which fail in controlling the water passage, or splenopulmonary asthenia qi after illness, which fails to regulate the water passage and to control the bladder.

MAIN POINTS FOR DIAGNOSIS

The common clinical symptoms of the problem is that

八、遗尿

【概述】

遗尿是指 3 岁以上的小儿睡眠中不自主排尿的病症,男孩多见。现代医学认为排尿主要是由于中枢神经系统反射的作用,随着大脑皮层逐渐发育完善,膀胱排尿就由大脑皮层控制,成为随意的动作。但由各种原因引起的大脑皮质功能紊乱而造成膀胱随意性排尿功能失调,就会导致遗尿病症的发生。至于因智力未健,排尿正常习惯尚未养成的 3 岁以下的小儿,或因白天嬉戏过度,或学龄前儿童夜间偶有遗尿者,则不属病变。

中医认为遗尿多因肾气不足,膀胱虚冷,不能制约水道,或病后脾肺气虚,不能通调水道,约束膀胱所致。

【诊断要点】

临床常见症状有患儿经

the affected children often pass water involuntarily in sleep, once several nights in mild cases, and several times a night in severe cases. Enuresis commonly occurs at a relatively fixed time at night, usually before midnight. Enuresis is more likely to occur in patients who are over-excited in the daytime, or in overcast and rainy days.

（1）Patients with deficiency of kidney qi may be accompanied by symptoms such as pallor complexion, mental retardation, soreness and weakness in the lumbus and the knees, cold limbs, and clear and profuse urine.

（2）Patients with splenopulmonary asthenia qi manifest symptoms like insufficiency of qi with less speech, lassitude, spontaneous perspiration and night sweating, sallow complexion, poor appetite, and loose stools.

（3）Patients with damp-heat in the liver meridian have symptoms like irritability, restless sleep, flushed face and reddened lips, bitter taste in the mouth, preference for sighing, yellow and foul urine.

BASIC MANIPULATIONS

The principle of tuina therapy: warming and nourishing the spleen and the kidney, and strengthening the kidney to arrest enuresis.

Knead Dantian 100 times, rub-knead the umbilicus and the lower abdomen 100 times respectively, press-knead Sanyinjiao（SP 6）100 times, knead Shenshu（BL 23）100 times, press-knead Mingmen（GV 4）30 times, press-knead Ganshu（BL 18）50 times, knead Guiwei 100 times, pinch the spine 3 - 5 times, rub transversely the lumbosacral region for about one minute until a hot sensation is gained.

MODIFIED MANIPULATIONS WITH SYNDROME DIFFERENTIATION

（1）Patients with Insufficiency of Kidney Qi: Additionally push Shenjing 300 times, push Sanguan 100

常睡眠中不自主排尿，轻则数夜一次，重则一夜数次。遗尿常发生于晚上相对固定的时间，以上半夜较多。如白天过于兴奋，或阴雨天则更易发生遗尿。

（1）肾气不足者可伴面色㿠白，智力迟钝，腰膝酸软，四肢欠温，小便清长。

（2）肺脾气虚者可伴少气懒言，四肢疲倦，自汗盗汗，面色苍黄少华，胃纳欠佳，大便溏薄。

（3）肝经湿热者可伴性情急躁，睡眠不宁，面赤唇红，口苦，喜叹息，小便黄臊。

【基本治法】

推拿治疗原则是温补脾肾，固涩下元。

揉丹田 100 次，摩揉脐部和小腹部各 100 次，按揉三阴交 100 次，揉肾俞 100 次，按揉命门 30 次，按揉肝俞 50 次，揉龟尾 100 次，捏脊 3～5 遍，横擦腰骶部约 1 分钟，以温热为度。

【随症加减】

（1）肾气不足者，加推肾经 300 次，推三关 100 次，按揉

times, and press-knead Yongquan (KI 1) 100 times.

(2) Patients with Splenopulmonary Asthenia Qi: Additionally press-knead Baihui (BL 9) 100 times, push Pijing 300 times, push Feijing 300 times, knead Wailaogong (EX-UE 8) 50 times, and push Sanguan 100 times.

(3) Patients with Damp-heat in the Liver Meridian: Additionally clear Ganjing 100 times, clear Xiaochang 100 times, reduce Liufu 100 times, press-knead Taichong (LR 3) 50 times, and rub the hypochondrium 50 times.

The therapy is given once a day, and ten days form one treatment course. Usually, the problem needs 2 - 3 treatment courses or more.

Patient education should be given to those children with enuresis. Encourage them to establish self-confidence, and make them have no fear and tension so as to avoid affecting their physical and mental health. Meanwhile help the child patients to develop a habit of passing water regularly. Patients with enuresis should avoid overfatigue in the daytime, not get overexcited, not drink water or other fluids before going to bed. During sleeps, wake them up to pass water before their usual urination time.

4. 2. 9　Infantile Convulsion

INTRODUCTION

Infantile convulsion is also called clonic convulsion or eclampsia in TCM, and is one of the acute and serious diseases commonly seen in infants. Modern medicine believes that infants' central nervous system is under development; when they are infected to develop inflammation or stimulated by high fever, functional disorders of their cranial nerves will occur. Infantile convulsion is in fact a manifestation of this disorder.

In TCM, convulsion is divided as acute convulsion

涌泉 100 次。

（2）肺脾气虚者，加按揉百会 100 次，推脾经 300 次，推肺经 300 次，揉外劳宫 50 次，推三关 100 次。

（3）肝经湿热者，加清肝经 100 次，清小肠 100 次，退六腑 100 次，按揉太冲 50 次，搓胁肋 50 次。

推拿每日 1 次，10 天为 1 个疗程。治疗常需 2～3 个疗程或更多。

对遗尿患儿应注意耐心教育，鼓励其建立自信心，勿使患儿产生恐惧紧张感，以致影响身心健康。注意培养患儿按时排尿的习惯。遗尿患儿，白天应避免其过度疲劳；临睡前不使其过度兴奋及不给饮水和其他流质，睡中应按其平素遗尿的时间，提前唤醒，让其小便。

九、惊风

【概述】

惊风又称抽风、惊厥，是小儿常见的急重病症之一。现代医学认为，该病是因小儿中枢神经系统发育不完全，每在感染炎症或高热刺激时而出现的脑神经功能紊乱的一种表现。

中医认为惊风可分为急、

and chronic convulsion. Acute convulsion chiefly results from invasion of six exogenous pathogenic factors, which transform heat into wind to cause the disease, or from accumulated milk and food, or excessive accumulation of phlegm-heat which lead to disorder of qi activity and further obstruction of the upper orifices. Chronic convulsion is developed from acute convulsion when it is not treated promptly, or caused by sudden fright, or occur after illness when infants are weak with excessive consumption of fluids and blood, which deprive their muscles, tendons and vessels of nourishment.

MAIN POINTS FOR DIAGNOSIS

Common symptoms of convulsion are contracture and spasm of the limbs and unconsciousness.

1. Acute Convulsion   It is manifested as high fever, flushed face, reddened lips, short breath, flapping of ala nasi, restlessness and irritability, tearless cry; further there will be loss of consciousness, up-staring of the eyes, clenching teeth, rigidity of the spine and the back, convulsion of the limbs and continuous tremor.

2. Chronic Convulsion   Symptoms are pallor complexion, lethargy, listlessness, clenched fists, intermittent attacks of powerless convulsion. Sometimes convulsion occurs suddenly in deep sleep, with extremely cold limbs.

BASIC MANIPULATIONS

The general principle of tuina therapy is relieving convulsion and inducing resuscitation.

(1) Nip Renzhong (GV 26), grasp Hegu (LI 4), nip Duanzheng, and nip Shixuan (EX-UE 11) in turn until the patient regains consciousness.

(2) Grasp Jianjing (GB 21), Weizhong (BL 40) and Chengshan (BL 57) in turn until convulsion stops.

慢惊风两种,急惊风多由感受六淫外邪,化热生风,或由乳食积滞,痰热内壅,进而导致气机逆乱,清窍蒙蔽而发病。慢惊风则由急惊风延误失治或突受惊吓,病后体虚,津血耗伤,筋脉失养而致。

【诊断要点】

惊风常见的共同症状是肢体抽搐、痉挛、神志不清等。

1. 急惊风型   多见高热,面红唇赤,气急鼻翕,烦躁不安,啼无涕泪,进而神志昏迷,两目上视,牙关紧闭,脊背强直,四肢抽搐,颤动不已。

2. 慢惊风型   多见面色苍白,嗜睡无神,两手握拳,抽搐无力,时作时止,有时可在沉睡中突发痉挛,四肢厥冷。

【基本治法】

推拿治疗惊风的总的原则是开窍镇惊。

(1) 掐人中、拿合谷、掐端正、掐十宣,各穴轮换操作,以清醒为度。

(2) 拿肩井、拿委中、拿承山,各穴轮换操作,以搐止为度。

(3) Clear Feijing, push-knead Danzhong (CV 17), Tiantu (CV 22) and Zhongwan (CV 12) 30 - 50 times respectively.

(4) Press-knead Zusanli (ST 36), and digitally-press Fenglong (ST 40) for 1 - 3 minutes respectively.

MODIFIED MANIPULATIONS WITH SYNDROME DIFFERENTIATION

（1）Acute Convulsion：Additionally grasp Fengchi (GB 20) 30 - 50 times, push-scrape downward Tianzhugu 100 - 300 times, perform manipulation of Qingtianheshui 100 times, and reduce Liufu 100 times.

（2）Chronic Convulsion：Additionally rub the abdomen clockwise and counterclockwise 100 - 300 times respectively, reinforce Pijing 100 times, clear Ganjing 100 times, reinforce Shenjing 100 times, push Sanguan 100 times, and pinch the spine 3 - 5 times.

Convulsion, especially acute convulsion, has a sudden and violent attack. If treated improperly, it will cause anoxia in the brain tissues and local parts of the body that may lead to sequelae. In even worse cases it may bring about asphyxia, and cause respiratory and circulatory failures. Therefore, "quick dealing with" is emphasized in its treatment. When infantile convulsion attacks, first use tuina therapy for emergency treatment, then send the patient to a hospital for further treatment.

4.2.10　Night Crying

INTRODUCTION

If the infant is normal in the daytime, but cries intermittently or continuously at night, and even the whole night, or cries at certain fixed times every night, it is called night crying. It is often observed in infants under six months old. Modern medicine holds that the infantile

---

（3）清肺经、推揉膻中、天突、中脘各 30～50 次。

（4）按揉足三里，点按丰隆各 1～3 分钟。

【随症加减】

（1）急惊风，加拿风池 30～50 次，向下推刮天柱骨 100～300 次，清天河水 100 次，退六腑 100 次。

（2）慢惊风，加顺、逆时针摩腹各 100～300 次，补脾经、清肝经、补肾经各 100 次，推三关 100 次，捏脊 3～5 遍。

惊风尤其是急惊风，起病突然、凶猛，处理不当可使脑组织和局部机体缺氧，将留下后遗症，严重的甚至引起窒息，发生呼吸和循环衰竭。因此，在治疗中强调一个"快"字，所以遇到小儿发生惊风时，可用推拿方法先救急，赢得时间后，还应抓紧时间去医院诊治。

十、夜啼

【概述】

凡小儿白天如常，入夜啼哭，间歇发作或持续不已，甚则通宵达旦，或每夜定时啼哭者，称为夜啼。本症常见于 6 个月以内的婴儿。现代医学

nervous system is under development and growth, some diseases may cause dysfunction of the nervous system to induce night crying. It may also be because of improper nursing, such as hunger, stuffiness, bites of insects, wet napkin, or over-tightly wrapping.

In TCM, night crying is mainly derived from splenogastric asthenia cold and stagnation of qi activities or hyperactivity of heart fire and disturbance of the heart by pathogenic heat or retention of milk or food, which internally injures the spleen and stomach. Night crying may be induced by fright and fear which cause mental restlessness.

MAIN POINTS FOR DIAGNOSIS

The illness is characterized by infants' frequent night crying for no apparent reasons.

1. Syndrome of Splenogastric Asthenia Cold Symptoms include pallor, white or blue complexion, listlessness with frightened expression, cold limbs, crying in lower voice, coiled belly while crying, preference for pressing its abdomen with hands, crying stopped by warmth, or diarrhea.

2. Syndrome of Hyperactivity of Heart Fire It is manifested as flushed face and red eyes, restlessness, loud crying, aversion to lamp light, preference for lying in a supine position, constipation, short and dark urine.

3. Syndrome of Fright and Fear Symptoms are sudden pale or sudden blue complexion, restlessness due to fright, crying on hearing any sound or in dreams with tense and wretched voice, preference for sleep being carried in parents' arms.

4. Syndrome of Milk-food Retention Symptoms are anorexia and milk-vomiting, acid regurgitation, distending pain and fullness in the abdomen, sour stinking stools, and disturbed sleep.

认为小儿神经系统发育不完全,可能因一些疾病导致神经功能紊乱而造成夜啼的发生。也可因生后护理失宜,如饥饿、闷热、虫咬、尿布浸湿、包扎过紧等不适所引起。

中医认为夜啼多因脾胃虚寒,气机凝滞;心火过盛,邪热扰心;乳食积滞,内伤脾胃;或惊恐骇惧,心神不宁等所致。

【诊断要点】

本症以患儿常在夜间无明显诱因而哭闹不止为特点。

1. 脾胃虚寒型 症见面色㿠白或青,神怯困倦,四肢不温,啼哭声细,哭时曲腹,喜用手按其腹,得温则哭止,或有腹泻。

2. 心火过亢型 症见面红目赤,烦躁不安,哭声响亮,厌见灯光,喜仰卧,便秘,小便短赤。

3. 惊骇恐惧型 症见面色乍白乍青,惊惕不安,每闻响声而啼,或梦中啼哭,声惨而紧,喜家长抚抱而睡。

4. 乳食积滞型 症见厌食吐乳,嗳腐泛酸,腹痛胀满,大便酸臭,睡卧不安。

BASIC MANIPULATIONS

The principle of tuina therapy: strengthening the spleen, regulating flow of qi, and allaying fear to stop crying.

Open Tianmen 30 times, separate yinying of the hand 50 times, clear Xinjing 300 times, reinforce Shenjing 100 times, knead Erren Shangma 200 times, knead Neilaogong 200 times, nip-knead Xiaotianxin 50 times, press-knead Baihui（GV 20）100 times, and knead Erhougaogu 30 times, press-knead Xinshu（BL 15）, Feishu（BL 13）and Ganshu（BL 18）on both sides for one minute respectively.

MODIFIED MANIPULATIONS WITH SYNDROME DIFFERENTIATION

（1）Syndrome of Splenogastric Asthenia Cold: Additionally, reinforce Pijing 300 times, knead Wailaogong（EX-UE 8）50 times, push Sanguan 100 times, rub the abdomen for 5 minutes, and press-knead Pishu（BL 20）and Zusanli（ST 36）50 times respectively.

（2）Syndrome of Hyperactivity of Heart Fire: Additionally clear Xiaochang 300 times, clear Tianheshui 100 times, and reduce Liufu 100 times.

（3）Syndrome of Fright and Fear: Additionally, nip Ganjing, Xinjing and Jingning 5 times respectively.

（4）Syndrome of Milk-food Retention: Additionally clear Pijing 100 times, clear Dachang 300 times, knead Banmen 100 times, arc-push Neibagua 100 times, and push the lower Qijiegu 50 times.

This therapy is operated once a day, and five days form a treatment course. On treating the problem with tuina therapy, night crying caused by intussusception, diarrhea, or some infectious diseases should be excluded first.

The affected infants should be kept in a proper temperature condition so as not to catch cold. Take care of

【基本治法】

推拿治疗夜啼的原则是健脾理气,镇惊止啼。

开天门 30 次,分手部阴阳 50 次,清心经 300 次,补肾经 100 次,揉二人上马 200 次,揉内劳宫 200 次,掐揉小天心 50 次,按揉百会 100 次,揉耳后高骨 30 次,按揉双侧心俞、肺俞、肝俞各 1 分钟。

【随症加减】

（1）脾胃虚寒型,加补脾经 300 次,揉外劳宫 50 次,推三关 100 次,摩腹 5 分钟、按揉脾俞、足三里各 50 次。

（2）心火过亢型,加清小肠 300 次,清天河水 100 次,退六腑 100 次。

（3）惊骇恐惧型,加掐肝经、心经、精宁各 5 次。

（4）乳食积滞型,加清脾经 100 次,清大肠 300 次,揉板门 100 次,运内八卦 100 次,推下七节骨 50 次。

推拿每日 1 次,5 日为 1 个疗程。在推拿治疗本病时,应排除因肠套叠、腹泻和一些感染性疾病而引起的啼哭。

患儿平时应寒暖适宜,避免受凉。并注意饮食卫生,定

infants' dietary hygiene, and their regularly sucking in appropriate quantity.

4. 2. 11   Myogenic Torticollis

INTRODUCTION

Myogenic torticollis is a disease marked with the head deviated to one side. It is often seen in infants. In modern medicine, myogenic torticollis is mainly because of malposition of the fetus in the uterus, which causes pressure against the sternocleidomastoid muscle on one side and obstruction of blood circulation leading to ischemic fibrosis of the muscle. And it may also be due to malposition of the fetus during delivery, which causes the sternocleidomastoid muscle to be pressed by the birth canal or by obstetric forceps so as to be injured and bleed with formation of hematoma. It further develops into contracture due to organization of the hematoma, which results in the occurrence of myogenic torticollis. In TCM, the pathological mechanism of the deviated head lies in disorders of qi and blood, obstruction of the meridians, and stagnation of qi as well blood stasis.

MAIN POINTS FOR DIAGNOSIS

（1）After the affected baby is born, a fusiform mass on one side of his or her neck can be observed, (some may disappear voluntarily in half a year), later gradual contracture of the muscles on the affected side takes place, and finally protrudes like a cord.

（2）The head is deviated to the affected side and bends forward, while the face turns to the healthy side. Or even the asymmetric sides of the face develops, that is, the healthy side is relatively large while the affected side small.

（3）If treatment is not given to the problem for a long time, the cervical vertebrae may protrude to the

时适量喂奶。

十一、肌性斜颈

【概述】

肌性斜颈是头向一侧偏斜的病症，常见于婴幼儿。现代医学认为本病症的发生多是因胎儿在子宫内位置不良，使一侧胸锁乳突肌受压而血液循行受阻，引起该肌缺血性肌纤维变性；或因分娩时胎位不正，胎儿胸锁乳突肌受产道或产钳挤压致伤出血，血肿机化形成挛缩，而导致斜颈的发生。中医认为气血逆乱，经脉不通，气滞血瘀是斜颈的发病机制。

【诊断要点】

（1）患儿出生后，颈部一侧可发现有梭形肿物（有的经半年后，肿物可自行消退），以后患侧的颈部肌肉逐渐挛缩紧张，突出如条索状。

（2）头部向患侧偏斜、前倾，颜面偏向健侧。甚至出现两侧面部不对称，健侧大而患侧小。

（3）如长期不治，颈椎可凸向健侧，甚至胸椎也可有代

healthy side, and compensatory lateral curvature of the thoracic vertebrae and ambiopia may even develop.

BASIC MANIPULATIONS

The principle of tuina therapy: relaxing muscles and tendons, promoting circulation of blood, softening and resolving hard mass.

(1) Have the infant lie on his back at the edge of the bed, and his head direct at the doctor, and the doctor sits at a chair in front of the bed. Hold the neck of the patient with one hand, and press-knead the affected side of his neck with the thumb, or the index, the middle and the ring fingers for 5 - 10 minutes, combined with finger-twisting to disperse the swelling lump gently. Apply more manipulations to the beginning and the ending parts of the sternocleidomastoid muscle on the affected side.

(2) Gently lift and grasp the sternocleidomastoid muscle on the affected side for 1 - 3 minutes, then wipe and pluck the tendons on the affected side along their directions with the thumb and the index finger 10 - 15 times.

(3) Pull or rotate the patient's head toward the healthy side repeatedly several times. The manipulation should be performed first lightly, then gradually heavily with an increasing amplitude; sudden, violent exertion of force beyond the physiological limitation should be avoided.

(4) Finally perform pressing-kneading manipulation to relax the affected area for 3 - 5 minutes.

MODIFIED MANIPULATIONS WITH SYNDROME DIFFERENTIATION

If the patient has been troubled by myogenic torticollis for quite a long time, the two sides of the face have been different in size, and the affected side of the neck has been hard, the following manipulations may be added

偿性侧弯,并发生复视。

【基本治法】

推拿治疗斜颈的原则是舒筋活血、软坚消结。

(1) 让婴儿仰卧床边,头向医者,医者坐于床前椅上,一手托住患儿颈枕部,另一手用拇指或食、中、无名指在患侧颈部作按揉法5~10分钟,且可配合对肿块轻轻地捻散。推拿重点在患侧胸锁乳突肌的起止点。

(2) 轻柔地提拿患侧的胸锁乳突肌1~3分钟,再用拇、食指分向理抹、弹拨患处筋腱10~15次。

(3) 将患儿头向健侧扳动或旋转,反复数次。用此法时要由轻到重,幅度由小到大,切不可骤然暴力而超出正常生理限度。

(4) 再用按揉法放松局部3~5分钟。

【随症加减】

患儿斜颈病程日久,颜面两侧大小不等,患侧颈部坚硬,除基本方法外,再加:

to the basic ones.

　　（1）Digitally-knead Taiyang（EX-HN 5），Yintang（EX-HN 3）and Dicang（ST 4）on the affected side of the face for one minute respectively.

　　（2）Digitally-press Hegu（LI 4）and Waiguan（TE 5）for one minute respectively.

　　（3）Pluck Yinlingquan（SP 9）and Juegu（GB 39）10 times respectively.

The treatment of myogenic torticollis is usually given once a day，10 – 15 minutes each time. One treatment course takes a month，and the number of courses is in direct proportion to the hardness of the muscles on the affected side. The manipulation should couple hardness with gentleness，and violent operation mustn't be done. What's more，the media talcum is used to protect children's skin. While the infant is in sleep，intentionally have his head turn to the healthy side to correct the malformation.

4.2.12　Subluxation of Capitulum Radii in Children

INTRODUCTION

It differs from the general dislocation of joints. It is only the smaller head of the radius that dislocates from its normal position，and no fissure of joint capsules occurs. The problem is often seen in children under six years old.

The head and the annular ligament of the radius in children are still under growth，excessively pulling children's forearms will easily cause the head of radius to slip out from its annular ligament，leading to its semi-dislocation. This disease often occurs when children play games arm-in-arm，and when their parents dress them，or lead them to walk，pulling their forearms with too much

　　（1）指揉患侧面部太阳、印堂、地仓穴各 1 分钟。

　　（2）点按合谷、外关各 1 分钟。

　　（3）弹拨阴陵泉、绝骨各 10 次。

　　推拿手法治疗斜颈，一般可每日治疗 1 次，每次 10～15 分钟，每 1 个月为 1 个疗程。推拿疗程的多少，与患侧肌肉的硬度成正相关。治疗时手法要刚柔相济，但忌粗暴，并用滑石粉作为介质以保护患儿皮肤。患儿睡眠时有意使儿头向健侧转动以帮助矫正畸形。

十二、小儿桡骨头半脱位

【概述】

　　小儿桡骨头半脱位与一般关节脱位不同，仅是桡骨小头离开了正常位置，并无关节囊破裂。多见于 6 岁以下儿童。

　　小儿桡骨头和桡骨环状韧带发育不全，若过度牵拉小儿前臂，易使桡骨头从环状韧带中滑出引起桡骨头半脱位。本病多在小儿手拉手游戏、家长给小儿穿衣或领小儿走路时过度牵拉前臂而发生。

force.

MAIN POINTS FOR DIAGNOSIS

（1）The patient has a history of getting his forearm pulled excessively.

（2）After the problem happens to him or her, the child will cry continuously and become restless. The affected arm dare not move, but rest beside the body, and the forearm is in a pronation position.

（3）There is local pain and tenderness, but no obvious swelling.

BASIC MANIPULATIONS

The principle of tuina therapy is mainly regulating muscles and tendons and getting reposition of the affected part.

Hold the elbow of the affected side with one hand and the thumb pressing on the head of the radius, hold the wrist of the affected side with the other hand, overextend the forearm slightly, then rotate it backwards (rotating forwards is needed in some patients), and finally flex the elbow joint of the affected side, reposition will be achieved. After reposition, hang up the affected side with a triangular bandage to benefit the restoration of the affected arm.

Usually, be careful not to pull children's upper limbs forcefully.

4.2.13 Myopia

INTRODUCTION

Myopia refers to the poor distant vision, and is one of the common ophthalmic diseases.

In modern medicine, myopia occurs mostly in the adolescent. Besides some with hereditary factors, most of them are related to the poor illuminating light, or bad reading habit, which causes the axis of the eyeball to be

【诊断要点】

（1）有牵拉前臂史。

（2）小儿桡骨头半脱位后哭闹不安,患肢不敢活动而垂于体侧,前臂呈旋前位。

（3）局部疼痛和压痛,但无明显肿胀。

【基本治法】

推拿治疗以理筋复位为主。

医者一手握住患儿的患侧肘部,以拇指压在桡骨头处,另一手握住患侧腕部,将前臂微微过伸和旋后(有的患者须旋前),然后将患侧肘关节屈曲即可复位。复位后,可用三角巾悬吊,以利恢复。

平时注意不要过于用力牵拉小儿上肢。

十三、近视

【概述】

近视系指远视力不好,是常见的一种眼科病症。

现代医学认为,近视的发生多在青少年时期,除部分有遗传因素外,大部分与灯光照明欠佳、看书习惯不良等有

lengthened and ametropia, leading to the converged focus of the parallel rays resting before the retina. In TCM, myopia was called "symptom of normal vision in short distance, but poor in long distance" in ancient times, which is mainly due to congenital deficiency, insufficiency of liver blood and kidney essence unable to supply the eyes and maintain normal vision.

MAIN POINTS FOR DIAGNOSIS

(1) Long-distance vague vision.

(2) Symptoms such as distension of the eyes, headache, ophthalmokopia will also appear after short-distance vision for a long time.

BASIC MANIPULATIONS

The principle of tuina therapy: nourishing the liver and the kidney, and dredging the meridians in the eye area.

(1) The child patient sits or lies on his back, the doctor pushes with one-finger manipulation from Yintang (EX-HN 3) to Shenting (GV 24) back and forth 3 - 5 times.

(2) The patient sits or lies on his back, the doctor pushes with one-finger manipulation from Yintang (EX-HN 3) to Taiyang (EX-HN 5) first to the left one, then to the right one 3 - 5 times.

(3) Push with one-finger manipulation around the orbits in a "∞" way 3 times.

(4) Press-knead Cuanzhu (BL 2), Jingming (BL 1), Yuyao (EX-HN 4), Chenqi (ST 1), Sibai (ST 2), Tongziliao (GB 1) and other points around the eyes for one minute respectively.

(5) Wipe the superior and the inferior orbits 10 - 20 times respectively.

(6) Grasp-pinch or press-knead Hegu (LI 4) and Fengchi (GB 20) 30 times each.

关,导致眼球的前后轴拉长而屈光不正,造成平行光线结成的聚光点落在眼视网膜之前。中医古称近视为"能近怯远症",认为主要由于先天禀赋欠强,肝血肾精不足,不能贯注于目而导致光华不能发越。

【诊断要点】

(1) 远视时视物模糊。

(2) 近视过久亦会出现眼胀、头痛、视力疲劳等症状。

【基本治法】

推拿治疗的原则是补益肝肾,疏通眼络。

(1) 患儿坐或仰卧,医者以一指禅推从印堂开始推到神庭,来回3~5遍。

(2) 患儿坐或仰卧,医者以一指禅推从印堂开始推到太阳,先左后右,来回 3~5遍。

(3) 用一指禅推沿"∞"绕眼眶推3遍。

(4) 按揉攒竹、睛明、鱼腰、承泣、四白、瞳子髎等眼周穴位各1分钟。

(5) 抹眼眶上下各10~20次。

(6) 拿捏或按揉合谷、风池穴各30次。

(7) The patient is in a prone position, press-knead Ganshu (BL 18) and Shenshu (BL 23) 50 times respectively.

(8) Shake the neck leftward and rightward slightly 3 - 5 times, and twist the neck gently leftward and rightward once each, and sounds are not necessarily made.

MODIFIED MANIPULATIONS WITH SYNDROME DIFFERENTIATION

If myopia with long-distance vague vision and fatigue in short-distance vision is accompanied by pain in the orbits and forehead, additionally digitally-press Yiming (EX-HN 13) 50 times, nip-press Duanzheng 100 times, reinforce Shenjing and Ganjing 300 times each.

The therapy is given once a day. After treatment, the doctor directs the patient to rotate his eyes toward one side along the orbits 18 times with his hand, then another 18 times toward the opposite side. Next ask the patient to stare as far as possible, and then look at the nearby area. Repeat the operation several times.

The patient should pay attention to the hygiene of utilizing his eyes, improve nutrition, and treat saprodontia, etc. thoroughly.

4. 2. 14　Infantile Health Care

Infantile tuina for health care is an effective method to prevent diseases. In the Tang dynasty, there was a record in the great medical book —"*Prescriptions Worth a Thousand Gold*"(Qianjinyaofang) written by Sun Simiao, a famous doctor. It says "Even though infants are not sick, massage with ointments can often be performed on their fontanel, palms, and soles in the early morning, which really has the effect in protecting infants from cold wind. " Therefore, it is evident that tuina is also of significance in infants' health care and prevention of diseases.

（7）患者俯卧，按揉肝俞、肾俞穴各 50 次。

（8）轻轻摇动颈椎左右各 3～5 次，左右轻扳各 1 次，不要追求响声。

【随症加减】

若见远视模糊，近视视力疲劳严重，伴眼眶、前额疼痛者，加点按翳明穴 50 次，掐按端正 100 次，补肾经、补肝经各 300 次。

推拿操作，每日 1 次，结束操作后，医者可以手引导患者双眼球先向一侧沿眼眶转动 18 周，然后再向相反方向转动 18 周。继而尽量远眺凝视，收视近处，反复数次结束。

患者应注意用眼卫生，加强营养，积极根治龋齿等病症。

十四、小儿保健

小儿推拿保健是一种有效的预防疾病的方法。远在唐朝名医孙思邈的著作《千金要方》中就有："小儿虽无病，早起常以膏摩囟上及手足心，甚辟寒风"的记载。可见运用推拿对小儿预防保健同样重要。

Methods of infantile tuina for health care are simple, convenient and effective, and acceptable to infants. They are also easy to be spread and popularized. Now several sets of commonly used tuina methods for infants' health care are introduced in the following.

4. 2. 14. 1 Methods for Health Care and Building Up the Constitution

MANIPULATIONS Press-knead Zhongwan (CV 12) for 3 minutes, rub the abdomen for 3 minutes, press-knead Zusanli (ST 36) on both sides 50 times each, and pinch the spine 3 - 5 times.

Usually this therapy is given in the morning or on an empty stomach, once a day. It has to stop when some acute diseases occur, and resumes after the infant recovers.

ACTIONS The therapy has the effect of strengthening the spleen and regulating the stomach, improving appetite, bettering the physique, and promoting growth and development.

4. 2. 14. 2 Methods for Preventing Common Cold

MANIPULATIONS Rub both palms against each other till they become hot, and scrub the face with the hot palms 80 times or until the cheeks become hot. Press Yingxiang (LI 20) 30 times with a finger, push-rub the chest and the back 3 - 5 times each, press-knead Hegu (LI 4) 30 times, and knead Wailaogong (EX-UE 8) 100 - 300 times.

This therapy is to be operated once a day, or twice a day when influenza is popularly spreading. While rubbing the chest or the back, put some sesame oil or talcum on these areas. Meanwhile catching cold should be avoided during treatment.

ACTIONS The therapy has effects of dispersing

小儿推拿保健方法,简便有效,小儿乐于接受,易于普及推广。现介绍几套常用的小儿推拿保健方法。

(一)强身保健法

【操作方法】 按揉中脘3分钟,摩腹3分钟,按揉双侧足三里各50次,捏脊3~5遍。

该法一般宜在清晨或空腹时进行,每天操作1次。患急性病期间可暂停,待愈后再恢复进行。

【作用】 健脾和胃,增进食欲,强壮身体,促进发育。

(二)预防感冒保健法

【操作方法】 搓掌(以双手掌对搓发热为度),趁掌热擦面80次(或面颊发热即止),指揉迎香穴30次,推擦胸背各3~5遍,按揉合谷30次,揉外劳宫100~300次。

本法可每日操作1次。流感严重流行时,可每日2次。擦胸背时可蘸少许麻油,或医用滑石粉等,注意防止受凉。

【作用】 宣肺利窍,通阳

lung qi and smoothing the orifices, activating yang and consolidating the exterior, and preventing the occurrence of common cold and bronchitis.

4.2.14.3 Methods for Protection of the Eyes

MANIPULATIONS Wipe the forehead with index fingers or separating-push the forehead from above Yintang (EX-HN 3) to both the sides 30 times. Press-knead Zanzhu (BL 2), Jingming (BL 1), the middle point of the brows, Tongziliao (GB 1) and Sibai (ST 2) 30 times respectively. Knead-wipe the orbits 30 times.

Usually these manipulations are performed after ophthalmokopia, such as after infants' learning, small children's reading, or watching TV.

ACTIONS They have the effects of dredging the meridians, activating circulation of qi and blood, relieving fatigue of the ocular muscles, regulating the vision, and preventing myopia.

The manipulations of infantile tuina for health care can be taught to operate by older children. Infants or those small children who have difficulty in performing these manipulations can be performed with their parents' help.

固表;预防感冒、支气管炎。

(三)眼保健法

【操作方法】 以示指抹前额或从印堂穴上分推前额 30 次,按揉攒竹、睛明、鱼腰、瞳子髎、四白各 30 次,揉抹眼眶 30 次。

本法一般可在用眼疲劳后进行,如幼儿教育、少儿学习后或收看电视节目后操作。

【作用】 疏经活络,运行气血;解除眼肌疲劳和调节视力,防止近视。

小儿推拿保健方法,年长儿童可教嘱自行操作,有困难的或婴幼儿也可由家长帮助进行。

5 Self-tuina

第五章　自我推拿

Tuina by using simple manipulations such as pushing, grasping, pressing, rubbing, kneading, thumping with one's own hands on certain points and particular areas of the body surface to attain the purpose of health care, rehabilitation and treating diseases is known as self-tuina. As an important component of Chinese tuina, self-tuina functions mainly because the stimulations generated by self-performed manipulations activate one's meridian points and the qi and blood systems to exert therapeutic effects. Meanwhile self-tuina process itself is actually an active exercise. Therefore, a satisfactory result will certainly be gained if one selects correct points and areas to be treated in accordance with syndrome differentiation and his individual health conditions, and conducts self-tuina therapy carefully, progressively and persistently.

Self-tuina therapy can be done in a sitting, standing or lying position as one's condition requires. The practitioner of self-tuina should perform manipulations calmly and attentively, breathe naturally, but not hold his breath. He should also take a proper posture, get manipulations, strength, mental activities and qi flow well-coordinated, viz. the mind and will should follow the movements of the hand to the manipulated areas, meanwhile coordinating with breath, direct qi in his mind to the meridians and points in the treated area. When manipulations like pressing are performed, force exerted should first be light, then gradually become heavy until one feels qi-arrival with a sore and distending sensation at the

通过自己的双手,采用推、拿、按、摩、揉、捶等简单手法在自身体表经穴与特定部位进行推拿,以达到保健、养生及治疗疾病的方法称为自我推拿。自我推拿是中国推拿的重要组成部分,它主要是因为自我手法的刺激,激发了自身的经穴、气血系统而发挥治疗作用的;同时,自我推拿的操作过程,本身也是一种主动的运动锻炼。所以,只要根据自身的具体情况,辨证地选择好治疗经穴与部位,认真操作,循序渐进,持之以恒地进行自我推拿,一定会取得理想的功效。

自我推拿在施术时,可根据自身的健康状态,选取坐位、站位或卧位。操作时要心平气和、精神集中,呼吸自然,不要憋气,在正确的体位下做到"手"到、"力"到、"心"到、"气"到,即要求意念也要随着手的动作转移至操作部位,并配合呼吸将"气"在意想中输送到受术部位的经穴。在施行按压类手法时,用力先轻渐重,以经穴处有酸胀等得气感

meridian points. When manipulations of circular rubbing or to-and-fro rubbing (Mofa or Cafa) are performed, the hands and the skin in the treated areas should be kept dry. Talcum powder or some other media may be applied if there is sweat. The force exerted should be proper, and the manipulations are operated until a warm or hot sensation is attained in the local area. Too heavy force and too long time of rubbing should be avoided, in case the skin is scratched. Self-tuina is usually conducted twice a day, one in the morning and the other in the evening; 20 - 30 minutes each time are enough.

At the initial stage of practicing self-tuina, general fatigue, especially aching pain and other discomforts in the hands may occur after doing massage for some time, which is a normal phenomenon because one's physical strength is not adaptabe to it. However, as one's manipulations become skillful, physical strength improves and exercises are bettered, these discomforts will voluntarily disappear, and one will feel warm all over the body, and light-hearted and relaxed mentally and physically if one sticks to practising self-tuina. What's more, as long as the joints in one's two upper extremities function normally, and after some time of practice, one will be able to perform self-tuina freely on any parts of his body.

The manipulations of local self-tuina and the commonly used manipulations of expectant self-tuina are briefly introduced in the following two sections of this chapter.

5. 1　Local Self-tuina

5. 1. 1　Self-tuina on the Head and the Face

MANIPULATIONS

1. Pushing the Forehead on Either Side Separately

为宜；在做摩擦类手法时，手与受术处皮肤要保持干燥，如有汗水可搽些爽身粉或使用介质，用力要适中，手法以局部产生温热感为度，不要加力太重，摩擦太久，以免擦破皮肤。自我推拿一般每日早、晚各做 1 次，每次在 20～30 分钟即可。

自我推拿在开始时，由于体力不适应，往往在做后觉得全身疲乏，特别是施术的双手会出现酸痛等不适感，这是正常现象。只要坚持进行，随着手法的熟练、体力的增长与功夫的长进，不但这些不适感会自行消失，而且还可在行功后感到通体温热，身心轻松愉快。再者，只要两个上肢的各个关节的运动功能基本正常，通过锻炼便可在自己身体的任何部位自由地进行自我推拿。

本章将分两节简要介绍人体各部自我推拿方法和五脏自我推拿方法。

第一节　分部推拿法

一、头面部

【操作方法】

1. 分推前额　以印堂至

Starting from the midline of the forehead, which runs from Yintang (EX-HN 3) to the anterior hairline, push from below to above with the radial sides of the second knuckle of the two bent index fingers towards the left and right Sizhukong (TE 23), Taiyang (EX-HN 5) and Touwei (ST 8) respectively 30 – 50 times.

2. Wiping the Temples　Press the temples forcefully with the whorled surfaces of the thumbs, and push forward and backward repeatedly about 30 times until a sore and distending sensation is generated.

3. Pressing-kneading the Back of the Head　Press Fengchi (GB 20) with the whorled surfaces or the tip of the thumbs tightly 10 times or more, then press-knead them rotationally, and finally press-knead the point Naokong (GB19) or Naohoukong (GB 19) for about 80 times until a sore and distending sensation is generated.

4. Patting the Vertex　Sitting upright with the eyes looking straight ahead, the teeth clenched, pat the fontanel area rhythmically with the palm about 10 times.

5. Rubbing the Face with the Hot Palms Generated by Rubbing (Cuoshouyumian)　Rub the hands against each other to get them hot first, put the palms closely against the forehead, rub-scrape forcefully downward to the mandible, push along the inferior margins of the mandible outward to Jiache (ST 6), continuing upward through the preauricular areas and the temples to the midline of the forehead. This procedure is to be repeated 20 – 30 times until a hot sensation on the face is achieved.

ACTIONS　It functions in invigorating the brain, improving intelligence and tranquilizing the mind. It proves to be effective in prevention and treatment of headache, dizziness, insomnia, amnesia, neurosis and facial paralysis.

前发际正中之连线为中线,两手食指屈成弓状,用第二指节的桡侧面为着力面,由下而上,自中线向前额两侧分别推至丝竹空、太阳、头维穴处,约30～50次左右。

2. 双抹两颞　以两手拇指螺纹面,紧按两侧鬓角处,由前向后反复用力推抹,约30次左右,以酸胀为宜。

3. 按揉脑后　以两拇指螺纹或指端,紧按风池穴,先用力按压10余次,再作旋转按揉,随后再按揉脑后空穴约80次左右,以酸胀为宜。

4. 拍击头顶　人正坐,眼睛睁开前视,牙齿咬紧,用手掌心在囟门穴处做有节律的拍击动作,约10次左右。

5. 搓手浴面　先将两手搓热,随后掌心紧贴前额,用力向下擦刮下颌,再沿下颌下缘向外至颊车,再向上经耳前、鬓角转推至前额中间,如此反复旋转推摩面颊,每次约20～30遍左右,以面部有热感为宜。

【作用】　健脑、益智、安神,可防治头痛、头晕、失眠、健忘、神经衰弱、面瘫等病症。

5.1.1.3　ADDITIONAL MANIPULATIONS

1. Health Care of the Eyes with Self-tuina

(1) Kneading Cuanzhu (BL 2): Place the whorled surfaces of the thumbs on Cuanzhu (BL 2) in the depressions proximal to the medial end of the eyebrows, and knead them with gradually-increasing force about 20 times until a sensation of soreness and distension is achieved.

(2) Kneading Jingming (BL 1): Put the whorled surface of the thumb and the index finger of the right hand respectively on the two points of Jingming (BL 1), which is located in the depression 0.1 cun above the inner canthus. Press downward forcefully and then pinch upward. Repeat the operation 20–30 times.

(3) Pressing-kneading Sibai (ST 2): Place the whorled surfaces of the index fingers on Sibai (ST 2), 1 cun below the midpoint of the lower orbit respectively, and press-knead about 20 times until a sore and distending sensation is generated.

(4) Scraping the Orbits: Bend the two index fingers, apply the radial surfaces of the second knuckles to the internal ends of the upper orbits, rub and wipe outward to either external end. Then do the same to the lower orbits. Repeat the manipulations about 20–30 times.

(5) "Ironing" the Eyes: Shut the eyes slightly, rub the hands against each other to get them hot, tenderly press and iron the eyes with the palmar bases for 30 seconds, and then knead them gently about 10 times.

(6) Kneading Taiyang (EX-HN 5): Place the whorled surfaces of the thumbs at the points Taiyang (EX-HN 5) on both sides of the face tightly, and press and knead them repeatedly about 30 times until a sore and distending sensation is achieved.

【附】

1. 眼部保健

加① 揉攒竹。以双手拇指螺纹面,分别按在双眉内侧头凹陷处的攒竹穴处,由轻而重反复轻揉约 20 次左右,以酸胀为宜。

② 揉睛明。以右手拇、食二指螺纹面,揉压在两目内眦角上0.1 cm凹陷中之睛明穴,先用力向下按压;然后向上挤捏,如此一按一挤,反复进行,每次约20～30 遍左右。

③ 按揉四白。以双手食指螺纹面,分别按在眼下眶正中下 1 寸处的四白穴,反复按揉20 次左右,以酸胀为宜。

④ 刮眼轮。双手食指屈曲,以第二指节的桡侧面紧贴上眼眶的内侧端,自内向外推抹至眼眶的外侧端,然后再如此推抹下眼眶,如此先上后下,自内向外反复刮推约20～30 次。

⑤ 熨眼。双目轻闭,先将两掌搓热,用双手掌根处轻压热熨双目 30 秒钟,再轻轻揉动 10 余次。

⑥ 揉太阳。以两手拇指螺纹面紧贴双侧太阳穴处,反复按揉 30 次左右,以酸胀为宜。

These manipulations can be used to treat and prevent myopia, blurred vision, glaucoma, optic atrophy and other eye diseases.

2. Health Care of the Nose Area with Selftuina

(1) Pressing-kneading Yingxiang (LI 20): Press Yingxiang (LI 20) on both sides of the nose with the whorled surfaces of the middle fingers, and press and knead them forcefully and repeatedly about 30 times until a sore and distending sensation is generated.

(2) Palm-twisting and Rubbing Both Sides of the Nose: Rub the palmar surfaces of the index or the middle fingers against each other till they become hot. Then put them immediately on the nasolabial grooves, palm-twist and rub up and down to get them hot. Do the operation about 30 times each time.

The manipulations are proved to be effective in preventing and treating common cold, nasal obstruction, nasal discharge, allergic or chronic rhinitis, and paranasal sinusitis, etc.

3. Health Care of the Ear Area with Self-tuina

(1) Pressing-kneading the Points Around the Ears: Press-knead the points around the ears, Ermen (TE 21), Tinggong (SJ 19), Tinghui (GB 2), Yifeng (TE 17) and others, with the tips of the thumb or the middle finger about 20 times each until a sore and distending sensation is generated.

(2) Rubbing the Helix: Pinch the helices gently with the whorled surfaces of the thumbs and the radial surfaces of the bow-curved index fingers, do kneading and rubbing up and down repeatedly about 20 - 30 times.

(3) Making Sounds in the Ears (Mingtiangu): Cover the two ears with the two palms, get the palmar bases directing forward and the fingers pointing backward, and

可防治近视眼、视物不清、青光眼、视神经萎缩等各种目疾。

2. 鼻部保健

加① 按揉迎香。以两手中指螺纹面，按压在双侧迎香穴处，用力反复按揉30次左右，以酸胀为宜。

② 搓擦鼻旁。先将两手食指或中指掌面相对搓热，趁热在鼻翼两侧的鼻唇沟处，上、下搓擦，以热为宜。每次擦30次左右。

可防治感冒、鼻塞流涕、过敏性鼻炎、慢性鼻炎、副鼻窦炎等病症。

3. 耳部保健

加① 按揉耳周诸穴。以双手拇指端或中指端为着力点，分别按揉耳周围的耳门、听宫、听会与翳风等穴，每穴按揉20次左右，以酸胀为宜。

② 摩擦耳轮。以双手拇指螺纹面与屈曲成弓状的食指桡侧面，轻轻捏住两侧耳轮，上下反复摩擦20～30次左右。

③ 鸣天鼓。以两手掌心掩住两耳孔，掌根在前，手指指向脑后，用食指搭在中指

the index fingers on the middle fingers. Flick-hit the protruded bones behind the ears with the index fingers about 20 times to produce booming sounds in the ears.

(4) Palm-twisting and Rubbing the Area in Front of the Ear: With the radial surface of the thumb or the palmar aspect of the index finger, rub and palm-twist the parts in front of the ears upward or downward repeatedly about 30 times until they become hot.

This operation can be used to treat and prevent tinnitus, dysacousis, deafness and otitis media.

5.1.2　Self-tuina on the Neck and Nape

MANIPULATIONS

(1) Pushing Fengchi (GB 20) and Dazhui (GV 14): Press-knead from Fengchi (GB 20) on both sides downward, via Tianzhu (BL 10) to the base of the neck with the tips of the index, the middle and the ring fingers of the two hands 5 - 10 times. Then press-knead from Fengfu (GV 16) downward to Dazhui (GV 14) with the tips of the index, the middle and the ring fingers of one hand 5 - 10 times. While getting to each point, have a stop and press-knead it 20 - 30 times.

(2) Pressing-kneading the Points on the Neck and Nape: Extend the middle finger of one hand backward to the back of the opposite side, and press-knead Dazhui (GV 14), Dazhu (BL 11), Shenzhu (GV 12), Fengmen (BL 12), Feishu (BL 13) each about 30 times until a sensation of soreness and distention is achieved. Then exchange the hand to do the same operation on the other side.

(3) Pushing Qiaogong: Push and wipe the right Qiaogong with the radial side or the whorled surface of the right thumb from the mastoid process behind the right ear downward, along the sternocleidomastoid muscle to point Quepen (ST 12). The whole process is repeated up and

上,向下弹击耳后高骨 20 次左右,使耳中隆隆作响。

④ 搓擦耳前。以双手拇指桡侧,或食指掌面,紧贴在耳前,由上而下、由下而上的反复搓擦约 30 次左右,以热为宜。

可防治耳鸣、重听、耳聋、中耳炎等病症。

二、颈项部

【操作方法】

(1) 推风池、大椎　先以双手食、中、无名指端,沿双侧风池向下,经天柱至项根按揉 5～10 遍左右;再以一手食、中、无名指端,自风府向下至大椎穴按揉 5～10 遍,在穴位处稍停按揉 20～30 次左右。

(2) 按揉颈项部穴位　用一手中指向后伸向对侧背后,按揉大椎、大杼、身柱、风门、肺俞等穴,每穴按揉 30 次左右,以酸胀为宜,左右交换。

(3) 推桥弓　先用右手拇指桡侧或螺纹面推右侧桥弓穴,自右耳后乳突处向下,沿胸锁乳突肌推至缺盆穴处,如此由上向下推抹 10 次;然后

down 10 times. Then do the same operation to the left Qiaogong with the left thumb.

(4) Pounding Jianjing (GB 21): Sit or stand and keep the upper body straight, clench the hand and pound Jianjing (GB 21) on the opposite side with it 20 - 30 times. Then do the same to the other Jianjing (GB 21) with the other hand.

(5) Rubbing Gaohuang (BL 43): Keep the upper body erect, abduct the two upper limbs to the horizontal level, and flex the elbows. Do the rotating movements of the shoulder joints, and make them extend backward as much as possible so as to use the encircling movements of the scapula to stimulate Gaohuang (BL 43) and other points on the interscapular regions on both sides.

(6) Rotating the Head: Slowly rotate and shake the cervical vertabrae clockwise with an increasing amplitude 10 times. Then rotate and shake it counterclockwise with the same requirements.

(7) Grasping-pinching the Cervical Muscles: Grasp-pinch the cervical muscles downward from the level of Fengchi (GB 20) to the level of Dazhui (GV 14) with the thumb and the whorled surfaces of the rest four fingers of one hand in a way of oppositely exerting force 10 - 20 times. Then grasp-pinch with both hands the muscles in the shoulder regions of the two sides in the same way 10 - 20 times.

ACTIONS These manipulations have the effects of relaxing the muscles and tendons, activating the meridians, lubricating the joints, bringing down blood pressure, relieving asthma, eliminating chest stuffiness and regulating flow of qi. They can be used to treat and prevent pain, soreness and distension in the back, cervical spondylopathy, stiff neck, cough, asthma, phlegm accumula-

用左手拇指推抹左侧桥弓,方法同前。

(4)捶击肩井 正坐或直立,上身挺直,一手握成空拳捶击对侧肩井穴 20～30 次,再以另一手用捶击另一侧肩井。

(5)摩膏肓 上身挺直,两上肢外展至水平位置,屈肘。作肩关节的环转动作,并尽量增大向后的伸展幅度,以利用肩胛骨的环转动作来刺激位于两侧肩胛间区的膏肓等穴。

(6)摇头晃脑 先按顺时针方向转摇颈椎 10 次,速度要慢,幅度由小渐大;然后按逆时针方向转摇颈椎 10 次,要求同前。

(7)拿捏项肌 以一手拇指和其余四指螺纹面相对用力拿捏项肌,由上向下,自风池穴水平至大椎水平,反复 10～20 遍;然后用双手以同样的方法拿捏两侧肩部肌肉各 20～30 次。

【作用】 舒筋通络,滑利关节,降压平喘,宽胸理气。可防治背痛酸胀、颈椎病、落枕、咳嗽、哮喘、痰结、虚劳、胸闷、胸痛、心悸、心绞痛等病症。

tion, consumptive disease, chest stuffiness, palpitation and angina pectoris.

5.1.3 Self-tuina on the Upper Limbs

MANIPULATIONS

(1) Pressing-kneading the Points on the Upper Limbs: Press-knead with the whorled surface of the thumb or the palmar aspect of the middle finger orderly Jianyu (LI 15), Jianjing (GB 21) around the shoulder joint, Quchi (LI 11), Shousanli (LI 10), Chize (LU 5), Quze (PC 3), Shaohai (HT 3), Xiaohai (SI 8) around the elbow joint, and Waiguan (TE 5), Neiguan (PC 6), Yangchi (TE 4), Yangxi (LI 5), Hegu (LI 4) on the forearm and around the wrist. Press-knead each point about 20 times until there is a sensation of qi arrival with soreness, distension and numbness. Massage the points on the right upper limb with the left hand, and vice versa.

(2) Pushing-rubbing the Upper Limbs: Rub with one palm the anterior, posterior, medial and lateral aspects of the opposite shoulder, elbow and wrist, 10 – 30 times each aspect, until they become hot. Then rub with one palm the lateral side of the opposite limb, from the dorsal carpal cross striation up along the direction of the meridians to Jianyu (LI 15) on the lateral aspect of the shoulder, then turn to the anterior side of the shoulder, and rub along the medial side of the upper limbs down to the intracarpal cross striation. Thus rub the lateral side upward and the medial side downward repeatedly about 30 times until they become hot.

(3) Rubbing and Finger-twisting the Palms and Knuckles: Rub the intermetacarpal muscles in the dorsal aspect of the left hand with the major thenar eminence of

三、上肢部

【操作方法】

（1）按揉上肢诸穴　用拇指螺纹面，或中指指面先后按揉肩关节附近的肩周诸腧穴，如肩髃、肩井穴，以及肘关节周围的曲池、手三里、尺泽、曲泽、少海、小海穴，前臂与腕关节周围的外关、内关、阳池、阳溪、合谷等穴，每穴按揉 20 次左右，以有酸、胀、麻等得气感为宜。左上肢诸穴由右手操作，右上肢诸穴由左手操作。

（2）推擦上肢　先用一手掌心分别将对侧上肢的肩、肘、腕关节的前、后、内、外各面擦热，每面擦 10～30 次左右，再沿经络循行方向，用一手掌心在对侧上肢的外侧，自腕背横纹处向上直擦至肩外侧之肩髃穴，再转向肩前方，沿上肢内侧向下直擦到腕内侧横纹处。如此在上肢的外侧由下而上，在上肢的内侧由上向下地反复推擦 30 遍左右，以擦热为宜。

（3）擦捻掌指　先用右手的大鱼际，将左手手背各掌骨间的肌肉分别擦热，再以右手

the right hand until they become hot. Then knead and finger-twist each of the interphalangeal joints of the left hand about 10 - 20 times each with the right thumb and the right index finger. Exchange the hands and repeat the above manipulations with the same requirements.

ACTIONS These manipulations have the effects of relaxing the muscles and activating the meridians, promoting blood circulation and removing blood stasis, expelling wind and dispersing cold, and lubricating the joints. It can be used to treat and prevent scapulohumeral periarthritis, subacrominal bursitis, tennis elbow, wrist tenosynovitis and other disorders of the upper limbs. It is also effective in relaxing the muscles in the upper limbs, relieving fatigue, improving the motor function of the upper limbs and preventing occupational injuries.

5. 1. 4 Self-tuina on the Chest and the Abdomen

MANIPULATIONS

(1) Pressing-kneading the Points on the Chest and the Intercostal Spaces: With the whorled surface of one middle finger, press and knead respectively Danzhong (CV 17), Zhongfu (LU 1), Rugen (ST 18) and Rupang about 20 times each. Then start from the infraclavicular intercostal spaces, and press-knead every intercostal space from above to below, inside to outside until a sensation of soreness and distension is obtained.

(2) Grasping the Muscles of Thorax: Put the thumb of one hand closely against the anterior aspect of the chest, the index and middle fingers tightly below the armpit, and have them lift and grasp up and down the anterior axillary fold, which is formed by the lateral side of the greater pectoral muscle, combined with gentle and slow pinching-kneading movements. Each operation is

拇、食二指,分别将左手的各个指间关节揉捻 10～20 次。左右交换,要求相同。

【作用】 舒筋通络,活血化瘀,祛风散寒,滑利关节。可防治肩周炎、肩峰下滑液囊炎、网球肘、腕部腱鞘炎等上肢各关节疾患,并有放松上肢肌肉、解除疲劳、增强上肢关节运动功能、预防职业性创伤等功效。

四、胸腹部

【操作方法】

(1) 按揉胸部诸穴及肋间

以一手中指螺纹面,先分别按揉膻中、中府、乳根、乳旁等穴,每穴 20 次左右,再自锁骨下肋骨间隙开始,从上而下,由内向外,用力按揉每个肋间隙,以酸胀为宜。

(2) 拿胸肌 一手拇指紧贴胸前,食、中两指紧贴腋下相对用力提拿由胸大肌外侧组成的腋前壁,一提一拿并加以缓慢柔和的捏揉动作,每次操作 5 遍左右。

performed about 5 times.

(3) Patting the Chest: Clench a hollow fist and use it to knock the chest along the thoracic median line and the breast median lines respectively downward about 10 times each without holding breath.

(4) Rubbing the Chest: Place the major thenar or the whole palm closely on the chest and rub horizontally to and fro about 20 times until it becomes hot.

(5) Pressing-kneading the Points on the Abdomen: With the palmar tip of the middle finger or the major thenar eminence or the palmar base exerting force, press and knead Zhongwan (CV 12), Zhangmen (LR 13), Tianshu (ST 25), Qihai (CV 6), Guanyuan (CV 4), Zhongji (CV 3), etc. respectively 20 - 30 times each until a sensation of qi-arrival is achieved.

(6) Rubbing-kneading the Abdomen: Place the palm of one hand or the overlapped hands on the abdomen, rub and knead it clockwise first and then counterclockwise for 5 - 10 minutes.

(7) Rubbing the Lower Abdomen: Put the palmar side of the hypothenar of both hands on Tianshu (ST 25), about 2 cun beside the navel, and do up and down rubbing movements about 30 times.

(8) Finger-pressing Qihai (CV 6), Guanyuan (CV 4) and Zhongji (CV 3): Finger-press Qihai (CV 6), Guanyuan (CV 4) and Zhongji (CV 3) with the tip of the middle finger 30 - 50 times respectively until a distending and numb sensation is transmitted to the pudendum.

ACTIONS These manipulations have the effects of relieving chest stuffiness and regulating flow of qi, strengthening the spleen and the stomach, and warming the kidney to invigorate yang. It can be used to treat

（3）拍胸　手握空拳,沿胸前正中线与两侧乳中线,自上向下,叩击胸部,在每条操作路线上叩击 10 次左右,叩击时不要屏气。

（4）擦胸　用一手大鱼际,或全掌紧贴胸部体表,横向用力来回摩擦 20 次左右,以产生热感为宜。

（5）按揉腹部诸穴　用中指端、大鱼际或掌根为着力面,分别按揉中脘、章门、天枢、气海、关元、中极等穴,每穴 20～30 次左右,以产生得气感为宜。

（6）摩揉腹部　以一手掌心或两手重叠摩揉腹部,先按顺时针方向,再按逆时针方向旋转摩运 5～10 分钟。

（7）擦少腹　以两手小鱼际掌侧贴紧脐旁 2 寸处的天枢穴,作上、下往返摩擦 30 次左右。

（8）点气海、关元、中极穴　以一手中指端分别点击气海、关元、中极穴,每 30～50 次左右,以向外生殖器有胀、麻等传导感为宜。

【作用】　宽胸理气,健脾和胃,温肾壮阳,可防治岔气、胸痛、胸闷、咳嗽、气喘、气机不畅、心悸、胃脘不适、消化不

diseases like pain and stuffiness in the chest, cough, asthma, unsmooth qi activity, palpitation, discomfort in the stomach, indigestion, constipation, abdominal pain, irregular menstruation and impotence.

5.1.5 Self-tuina on the Back and the Lumbus

MANIPULATIONS

(1) Patting the Back: Pat the opposite side of the back with a hollow palm left and right alternately about 30 times each side.

(2) Pressing-kneading the Points on the Lumbodorsal Regions: Clench the fists of both hands and use the prominence of the metacapophalangeal joints of the index fingers to press-knead Ganshu (BL 18), Pishu (BL 20), Weishu (BL 21), Shenshu (BL 23), Zhishi (BL 52), Yaoyan (EX-B 6) respectively about 30 times each point until a sore and distending sensation is achieved.

(3) Pounding and Vibrating the Lumbar Region: Knock and beat the lumbar region lightly, with the back sides of the two fists, downward along the line from Shenshu (BL 23) to Pangguangshu (BL 28), still the line from Zhishi (BL 52) via Yaoyan (EX-B 6) to Baohuang (BL 53), and another line from Mingmen (GV 4) to the lumbosacral joint respectively 5 - 10 times, each time to produce vibrations to the lower back.

(4) Rubbing the Back and the Lower Back: Press both palms closely to the skin on the lumbodorsal region, rub up and down from the ninth thoracic vertebra to the sacro-iliac joint until the areas become hot.

(5) Flexing, Extending and Rotating Back and the Lumbus: Slowly have the lumbus and the back flex forward, extend backward, flex laterally and rotate left and right with increasing amplitude.

ACTIONS These manipulations have the effects of

良、大便秘结、腹痛、月经不调、阳痿等病症。

五、腰背部

【操作方法】

(1) 拍背 以一手虚掌,向后伸向对侧背后,拍打背部10 次左右。左右交替操作。

(2) 按揉腰背部诸穴 两手握拳,用食指掌指关节突起处用力,分别按揉肝俞、脾俞、胃俞、肾俞、志室、腰眼诸穴,每穴按揉 30 次左右,以酸胀为宜。

(3) 捶振腰区 两手握拳,以拳背自上而下轻轻捶击,分别沿肾俞至膀胱俞一线,志室经腰眼至胞肓一线与命门至腰骶关节一线,叩击捶振腰部 5~10 遍。

(4) 擦腰背 用两手掌紧按腰背部皮肤,自第九胸椎水平向下至骶髂关节处,上下往返摩擦,以局部发热为宜。

(5) 转摇腰背 慢慢地做腰背的前屈、后伸、左右侧屈、左右旋转等活动,幅度由小渐大。

【作用】 镇静安神,补肾

tranquilizing the mind and relieving mental stress, reinforcing the kidney to strengthen the lumbus, relaxing the muscles and tendons, promoting blood circulation, and lubricating the joints. It can be used to treat pain and soreness in the lumbar region caused by various factors, general fatigue, insomnia, impotence, frequency of micturition, lumbar muscle strain, protrusion of the lumbar intervertibral disc, irregular menstruation, diarrhea. It can also relax the lumbar muscles, relieve fatigue, and strengthen the motor function of the lumbar region.

5.1.6　Self-tuina on the Lower Limbs

MANIPULATIONS

（1）Pressing-kneading the Points on the Lower Limb: With the palmar surface or the tip of the thumb or the tip of the middle finger, press-knead Juliao (GB 29), Huantiao (GB 30), Futu(ST 32), Zusanli (ST 36), Yanglingquan (GB 34), Chenshan (BL 57), Sanyinjiao (SP 6) from top to bottom respectively about 20 times each point until qi-arrival sensation is gained.

（2）Pressing-kneading the Thigh: Use the palmar roots of both hands to press-knead the muscles in the lateral, medial and anterior aspects of the thighs respectively from above to below 3 - 5 times to achieve a sensation of soreness and distension.

（3）Pressing-kneading the Patella: Extend the lower limb naturally and relax the muscles, grasp-pinch and press-knead the patella with the palmar side of the thumb and the radial surface of the arc-curved index finger about 20 times.

（4）Grasping the Shank: Gently lift, grasp, pinch and knead the gastrocnemius muscle with the tips of a thumb, an index finger and a middle finger up and down to the Achilles tendon about 10 times until a sore and disten-

健腰，舒筋活血，滑利关节。可防治各种原因引起的腰部酸痛、无力、失眠、阳痿、尿频、腰肌劳损、腰椎间盘突出症、月经不调、腹泻等病症，并有放松腰部肌肉、恢复疲劳、增强腰部运动功能等功效。

六、下肢部

【操作方法】

（1）按揉下肢诸穴　先用拇指指面、指端或中指端，自上而下分别用力按揉居髎、环跳、伏兔、足三里、阳陵泉、承山、三阴交等穴，每穴按揉 20 次左右，以有得气感为宜。

（2）按揉大腿　以两手掌根，自上而下，分别用力按揉大腿外侧、内侧与前侧肌肉3～5遍，以酸胀为宜。

（3）按揉髌骨　下肢自然伸直，肌肉放松。以一手拇指指面及屈成弓状的食指桡侧面，拿捏并按揉髌骨 20 次左右。

（4）拿小腿　以一手拇指与食、中指指端，提拿捏揉腓肠肌，自上而下直至跟腱，用力柔和，每次操作 10 遍左右，

ding sensation is gained.

(5) Patting and Striking the Lower Limb: Pat and strike the lower limb hard with the palm or palmar bases of both hands from the root of the thigh down to the ankle joint about 10 - 15 times.

(6) Rubbing the Point Yongquan (KI 1): Quickly and forcefully rub Yongquan (KI 1) on the opposite sole with the palmar side of the hypothenar about 30 times until it becomes hot. Exchange the feet and do the same as the above.

(7) Shaking the Ankle Joint: Sit upright with the leg bent to have its radial side facing up. Hold the part above the ankle with one hand, and the metatarsophalangeal part with the other hand. Rotate the ankle joint clockwise and counterclockwise and shake it about 20 times.

ACTIONS These manipulations have the action of relaxing the muscles, activating the meridians, relieving blood stasis to promote blood circulation, expelling wind and dispersing cold, and lubricating the joints. It can be used to prevent and treat injury of the superior clunial nerves, strain of the gluteal fascia, swelling and pain in the knees, cramping of m. gastrocnemius, injury of the ankle joint and so on. They also have the function of relaxing the muscles of the lower limbs, relieving fatigue, improving the motor function of the lower limb joints and preventing various kinds of occupational injuries. Besides, pressing-kneading Zusanli (ST 36) and Sanyinjiao (SP 6) and rubbing Yongquan (KI 1) in combination with self-tuina operated on the abdomen, head and face has the effect of health care of the digestive, urinary, reproductive and central nervous systems.

The regional self-tuina therapy introduced above can be conducted in different ways for different purposes. For

以酸胀为宜。

（5）拍击下肢　以两手掌心或掌根，自大腿根部起，从上而下，相对用力拍击下肢，直至踝关节处，约 10～15 遍左右。

（6）擦涌泉　用一手小鱼际掌侧面，快速用力摩擦对侧足心的涌泉穴 30 次左右，以发热为宜，两足交替进行。

（7）摇踝关节　正坐搁腿，一手抓踝上，一手握住足跖趾部，作顺时针及逆时针方向的旋转摇动踝关节，约 20 次左右。

【作用】　舒筋通络，活血化瘀，祛风散寒，滑利关节。可防治臀上皮神经损伤、臀筋膜劳损、膝关节肿痛、腓肠肌痉挛、踝关节损伤等病症。并有放松下肢肌肉、恢复疲劳、增强下肢各关节运动功能、预防各种职业性损伤等功效。另外，按揉足三里、三阴交，擦涌泉等法配合腹部及头面部自我推拿，对胃肠消化系统、泌尿生殖系统与中枢神经等有保健作用。

以上介绍的分部自我推拿法可用于多方面。如作为

general health care, one can massage all parts of the body once a day in the order of the head first, then the neck, the upper limbs, the chest and abdomen, the lumbodorsal region, and finally the lower limbs. For regional health care of the limbs or five sensory organs, one can give manipulations to a certain region or a certain part as required. Moreover, for those who are troubled with some occupational diseases due to their jobs, they are most likely to have regional fatigue or injury, so their working efficiency is affected. They may choose some related parts to be massaged to prevent occupational diseases and promote their working efficiency. Long-distance runners or people who have to stand working, for example, may self-massage their lower limbs before or after work or training. Single self-tuina manipulations of different kinds can be adopted selectively in accordance with one's own health conditions.

5.2 Self-tuina for Regulation of Five Zang Organs

5.2.1 Manipulations for Soothing the Liver and Regulating Flow of Qi

The principal function of the liver is to promote the unobstructed and free circulation of blood and qi. This function reflects its physiological features of controlling ascending and moving, which is manifested in the way of regulating the general activities of qi, smoothing the meridians and collaterals, promoting normal physiological function of the visceral organs, accelerating the general circulation of qi, blood and body fluid, and strengthening

全身性保健推拿,可按头部、颈项、上肢、胸腹、腰背、下肢的顺序,每天全部操作 1 遍;也可根据需要选做其中的一部分或某一部位的操作,以作为肢体或五官的局部保健治疗。另外,如因从事某种职业而使身体的某些部位容易疲劳,或发生劳损而影响工作效率与好发职业病的人,则可选择其中相关的部位进行自我推拿,以提高工作效率或预防职业病。如长跑运动员或取站姿工作的人,可在每天训练与工作的前后做下肢部的自我推拿操作。再者,分部自我推拿中的各种单一的操作方法,也可根据自身的情况,有选择地采用。

第二节 五脏调理推拿法

一、疏肝理气法

肝脏主要具有疏泄的功能,这种功能反映了肝脏主升、主动的生理特点,表现在能调畅全身气机,使经络和利,并促进各脏腑器官的生理活动发挥正常,更能推动全身气血和津液的运行及增强脾胃的运化功能。因此,如果肝

transporting and transforming function of the spleen and the stomach. Therefore, if disorders of the liver's main function occur, qi activities of the whole body will be hindered. As a result, some pathological changes will take place, such as obstruction of flow of qi, stagnation of qi, hyperactivity of qi, and further affect the function of storing blood, distribution and metabolism of body fluid, and transportation and transformation of the spleen and the stomach. Interiorly the liver is connected with the gallbladder through the meridians. Its functions can be manifested through Jin (tendons and muscles) and the eyes. This is because the liver is in charge of the tendons and has the meridians and vessels to communicate upward with the eyes. When the liver functions normally in promoting and soothing the flow of qi and the liver-qi is sufficient, the tendons will be strong and powerful, the nails will be hard and tough, and the eyes, clear and bright. Otherwise, Jin will be feeble, flaccid and shrunk, and the vision will be blurred. In one word, the liver is interiorly-exteriorly related with the gallbladder, it controls the tendons beneath the body surface and is reflected on the eyes. Liver diseases in TCM, chiefly refer to some digestive diseases in modern medicine, including hepatitis, infection of the biliary tract, cholecystitis, gallstones, some disorders of the nervous system like the intercostal neuralgia, tendon problems like spasm in the hands and feet, hypertension caused by hyperactivity of liver yang, and some eye troubles. So frequently performing manipulations of health-care massage for soothing the liver and regulating flow of qi will certainly be effective in preventing and treating the diseases mentioned above.

5.2.1.1 Soothing Qihui (the influential acupoint of qi)

Overlap the two hands, place them on Danzhong (CV

的疏泄功能失常,人体各部的气机活动就会受到阻碍,进而形成气机不畅、气机郁结、气机亢逆等病理变化,并进一步影响藏血和津液的输布代谢、脾胃的运化功能。肝在体内有经脉和胆相联系,其功能的盛衰在体表可从筋及眼睛表现出来,这是因为肝主筋,并有经脉上联于目,疏泄正常,肝气充足,则筋强力壮,爪甲坚韧,眼睛明亮,否则筋软弛缩,视物不清。总之,肝与胆相表里,在体主筋,开窍于目。中医学所说的肝病范畴,对照现代医学病名,主要包括了部分消化系统疾病,如肝炎,胆道感染、胆囊炎、胆结石等和一些神经系统疾病如肋间神经痛等,以及手足拘挛等筋腱疾病,肝阳上亢导致的高血压,有关眼睛的疾病等等。因此,经常施行疏肝理气的保健按摩方法,对上述疾病可有良好的防治作用。

(一) 舒气会

双掌相叠,置于两乳中间

17) (which is one of the eight influential acupoints) between the breasts, and rub up and down 30 times.

5.2.1.2　Alleviating Depression in the Chest

Take a sitting position, place the hollow palm of the right hand over the right breast, pat with a proper force, while moving gradually and horizontally to the left, back and forth 10 times. Then exchange into the left hand and do the operation alternately.

5.2.1.3　Soothing the Intercostal Spaces

Take a sitting position, put both palms transversely under the armpits with the fingers separating at an equal distance to the intercostal space. Push the right palm leftward to the sternum first, and then push the left palm rightward to the sternum, too. Do the manipulation up and down alternately to get both palms to the level of the umbilicus 10 times. Be careful to have the fingers press closely against the intercostal parts and exert force evenly. It is advisable to produce a warm and hot sensation in the chest and ribs.

5.2.1.4　Grasping the Muscles in the Lumbar Region

Being in a sitting position, clamp the muscles in both sides of the lumbus with Hukou (the parts between the thumb and the index finger), and pinch-grasp them downward to the illiac regions repeatedly 10 times.

5.2.1.5　Rubbing the Lower Abdomen

Take a sitting or lying position, place the two hands under the hypochondriac regions, push and rub obliquely through the lower abdomen to the pubis back and forth 20 times.

5.2.1.6　Regulating the Triple Energizer (Lisanjiao)

Being in a sitting or lying position, cross the four fingers of the two hands, place them horizontally on Danzhong (CV 17) with the palmar bases on the medial

的膻中穴(本穴为八会穴之气会),上下擦动30次。

(二)宽胸法

坐位,右手虚掌置于右乳上方,适当用力拍击并渐横向左侧移动,来回10次。左右交换。

(三)疏肋间

坐位,两手掌横置两腋下,手指张开,指距与肋间隙等宽,先用右掌向左分推至胸骨,再用左掌向右分推至胸骨,由上而下,交替分推至脐水平线,反复10次。注意手指应紧靠肋间,用力宜均匀,以胸肋有温热感为佳。

(四)拿腰肌

坐位,双手掌虎口卡置于两侧腰胁部肌肉,由上而下至骶部捏拿腰胁肌肉,往返操作10次。

(五)擦少腹

坐或卧位,双手掌分置两胁肋下,同时用力斜向少腹推擦至耻骨,往返操作20次。

(六)理三焦

坐或卧位,两手四指相交叉,横置按于膻中穴,两掌根按置两乳内侧,自上而下,稍

sides of the breasts, push with greater force downwards to the end of the abdomen 20 times.

5.2.1.7　Plucking Yanglingquan (GB 34)

Take a sitting position, place the two thumbs respectively on Yanglingquan (GB 34), the converging acupoint of tendon, one of the eight influential acupoints, on both sides. With the help of the other four fingers, first press-knead these points for one minute, and then pluck transversely the tendons around the point forcefully 5 - 10 times until a sore and numb sensation is radiating out.

5.2.1.8　Vibrating the Chest (musculi pectoralis major)

Take a sitting position, first grasp and pinch the left musculi pectoralis major with the right hand from under the armpit 10 times, and then do the same operation with the left hand. Next cross the fingers of the hands and put them on the occiput, keep the two elbows at a horizontal level, and sway them backward as hard as possible. Inhale while swaying backward and exhale while swaying forward. Operate 10 times in this way.

5.2.1.9　Moving the Eyes

Look ahead with the head upright and the lumbus straight, turn the eye-balls clockwise slowly 10 times, and then stare ahead for a while, and finally turn them counter-clockwise another 10 times.

5.2.1.10　Heaving Sighs

Relax the whole body, inhale deeply, and then exhale as much as possible. Make a sound of "Xu" (sh) when exhaling, and stare as hard as possible. Repeat the process 10 times.

5.2.2　Manipulations for Relieving Mental Stress and Easing the Mind

Physiologically, the heart controls blood and the ves-

用力推至腹尽处,共推 20 次。

(七) 拨阳陵

坐位,两手拇指分按置于两侧阳陵泉穴(八会穴之筋会穴),余四指辅助,先行按揉该穴 1 分钟,再用力横向弹拨该穴处肌腱 5～10 次,以酸麻放射感为好。

(八) 振胸膺

坐位,先用右手从腋下捏拿左侧胸大肌 10 次,再换手如法操作。然后双手叉指抱持于后枕部,双肘相平,尽力向后摆动,同时吸气,摆前时呼气,一呼一吸,操作 10 次。

(九) 运双目

端正凝视,头正腰直,两眼球先顺时针方向缓缓转动 10 次,然后瞪眼前视片刻,在逆时针方向如法操作。

(十) 叹息法

全身放松,先深吸气后,再尽量呼气,于呼气时发出"嘘"(xū)音,并尽力瞪目,重复 10 次。

二、宁心安神法

中医认为,心主血脉,为

sels, and is essential to life activities according to TCM. The significance of heart in controlling blood and the vessels is that blood depends on beating of the heart to be transported to all parts of the body and functions in nourishing. Meanwhile, the blood vessels also rely upon the driving force of the heart's transportation of blood to maintain their fullness and smoothness. Therefore, only when the heart controls blood well, blood can flow smoothly in the blood vessels, circulates constantly, nourishes the whole body and ensures the normal life activities. The heart is interiorly associated with the small intestine through the meridians, and the conditions of its function can be reflected through one's spirits, consciousness, mental activities, pulse or tongue condition. For example, when heart qi is vigorous and blood vessels are full, one will be in high spirits, act agilely, have a quick mind, forceful and easing-up pulse and a reddish and moist tongue proper. Otherwise, one may be spiritless with sluggish reaction, unsmooth and cacorhythmic pulse, and a purplish and pale tongue. In one word, the heart is connected with the small intestine, controls pulses interiorly, and is reflected exteriorly on the tongue. Compared with the medical terms in modern medicine, the range of heart diseases in TCM includes diseases of the cardiovascular system such as various disorders of the heart, arteriosclerosis, angitis, diseases of nervous system like neurasthenia, neurosis, insomnia as well as intracraniocerebral and extracraniocerebral diseases, intestinal malabsorption and diseases in the tongue body. Therefore, frequently performing these health-care manipulations will have very good effects on preventing and treating diseases mentioned above.

人体生命活动的关键所在。心主血脉的意义在于,血液依赖心脏的搏动而输送到全身,发挥其濡养的作用。而运送血液的全身脉管也要依赖心脏运送血液的推动力量,保持着充盈和畅通。因此,心主血脉的功能健全,血液才能在脉管内正常运行,周流不息,营养全身而保证生命的正常活动。心脏在体内有经脉和小肠相联系,其功能的盛衰在体表可以通过人的精神、意识、思维活动以及脉象和舌象表现出来。如心气旺盛,血脉充盈,则可见人的精神振作,思维敏捷,动作灵活,脉搏和缓有力,舌质淡红润泽。反之,则见人的精神委靡,反应迟钝以及脉涩不畅,节律不整,舌质紫暗或苍白等。总之,心与小肠相表里,在体主脉,开窍于舌。中医学所说心病的范畴,对照现代医学病名,可包括心血管系统疾病,如心脏的各种疾患、动脉硬化、脉管炎等,神经系统疾病如神经衰弱、神经官能症、失眠,以及颅脑内外疾患等;小肠吸收不良,舌体病等。因此,经常操练宁心安神的保健按摩方法,可对上述各类疾病的防治有良好的作用。

5.2.2.1 Making Sounds in the Ears (Ming-tiangu)

See the part of the Head and the Face Regions in Self Tuina Therapy.

5.2.2.2 Kneading Shenmen (HT 7)

Take a sitting position, overlap the index finger and the middle finger of the right hand and put the index finger on Shenmen (HT 7) of the left hand. Press-knead the point for one minute. Then exchange into the right hand and press-knead the acupoint in the same way alternately. If necessary, Neiguan (PC 6) on both sides may be pressed additionally.

5.2.2.3 Pinching Zhongchong (PC 9)

First use the right thumb and index fingers to clamp the tip of the left middle finger, where the point Zhongchong (PC 9) is. Press and nip it with slightly great force several times, and then pluck and release it at once. Do the operation 10 times. Then exchange the hands and continue the same manipulations alternately.

5.2.2.4 Digitally-pressing Jiquan (HT 1)

Place the right four fingers on the medial side of the left muscli pectoralis major, and press the right thumb on the lateral side of the muscle, so the index and the middle fingers will naturally digitally-press on the point Jiquan (HT 1) under the left armpit. While pinching-grasping the muscli pectoralis major, digitally-press Jiquan (HT 1) with the right index and the middle fingers about 10 times. Then exchange the hands and continue the operation in the same way alternately.

5.2.2.5 Grasping the Heart Meridians

Place the right thumb on the left armpit, and the other four right fingers on the anterior, medial aspect of the upper limb. Do grasping-pinching and pressing-kneading manipulations at the same time along the medial aspect of

（一）鸣天鼓

见"分部推拿之头面部"。

（二）揉神门

坐位,右手食、中指相叠,食指按压在左手的神门穴上,按揉 1 分钟,左右交换。可加按双侧内关穴。

（三）捏中冲

先用右手拇、食指夹持左手中指尖(中冲穴所在处),稍用力按捏数次,随之拨放,操作 10 次。左右交换。

（四）点极泉

先以右手四指置左侧胸大肌内侧,拇指置按胸大肌外侧,同时食、中指自然点按在腋下极泉穴,边捏拿胸大肌,边以食、中指点揉极泉穴,操作 10 次。左右交换。

（五）拿心经

右手拇指置左侧腋下,其余四指置上臂内上侧,边做拿捏,边做按揉,沿上臂内侧渐次向下操作至腕部神门穴处

the upper limb down to Shenmen (HT 7) on the wrist 10 times. Exchange the hands and continue the operation in the same way alternately.

5.2.2.6 Performing Swinging and Patting Manipulations

Sit and part the feet as wide as the shoulders, relax the body naturally, and stretch out the hands. Turn the waist to pull the arms to swing, and the swinging arms pull the elbows and the hands to swing naturally. One arm swings forward and the other backward. When one arm swings in front of the body, pat the anterior area of the chest on the opposite side with the palmar aspect of the hand. When it swings to the back, pat the posterior cardiac area on the other side with the dorsal aspect of the hand. Initially, the patting force should be light and mild, and it can be increased properly if no adverse reaction occurs. Do swinging and patting about 20 times each.

5.2.2.7 Rubbing the Chest

Press the right palm on the middle part between the breasts with the tip of the fingers pointing obliquely forward and downward. Push and rub the cardiac region, rounding from the inferior margin of the left breast back to the original area, then continue the manipulation with the palmar root of the right hand directing forward from the inferior margin of the right breast back to the middle part again. Thus push and rub in a "∞" or a transverse 8-shaped route about 20 times.

5.2.2.8 Stirring the Tongue in the Mouth (Jiaocanghai)

Rotate the tongue outside the upper and lower gums in the oral cavity first from left to right, then from right to left about 10 times respectively. Swallow the saliva produced by the movements of the tongue at three times.

止,如此 10 次。左右交换。

(六) 甩拍法

站立位,两足分开同肩宽,身体自然放松,两手掌自然伸开,以腰转动带胳膊,肘部带动手,两臂一前一后自然甩动。到体前时,用手掌面拍击对侧胸前区;到体后时,以掌背拍击对侧背心区。初做时,拍击力量宜轻,若无不适反应,力量可适当加重,每次甩打拍击 20 次左右。

(七) 摩胸膛

右掌按置两乳正中,指尖斜向前下方,先从左乳下环行推摩心区复原,再以掌根在前,沿右乳下环行推摩,如此连续呈"∞"(横 8 字)形,操作 20 次。

(八) 搅沧海

舌在口腔上、下牙龈外周从左向右,从右向左各转动 10 次。产生津液分 3 口缓缓咽下。

5.2.2.9　Rubbing Yongquan（KI 1）

Place one palm horizontally on Yongquan（KI 1）of one foot, rub it to and fro about 50 times. Do the same to the other side.

5.2.2.10　Methods for Tranquilizing the Mind

Close the eyes, breathe calmly and naturally and relax the whole body. While inhaling, the tongue touches the upper palatine; while exhaling, make a sound like "Ke" and the tongue leaves the upper palatine along the air flow. Breathing should be deep, long, moderate. Conduct 10 times of one inhale and one exhale.

5.2.3　Manipulations for Reinforcing the Spleen and Strengthening the Stomach

The spleen is in charge of transportation and transformation, which refers to its important functions of digestion, absorption and transportation of nutrients, and promotion of metabolism of the body fluid in the body. The exertion of visceral normal function and one's health condition mainly depend upon this function of the spleen. Therefore, the spleen is also known as the foundation of acquired constitution in TCM. The spleen also has the function of governing blood circulation and preventing it from overflowing out of the blood vessels, but this function could be fulfilled only when the splenic function in transportation and transformation is vigorous. The spleen is interiorly connected with the stomach through the meridians. And the strong or weak conditions of its function are reflected exteriorly through the muscles in the limbs, the lips, and taste in the mouth. Therefore, if the spleen functions normally in transportation and transformation, the essence of food will be absorbed constantly, blood and qi will be generated, nutrients will be sufficient and the lips will be red, lustrous and moist. Otherwise, one will

（九）擦涌泉

单掌横置涌泉穴处，来回擦 50 次，左右同。

（十）养心法

闭目、静息，全身放松，吸气时舌抵上腭，呼气时，轻轻发音"呵"（kē）字，随气流舌离上腭。呼吸要深长、柔和，一呼一吸为一次，共 10 次。

三、健脾益胃法

脾主运化，指脾有消化、吸收、运输营养物质和促进水液代谢等方面的重要作用，人体各脏器功能的发挥，身体的健康程度，大多取决于脾的这一功能，所以中医称"脾为后天之本"。脾还能统摄血液使其不致溢出脉外，而这种统摄能力只有在脾运化旺健时才能具有。脾在体内有经络和胃相联系。其功能的盛衰在体表从四肢肌肉、口唇、口味上表现出来。脾的健运功能正常，饮食精微不断吸收，化生气血，营养方可充足，口唇红润光泽。反之，则形体消瘦肌肉萎软，口淡无味或异味，口唇淡白枯槁。总之，脾与胃相表里，在体主肉，开窍于口。中医学所说的脾胃病的范畴，

have an emaciated physique, weak and withered muscles, dysgeusia and tastelessness or abnormal smell in the mouth, and pale and withered lips. In general, the spleen is interiorly-exteriorly connected with the stomach, controls the muscles of the body and its condition is reflected on the mouth. The splenogastric diseases covered in TCM include, in modern medicine, diseases of the digestive system such as gastritis, gastric or duodenal ulcer, indigestion, enteritis, diarrhea, constipation, also include myodystrophy, amyotrophy, oral disorders, and anemia, thrombopenia and other blood system diseases. Manipulations for reinforcing the spleen and nourishing the stomach for health care have very good therapeutic effects in preventing and treating the above-mentioned diseases.

5.2.3.1　Stirring the Tongue in the Mouth (Jiaocanghai)

See the part of Manipulations for Relieving Mental Stress and Easing the Mind

5.2.3.2　Rubbing the Epigastrium

Overlap the two palms, place them on Shenque (CV 8), and rub the epigastrium clockwise 30 times with continuously enlarging circle first. Then rub it counterclockwise another 30 times with gradually reducing circle.

5.2.3.3　Swaying the Stomach

Sit or lie, put the right palm on Zhongwan (CV 12), and slightly push the stomach leftward first with the palmar root. Then push it back rightward with the five fingers with greater force. Do this to-and-forth pushing 10 times.

5.2.3.4　Vibrating Zhongwan (CV 12)

Sit or lie on one's back, put the overlapped hands on the point Zhongwan (CV 12), and do vibrating manipulation to it for one minute.

对照现代医学病名,可包括消化系统疾病,如胃炎、胃及十二指肠溃疡、消化不良、肠炎、腹泻、便秘等,还包括肌营养不良、肌肉萎缩、口腔疾病,以及贫血、血小板减少等血液系统疾病。采用健脾益胃的保健按摩方法,可对上述各种疾病有良好的防治作用。

(一)搅沧海

见"宁心安神法"。

(二)摩脘腹

双掌相叠,置于神阙穴处,先逆时针,从小到大摩脘腹30圈,然后再顺时针,从大到小摩脘腹30圈。

(三)荡胃腑

坐或卧位,以右手掌按置于中脘穴上,先以掌根稍用力将胃脘向左推荡,继之再以五指将胃脘稍用力推荡向右,往返10次。

(四)振中脘

坐或仰卧,双掌相叠于中脘穴处,以振动手法操作1分钟。

5.2.3.5   Pinching the Three Lines (Niesanxian)

Sit or lie on the back, select three vertical lines from the two mammilla and Danzhong（CV 17）downward. Pinch-grasp the three lines with both hands one by one from up to below, which is counted as once, and operate 5 times in all. In addition, knead-pinch the muscles in the epigastric area.

5.2.3.6   Separating Yin and Yang

Sit or lie on the back, put the four fingers of either hand closely together except the thumbs, have the two middle fingers against each other and place below the xiphoid. Press the whole palms tightly on the skin, push separately along the ribs toward each hypochondrium, and move to the lower abdomen gradually. The whole procedure is conducted 10 times.

5.2.3.7   Soothing the Intercostal Spaces

See the part of Manipulations for Soothing the Liver and Regulating Circulation of qi.

5.2.3.8   Regulating the Triple Energizer (Lisanjiao)

See the part of Manipulations for Soothing the Liver and Regulating Circulation of qi.

5.2.3.9   Pressing Zusanli (ST 36)

Overlap the index and the middle fingers of the two hands, and press-knead Zusanli（ST 36）on both sides with them respectively 50 times.

5.2.3.10   Kneading Xuehai (SP 10)

Take a sitting position, place the thumbs on Xuehai（SP 10）on the thighs respectively, and press-knead rotationally for one minute.

5.2.4   Manipulations for Activating the Lung and Regulating Qi

Physiologically, the lung is considered to control flow

（五）捏三线

坐或仰卧,自两乳头和膻中穴向下取 3 条垂直线,以双手逐线自上而下捏拿、揉捏脘腹部肌肉,3 线操作为 1 次,共做 5 次。

（六）分阴阳

坐或仰卧,两手除拇指外其余四指并拢,中指相对于剑突下,全掌紧按皮肤,然后自内向外,沿肋弓向胁肋处分推,并逐渐向小腹移动,共操作 10 次。

（七）疏肋间

见"疏肝理气法"。

（八）理三焦

见"疏肝理气法"。

（九）按三里

双手食、中指相叠,按揉足三里穴 50 次。

（十）揉血海

坐位,双拇指分按于两侧腿部的血海穴上,作旋转按揉 1 分钟。

四、宣肺通气法

中医认为肺的生理功能

of qi and respiration in TCM, which refers to the fact that the lung is the place of air exchange, and through respiration of the lung, clean air in the nature is breathed into the body while the metabolized air is breathed out, and thus the air exchange is accomplished. By getting rid of the stale and taking in the fresh continuously, the lung promotes the formation of qi and regulates in-and-out, up-and-down activities of qi, and in so doing, maintains the metabolism of the body in smooth and normal functioning. Furthermore, the lung also has the function of activating dispersion of qi and essence, clarifying and descending pulmonary qi, and dredging and regulating water channels. The normality of all the lung functions can keep respiration, nutrition, metabolism of body fluid in good condition so as to maintain one's health. Otherwise, pathological manifestations as dyspnea, stuffiness in the chest, cough, or even edema will develop. Interiorly the lung is associated with the large intestine through the meridians, and exteriorly its functional asthenia and sthenia are reflected by luster and pathological changes of the skin and functions of the nose. In a word, the lung is interiorly-exteriorly connected with the large intestine, controls the skin and hairs exteriorly and is reflected on the nose. The range of the lung diseases discussed in TCM is equivalent to, in modern medicine, that of diseases of the respiratory system such as cough, cold, asthma, pneumonia and emphysema, those of the large intestine like enteritis and constipation, urticaria and other dermatosis as well as rhinitis and other nasal disorders. Self-massage for health care can be used to prevent and treat the diseases mentioned above effectively.

5.2.4.1 Opening the Point Feimen

The lung has its hila which are respectively located 1 cun lateral to the thoracic middle line, and are on a level

是"主气、司呼吸",是指肺为体内外气体交换的场所。通过肺的呼吸,吸入自然界的清气,呼出体内的浊气,实现了体内外气体的交换,通过不断的呼浊吸清,吐故纳新,促进气的生成,调节着气的升降出入运动,从而保证了人体新陈代谢的正常运行。肺还有"宣发、肃降、通调水道"的作用。这些功能的正常,可使人体呼吸、营养、水液代谢保持良好的状态,从而使人体保持健康。反之,则出现呼吸不利、胸闷、咳喘,甚至水肿等病态。肺在体内有经脉和大肠联系,其功能的盛衰在体表可通过皮肤的润泽、病变以及鼻部正常与否表现出来。总之,肺与大肠相表里,在体主皮毛,开窍于鼻。中医学所说肺病的范畴,对照现代医学病名,可包括呼吸系统的病变,诸如感冒、咳嗽、哮喘、肺炎、肺气肿等,某些大肠疾病如肠炎、便秘,以及荨麻疹等皮肤病和鼻炎等鼻部的疾病。采用保健按摩的方法,可以对上述各种疾病进行有效的防治。

(一)开肺门

双手拇指分别置于双侧的肺门穴(肺有肺门,位于胸

with the junction of the manubrium of the sternum and the sternal body. Place the two thumbs on Feimen on both sides respectively, and press-knead them for one minute. Then overlap the palms, put them on Danzhong (CV 17), and push-rub horizontally toward either side of the chest 20 times.

5.2.4.2　Hooking Tiantu (CV 22)

Place the tip of an index finger on Tiantu (CV 22), hook, digitally-press and knead it downward for one minute.

5.2.4.3　Regulating Lung Qi

Place the thumbs on Zhongfu (LU 1) on both sides, push-knead upward to Yunmen (LU 2) until a sensation of soreness and distension is achieved. Then put the thumbs, index and middle fingers on the first, second and third intercostal spaces respectively, and push-rub to and fro for one minute.

5.2.4.4　Pressing Fengchi (GB 20)

Sit, put the thumbs on Fengchi (GB 20) on both sides respectively, place the two little fingers on Taiyang (EX-HN 5), and the other fingers on the lateral sides of the head. Simultaneously press and knead Fengchi (GB 20), Taiyang (EX-HN 5) and the two sides of the head forcefully for one minute.

5.2.4.5　Rubbing Dazhui (GV 14)

Sit, place the palm horizontally on Dazhui (GV 14), rub it back and forth with the major thenar eminence and the index and the middle fingers until it becomes hot.

5.2.4.6　Grasping Hegu (LI 4)

Sit, grasp, press and knead the left Hegu (LI 4) with the right thumb and the right index finger oppositely for one minute. Then exchange the right hand for the left one and do the same operation.

部正中线旁开 1 寸，胸骨柄、体联结部相平处）按揉 1 分钟。然后双掌重叠置于膻中穴部，横向两侧胸膺部推擦 20 次。

（二）勾天突

以手食指尖置天突穴处，向下勾点、揉动 1 分钟。

（三）调肺气

双手拇指按置于中府穴处，向上推揉至云门穴，以酸胀为度。然后拇、食、中指平放一、二、三肋间，往返推擦 1 分钟。

（四）按风池

坐位，两手拇指按在两侧风池穴上，两手小指各按在太阳穴处，其余手指各散置头部两侧，然后两手同时用力按揉风池、太阳及头侧部 1 分钟。

（五）擦大椎

坐位，单掌横置于大椎穴，以大鱼际及食、中指往返擦动，以热为度。

（六）拿合谷

坐位，右手拇、食指相对拿按、揉动左侧合谷穴 1 分钟。左右交换。

5.2.4.7　Clearing the Feijing

Sit or stand, place the right palm above the left breast, and rub it rotationally until the area becomes hot. Then along the anterior side of the left shoulder, the anterior and upper part of the medial side of the left upper arm, and the radial side of the forearm, push-rub downward to the dorsal side of the left wrist, thumb and index finger. Do the manipulations to and fro 20 times, then change into the left palm and do the same as above.

5.2.4.8　Vibrating the Chest

See the part of Manipulations for Soothing the Liver and Regulating Flow of Qi.

5.2.4.9　Rubbing Yingxiang (LI 20)

Place the major thenar eminence on Yingxiang (LI 20) on either side. Rub them up and down. Meanwhile, breathe and whiff quickly until it is hot.

5.2.4.10　Manipulations of Dispersing the Superficies

Sit or stand, screw a dry towel into a column, and take the ends with both hands. Flex the elbows, get the towel on the back with the right hand above and the left one below, rub along the two sides of the spinal column up and down until they become hot. First one side then the other alternately.

5.2.5　Manipulations for Reinforcing the Kidney and Replenishing Vital Essence

The kidney, as an indispensable organ, is called "the congenital fundamentals" in TCM and is the driving source of life. It is located in the lumbar region, so the loin is compared to " the house of the kidney". Physiologically, the kidney mainly stores the essence of the human body, controls its growth and reproduction, and regulates metabolism of water and fluid in the body, which enables clean substances to ascend to the lung and to be distribu-

（七）清肺经

坐位或立位,右掌先置左乳上方,环摩至热后,以掌沿着肩前、上臂内侧前上方、前臂桡侧至腕、拇、食指背侧,往返推擦 20 次。左右交换。

（八）振胸膺

见"疏肝理气法"。

（九）擦迎香

双手大鱼际分按两侧迎香穴处,上下擦动,边擦边快速呼吸,喷气,以热为度。

（十）疏表法

坐或站位,以干毛巾拧成拄状,双手抓住两头,屈肘,右手在上,左手在下,过肩沿脊柱两侧上下擦动,先擦一侧,以热为度。左右交换。

五、固肾益精法

肾在人体中,是极为重要的脏器,中医称肾为"先天之本",是人体生命的动力源泉。肾位于腰部,有"腰为肾之府"之喻。肾的主要生理功能是贮藏人体的精气,主管人体的生殖与发育,并可调节人体的水液代谢,使其清者上升于肺

ted all over the body, and the used substances to descend to the bladder and to be discharged out of the body. Besides, the function of the kidney in promoting inspiration is significant to respiration of the human body because the inhaled air can come down only under the aids of the kidney though respiration is controlled by the lung. Therefore, there are the sayings "the lung controls respiration, while the kidney promotes inspiration" in TCM. The kidney is associated with the bladder through the meridians interiorly, and its functional conditions are exteriorly reflected by solidity of the bones, luster of the hair, spirits of the human being, and the hearing ability. In one word, the kidney is interiorly-exteriorly connected with the bladder, controls the bones of the body, is reflected on the ears and opens to the external urethral orifice and the anus. The range of nephritic diseases studied in TCM, compared with that in modern medicine, chiefly refers to diseases in the urogenital system, including nephritis, cystitis, urinary infection, prostatitis, seminal emission, prospermia, male and female infertility, some gynecological diseases like amenia, leukorrhea, some skeletal diseases, lumbar pain, toothache, some diseases of the nervous system and some hypofunctional problems like aversion to cold, listlessness, and some ear diseases like tinnitus, deafness. All these diseases can be prevented or treated with a satisfactory result by performing Manipulations for Reinforcing the Kidney and Replenishing Vital Essence.

5.2.5.1 Digitally-pressing Shenshu (BL 23)

Sit, use the two thumbs to clasp the lumbar and hypochondriac region, place the overlapped index and middle fingers on Shenshu (BL 23) on either side, and press-knead with slightly force for one minute.

而宣发全身,浊者则下降于膀胱而排出体外。此外肾的纳气功能,对人体呼吸亦有重要意义,因为人体呼吸虽是肺所主,但吸入之气,还必须下纳于肾脏,所以有"肺主呼气,肾主纳气"的说法。肾在体内有经脉和膀胱相联系。肾功能的盛衰在体表可从骨骼的坚强,毛发的荣枯,人外在的精神状态以及耳朵的听觉等表现出来。总之,肾与膀胱相表里,在体主骨,开窍于耳及二阴。中医学所说肾病的范畴,对照现代医学的病名,主要是泌尿生殖系统疾病,包括肾炎、膀胱炎、尿路感染、前列腺炎、遗精、早泄、男女不育症和闭经、带下等妇科疾病;骨骼的疾病,腰痛、齿痛;还有神经系统和一些功能低下的疾病,如怕冷、精神委靡,以及耳鸣、耳聋等耳部病变。选用保健按摩的方法可以对以上所说的各种疾病有较好的防治作用。

(一)点肾俞

坐位,双手拇指夹持腰胁部,食、中指相叠分按在双侧肾俞穴上,稍用力按揉1分钟左右。

5.2.5.2　Knocking the Lumbar and Spinal Regions

Sit or stand upright, clench the two hands to make hollow fists, and knock the two sides of the lumbar-spinal areas with the radial aspects of the soft fists from the place as high as possible down to the sacral region. The knocking is combined with bending forward movements of the lumbus, and done up and down 20 times.

5.2.5.3　Rubbing the Lumbar and Sacral Regions

Sit with the upper body bending slightly forward. Flex the elbows, try to place the palms as high on the lumbodorsal region as possible, rub quickly down to the sacrum by exerting force with the whole palm, especially the minor thenar eminence until a hot sensation is obtained.

5.2.5.4　Rubbing Guanyuan (CV 4)

Sit, and press the left palm on Mingmen (GV 4) horizontally. Rub the abdomen with the right hand around Guanyuan (CV 4), first counter-clockwise for 50 times, then clockwise another 50 times, and finally press the point inward and downward along with breathing 10 times.

5.2.5.5　Grasping the Medial Aspect of the Thigh

Take a sitting position. First get the right thumb separating from the rest fingers, grasp and knead the muscles in the medial side of the left thigh from the top down to the knee 10 times. Then grasp and knead the right thigh with the left hand another 10 times. Push-rub the medial side of the left thigh to the knee with the right palm until it becomes hot. Exchange the hand and the thigh and repeat the above operation.

5.2.5.6　Rubbing the Lower Abdomen

See the Part of Manipulations for Soothing the Liver

（二）叩腰脊

坐或直立位，两手握空拳，用拳眼叩击腰脊两侧，上自尽可能高的部位开始，下至骶部，叩击时可配合腰部的前屈活动，往返 20 次。

（三）擦腰骶

坐位，上身微前倾。屈肘，两手掌尽量上置于两侧腰背部，以全掌尤以小鱼际着力，向下至尾骶部快速擦动，透热为度。

（四）摩关元

坐位，左掌横按在命门穴，右掌以关元穴为圆心，先作逆时针摩腹 50 次，再作顺时针摩腹 50 次。然后随呼吸向内下按压关元 10 次。

（五）拿阴股

坐位，先以右手拇指与四指分开，从左侧大腿内侧上端起，边拿揉股内侧肌肉边向下移，直至膝部，操作 10 次，左右交换。再以右掌面推擦左大腿内侧至膝，以热为度，左右交换。

（六）擦小腹

见“疏肝理气法”。

and Regulating Flow of Qi.

5.2.5.7　Manipulations of Replenishing the Marrow

Take a sitting position. Press the right thumb on the left Sanyinjiao (SP 6), and the right index and the middle fingers on Juegu (GB 39), which is the marrow influential point of the eight influential points, and press-knead them with slightly force for one minute. Then move down to the Achilles tendon with the thumb on Taixi (KI 3) and the index and the middle fingers on Kunlun (BL 60), press and knead them forcefully for one minute. Change into the left hand and the right leg, and do the same manipulations.

5.2.5.8　Rubbing Yongquan (KI 1)

See the Part of Manipulations for Relieving Mental Stress and Easing the Mind.

5.2.5.9　Manipulating the Two Ears (Xishuanger)

Take a sitting position. Put the two palms on both the ears horizontally with the thumbs directing downward, and push-rub backward with even force. As the palms return back, bring the auricles down onto the ears, and push and rub them forward. Operate the whole procedure back and forth 20 times. Then pinch the earlobes with the thumbs and the index fingers, shake them several times. Finally, insert the index fingers into the ear orifices, quiver them quickly several times, and withdraw them suddenly. Repeat the whole procedure.

5.2.5.10　Contracting the External Genitalia and the Anus

Relax the whole body and keep it in a placid state. Do the abdominal respiration (namely, the abdomen sticks

（七）增髓法

坐位,右手拇指按于左侧的三阴交穴,食、中指按于绝骨穴(八会穴之髓会),同时稍用力按揉 1 分钟后,向下移动至跟腱处,拇指按于太溪穴,食、中指按于昆仑穴,亦用力按揉 1 分钟。左右交换。

（八）擦涌泉

见"宁心安神法"。

（九）洗双耳

坐位,用两手掌横置按于两耳上(拇指向下),均匀用力向后推擦,回手时将耳背带倒再向前推擦,往返操作 20 次。然后双手拇、食指捏住两耳垂做索抖法数次,再用两食指插入耳孔,行快速震颤法数下,猛然拔出,重复操作。

（十）缩二阴

处于安静状态下,全身放松,用顺腹式呼吸法(即吸气

out when inhaling and shrinks in when exhaling). Contract the external genitalia and the anus with force while
exhaling, and relax them while inhaling. Repeat the
whole process 10 times.

时腹部隆起,呼气时腹部收
缩),并在呼气时稍用力收缩
前阴和肛门,吸气时放松,重
复10次。

Postscript

The compilation of *A Newly Compiled Practical English-Chinese Library of TCM* was started in 2000 and published in 2002. In order to demonstrate the academic theory and clinical practice of TCM and to meet the requirements of compilation, the compilers and translators have made great efforts to revise and polish the Chinese manuscript and English translation so as to make it systematic, accurate, scientific, standard and easy to understand. Shanghai University of TCM is in charge of the translation. Many scholars and universities have participated in the compilation and translation of the Library, i.e. Professor Shao Xundao from Xi'an Medical University (former Dean of English Department and Training Center of the Health Ministry), Professor Ou Ming from Guangzhou University of TCM (celebrated translator and chief professor), Henan College of TCM, Guangzhou University of TCM, Nanjing University of TCM, Shaanxi College of TCM, Liaoning College of TCM and Shandong University of TCM.

The compilation of this Library is also supported by the State Administrative Bureau and experts from other universities and colleges of TCM. The experts on the Compilation Committee and Approval Committee have directed the compilation and translation. Professor She

后　记

《(英汉对照)新编实用中医文库》(以下简称《文库》)从2000年中文稿的动笔,到2002年全书的付梓,完成了世纪的跨越。为了使本套《文库》尽可能展示传统中医学术理论和临床实践的精华,达到全面、系统、准确、科学、规范、通俗的编写要求,全体编译人员耗费了大量的心血,付出了艰辛的劳动。特别是上海中医药大学承担了英语翻译的主持工作,得到了著名医学英语翻译家、原西安医科大学英语系主任和卫生部外语培训中心主任邵循道教授,著名中医英语翻译家、广州中医药大学欧明首席教授的热心指导,河南中医学院、广州中医药大学、南京中医药大学、陕西中医学院、辽宁中医学院、山东中医药大学等中医院校英语专家的全力参与,确保了本套《文库》具有较高的英译水平。

在《文库》的编撰过程中,我们始终得到国家主管部门领导和各中医院校专家们的关心和帮助。编纂委员会的国内外学者及审定委员会的

Jing, Head of the State Administrative Bureau and Vice-Minister of the Health Ministry, has showed much concern for the Library. Professor Zhu Bangxian, head of the Publishing House of Shanghai University of TCM, Zhou Dunhua, former head of the Publishing House of Shanghai University of TCM, and Pan Zhaoxi, former editor-in-chief of the Publishing House of Shanghai University of TCM, have given full support to the compilation and translation of the Library.

With the coming of the new century, we have presented this Library to the readers all over the world, sincerely hoping to receive suggestions and criticism from the readers so as to make it perfect in the following revision.

Zuo Yanfu

Pingju Village, Nanjing

Spring 2002

专家对编写工作提出了指导性的意见和建议。尤其是卫生部副部长、国家中医药管理局局长佘靖教授对本书的编写给予了极大的关注,多次垂询编撰过程,并及时进行指导。上海中医药大学出版社社长兼总编辑朱邦贤教授,以及原社长周敦华先生、原总编辑潘朝曦先生及全体编辑对本书的编辑出版工作给予了全面的支持,使《文库》得以顺利面世。在此,一并致以诚挚的谢意。

在新世纪之初,我们将这套《文库》奉献给国内外中医界及广大中医爱好者,恳切希望有识之士对《文库》存在的不足之处给予批评、指教,以便在修订时更臻完善。

左言富

于金陵萍聚村

2002 年初春

A Newly Compiled Practical English-Chinese Library of Traditional Chinese Medicine

(英汉对照)新编实用中医文库